Managing diabetes,
managing medicine

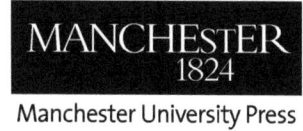
Manchester University Press

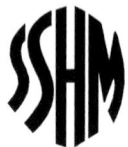

SOCIAL HISTORIES OF MEDICINE

Series editors: David Cantor and Keir Waddington

Social Histories of Medicine is concerned with all aspects of health, illness and medicine, from prehistory to the present, in every part of the world. The series covers the circumstances that promote health or illness, the ways in which people experience and explain such conditions, and what, practically, they do about them. Practitioners of all approaches to health and healing come within its scope, as do their ideas, beliefs, and practices, and the social, economic and cultural contexts in which they operate. Methodologically, the series welcomes relevant studies in social, economic, cultural, and intellectual history, as well as approaches derived from other disciplines in the arts, sciences, social sciences and humanities. The series is a collaboration between Manchester University Press and the Society for the Social History of Medicine.

Previously published

The metamorphosis of autism: A history of child development in Britain *Bonnie Evans*

Payment and philanthropy in British healthcare, 1918–48 *George Campbell Gosling*

The politics of vaccination: A global history *Edited by Christine Holmberg, Stuart Blume and Paul Greenough*

Leprosy and colonialism: Suriname under Dutch rule, 1750–1950 *Stephen Snelders*

Medical misadventure in an age of professionalization, 1780–1890 *Alannah Tomkins*

Conserving health in early modern culture: Bodies and environments in Italy and England *Edited by Sandra Cavallo and Tessa Storey*

Migrant architects of the NHS: South Asian doctors and the reinvention of British general practice (1940s–1980s) *Julian M. Simpson*

Mediterranean quarantines, 1750–1914: Space, identity and power *Edited by John Chircop and Francisco Javier Martínez*

Sickness, medical welfare and the English poor, 1750–1834 *Steven King*

Medical societies and scientific culture in nineteenth-century Belgium *Joris Vandendriessche*

Managing diabetes, managing medicine: Chronic disease and clinical bureaucracy in post-war Britain *Martin D. Moore*

Vaccinating Britain: Mass vaccination and the public since the Second World War *Gareth Millward*

Madness on trial: A transatlantic history of English civil law and lunacy *James E. Moran*

Managing diabetes, managing medicine

Chronic disease and clinical bureaucracy in post-war Britain

Martin D. Moore

Manchester University Press

Copyright © Martin D. Moore 2019

The right of Martin D. Moore to be identified as the author of this work has been asserted by him in accordance with the Copyright, Designs and Patents Act 1988.

An electronic version of this book is also available under a Creative Commons (CC-BY) licence, thanks to the support of the Wellcome Trust, which permits distribution, reproduction and adaptation provided the author and Manchester University Press are fully cited. Details of the licence can be viewed at https://creativecommons.org/licenses/by/4.0/

Published by Manchester University Press
Altrincham Street, Manchester M1 7JA

www.manchesteruniversitypress.co.uk

British Library Cataloguing-in-Publication Data
A catalogue record for this book is available from the British Library

ISBN   978 1 5261 1307 8   hardback
ISBN   978 1 5261 1309 2   open access

First published 2019

The publisher has no responsibility for the persistence or accuracy of URLs for any external or third-party internet websites referred to in this book, and does not guarantee that any content on such websites is, or will remain, accurate or appropriate.

Typeset
by Toppan Best-set Premedia Limited

Contents

List of figures and tables	vi
Acknowledgements	vii
List of abbreviations	x
Introduction: managing diabetes, managing medicine	1
1 Chronicity and the care team in Britain's New Jerusalem	46
2 Diabetes, risk management, and the birth of modern primary care	79
3 The making of integrated care	114
4 Retinopathy screening and the new politics of prevention	149
5 Constructing standards at a time of crisis	179
6 Making managerial policy in the neoliberal moment	213
Epilogue	241
Bibliography	266
Index	302

Figures and tables

Figures

2.1	Representation of English NHS as envisioned after 1974 reorganisation	100
2.2	Representation of Scottish NHS as envisioned after 1974 reorganisation	101
2.3	Representation of Welsh NHS as envisioned after 1974 reorganisation	102
3.1	Standard outpatient clinic review form, c.1968	124
3.2	Components of a new record card for GP diabetes care, c.1977	127
3.3	The community care co-operation booklet, c.1980s	130

Tables

4.1	Estimated costs of different screening modalities	164

Acknowledgements

This book has been the product of a long journey, during which I have accrued more debts than I can acknowledge in such a short space. I can only hope that over time I have been a decent enough person and scholar to have expressed my gratitude to my creditors. There are, however, some thanks that I wish to express more formally here.

This monograph was made possible by the support of the Economic and Social Research Council (Grant Reference ES/H010912/1) and the Wellcome Trust (Grant Reference 100601/Z/12/Z). First and foremost, I would like to thank these institutions for their belief in my research and their generosity over the past six years. During this period, I have also benefited from the immense assistance of staff at several fantastic institutions, and I would like to express my thanks to librarians and archivists at The National Archives, the National Records of Scotland, the Royal College of General Practitioners Archives, and the Wellcome Library, as well as to Claire Keyte and members of the Centre for Medical History at the University of Exeter. The team at Manchester University Press have offered expert advice during the production of this monograph. Particular thanks are owed to my two anonymous reviewers, and to Emma Brennan, Tom Dark, Rob Byron, and Keir Waddington. Their input has greatly improved the text, and I am deeply appreciative of their perseverance and support in the presence of my incompetence.

The present work has been greatly enhanced by the permission to reproduce materials and images from a range of sources. A deep gratitude is owed to Routledge for their kind permission to reuse work from Martin D. Moore, 'Reorganising chronic disease management: diabetes and bureaucratic technologies in post-war British general practice', in M. Jackson (ed.), *The Routledge History of Disease* (London: Routledge, 2017), pp. 453–72. This chapter was central in forming ideas developed within this monograph and is cited throughout. My thanks also to the reviewers of this piece and its editor, Mark Jackson, for their comments. I am similarly grateful to The National Archives for allowing reproduction of a standard outpatient clinic form (Fig. 3.1) and components from a community co-operation booklet (Fig. 3.3), as well as to the *Journal of the Royal College of General Practitioners* (now the *British Journal of General Practice*) for permission to reproduce components from a structured record card for GP diabetes care (Fig. 3.2). I would also like to thank the researchers and proprietors of the Diabetes-Stories project for permitting me to use materials from their wonderful archive, and I am likewise greatly indebted to the many wonderful research participants who gave up their time and energies to allow me to interview them for this book. Their testimonies have been essential in opening-up new areas of investigation, and have helped me to rethink many of my prior conceptual assumptions and readings of archival and published material. I hope I have done them justice here.

My penultimate thanks must go to the colleagues whose insight and feedback have enriched the following pages. I am grateful to Emily Andrews for our discussions about the cultural and political value of data and management systems, and to Jane Hand for conversations about chronic disease and post-war British public health. Over the past three years, moreover, I have had the greatest support from friends and colleagues on the Wellcome Trust-funded 'Balance' project and at the University of Exeter. Thanks go to Fred Cooper, Ali Haggett, Nicos Kefalas, Ayesha Nathoo, and Rebecca Williams for their comments on material, advice on publication, and friendship during my move to a new institution. Special mentions must also go to Natasha Feiner for her comments on the whole manuscript, to Mark Jackson for his intellectual and moral support during the production of this monograph, to Roberta Bivins for her unwavering faith and helpful black marker pen, and to my new colleagues on the Waiting Times project – especially Lisa Baraitser and Laura Salisbury – for their patience and help in thinking about time and temporality in new ways. Finally, Harriet Palfreyman and Gareth Millward deserve special recognition for offering consistent feedback on copious drafts, and for reading and commenting on the whole manuscript on numerous occasions. I also owe them an inexpressible debt for their friendship during some challenging times. To all these fantastic people, I hope what follows goes some way to justifying your hard work and considerable investment. And of course,

Acknowledgements

I apologise if my stupidity or stubbornness have led me to ignore some of your advice. All errors and inadequacies that remain are my own.

My final and greatest thanks, however, must – and will always – go to Lucy, without whom there would be nothing to publish. You have been a constant source of advice, love, laughter, and inspiration, and I am lucky enough to have had your support and forgiveness at all times, despite my frustrating inability to meet deadlines or be anywhere on time. This work is dedicated to you.

Abbreviations

BDA	British Diabetic Association
BMJ	*British Medical Journal*
CHSC	Central Health Services Council
CSAG	Clinical Standards Advisory Group
DEC	diabetic eye centre
DHSS	Department of Health and Social Security
FHSA	Family Health Services Authority
GP	general practitioner
GOS	General Ophthalmic Service
HbA1c	glycosylated haemoglobin
JCGP	*Journal of the College of General Practitioners*
JRCGP	*Journal of the Royal College of General Practitioners*
MOH	Medical Officer of Health
MRC	Medical Research Council
NHS	National Health Service
NICE	National Institute for Clinical Excellence
NSF	National Service Framework
QOF	Quality and Outcomes Framework
RCGP	Royal College of General Practitioners
RCP	Royal College of Physicians of London
RHA	Regional Health Authority
RHB	Regional Hospital Board
SHHD	Scottish Home and Health Department
SMD	Special Medical Development
TNA	The National Archives, London
WHO	World Health Organization
WTE	whole time equivalent

Introduction: managing diabetes, managing medicine

In April 1990, the Conservative government issued a new contract to general practitioners (GPs) working within the British National Health Service (NHS). The negotiations around the contract had been troubling for GPs. Whilst not the sole point of dispute, many practitioners found novel performance-related pay provisions to be particularly unwelcome departures from previous arrangements. Despite gaining concessions, GPs rejected multiple offers until a frustrated administration decided to simply impose the contract.[1] So far as remuneration was concerned, the government felt strongly that new incentive payments and targets were essential. They would, the government believed, simultaneously raise standards of service and enable primary care to confront a range of public health concerns, not least those associated with 'chronic disease'.[2]

The management of diabetes mellitus was one area of chronic disease care that the contract sought to improve. Political interest in diabetes had developed slowly over the twentieth century. Prominent British clinicians had warned that 'deaths from diabetes were as numerous as those from all infectious diseases put together' during the 1930s, and estimates of the condition's prevalence rose steadily over the post-war period.[3] Likewise, medical professionals regularly referred to increases in workload and escalating consultations for the disease during the 1970s and 1980s; new technologies and understandings of risk management had extended the boundaries of treatment, whilst greater life expectancy and disease detection buttressed changes of demography, employment, leisure, and diet that probably underpinned increased incidence.[4] Strong policy networks had been established around the condition by the early 1990s, and lobbyists drew government attention to diabetes' growing financial and human costs. Responding to these concerns, the GP contract included incentive payments for special diabetes management clinics.[5] Focused treatment within primary care would, the Department of Health hoped, provide a cost-effective way to reduce troubling rates of diabetes' long-term ocular, renal, hepatic, neuropathic, and cardiovascular complications.

Notably, the contract itself contributed to the government's broader programme of reform for the NHS. Imbued with 'neoliberal' views about the political importance of competition in national life, the innovative policies introduced market-like mechanisms of devolved budgeting and contracting to the NHS. They also put into operation widely held beliefs that subjecting medical practitioners to managerial instruments would reduce costs and improve quality of care.[6] Under the new arrangements, for instance, receipt of financial incentives for diabetes management was contingent upon health authorities reviewing practice records. If satisfied that care aligned with locally agreed protocols – documents that codified the facilities, tests, and treatment processes considered necessary for good patient management – authorities would approve payment to GPs.[7] Similar practices were extended to other areas of healthcare. Concurrent service reforms required all purchasing authorities to benchmark performance indicators for new contracts, and all practitioners were compelled to undertake medical audit to highlight areas for improvement.

Although mandated by British health departments, these activities were to remain predominantly professionally led. Local committees comprising hospital clinicians, GPs, and technical staff would support audit activity, whilst the Royal Colleges and elite specialist organisations produced national care guidelines and minimum datasets to inform local developments. Crucially, in terms of diabetes management, these bodies intended their standards to be used by hospital doctors as much as by primary care teams, and they stressed the need for local systems to bridge the community–hospital divide. Through these and similar measures, managed medicine became central, not just to diabetes care, but also to the NHS.

Looking closely at the measures introduced for diabetes care, we can see how the reforms of the early 1990s consolidated a post-war transformation in British medicine. Across the twentieth century, doctors considered diabetes an incurable condition, one characterised by a chronic state of raised blood sugar and subject to lifelong management to abate symptoms and correct disturbed metabolic functions. Patients were responsible for performing daily acts of treatment and self-surveillance, with practitioners setting the parameters of therapy, assessing ongoing care, providing patient education, and monitoring for the earliest signs of devastating (though increasingly treatable) complications. Between the 1930s and the 1950s, clinicians, civil servants, and politicians agreed that good long-term diabetes care rested on two foundations: firstly, that patients were provided regular access to experienced, specially trained doctors for clinical review and ongoing advice; and secondly, that these doctors were employed within well-staffed and fully equipped hospital facilities to enable comprehensive disease surveillance. Specialist outpatient clinics embodied the ideal, most efficient arrangement of resources, and questions of organisation generally concerned how best to geographically distribute clinics to maximise patient contact.[8] So far as managing medical practice was concerned, clinical decision-making might have been supported by a range of informal practices (peer advice, training in a firm, even the formatting of records), but medical skill provided the basis for good care. It was a belief echoed across different areas of medicine: 'there are wide fields ... of individual judgement and skill in general medical practice', declared one report in the 1930s, 'that disciplinary action cannot enter and where attempts at minute control and supervision would be harmful'. Rather, it concluded, 'the quality of the service will depend mainly on the quality of the entrants.'[9]

By the 1990s, however, faith in specialist practitioners, individual skill, and organised clinics to guarantee good care had disappeared. Laboratories, experience, and education were still important features of medical and political discourse. Now, though, neither policy-makers nor specialist practitioners considered them sufficient safeguards of quality. Instead, management of professional care teams – and thus of disease management itself – had come to be seen as the key to better patient care and improved public health. Over the preceding eighty years, doctors and their care teams had mobilised a range of tools – from patient registers and recall systems to specialist records and care protocol – to place patients with diabetes under increasing surveillance. By the end of the century, these same tools were consciously used to specify, divide, and integrate the responsibilities of spatially dispersed teams, as well as to subject the very timing and processes of patient management to codification and review. Although unconnected to mechanisms of punishment, these instruments were designed to be disciplinary: once integrated into practice, they were to set the rhythms and content of care, and to make deviations visible to practitioners and their peers for justification or correction.[10] Managerialism, moreover, was more broadly expressed through new structures of national and international clinical government, in temporary and enduring institutions dedicated to advising on, and auditing, the new structures of managed care.[11]

Today, objective-setting, standards production, guidelines, and auditing are widespread features of risk management and organisational governance.[12] Particularly in medicine, it appears almost common sense that 'best practice' should be methodically laid out in evidence-based guidelines or national frameworks, that state agencies should encourage adherence to these standards, and that a range of state and non-state bodies consistently review performance.[13] Institutions have grown up, in Britain and around the world, to support, guide, and monitor not just medicine, but the management of medicine.[14] Indeed, it is the knowledge that such activities produce, rather than the technology of bureaucratic management itself, that draws popular comment.[15]

Yet programmes for structuring and reviewing care embody a very specific iteration of medicine, one which emerged slowly during the post-war period, and which became established during the early 1990s. This approach to medical practice was predicated upon a radical restructuring of trust in professionals that took place during the late twentieth century.[16] Where once politicians, employers, and the public professed faith in the self-regulation and tacit knowledge of trained practitioners, they now demanded formal mechanisms of oversight, rituals of verification, codified standards documents, and incentive payments.[17] As was the case in finance and associated areas of welfare provision, the remaking of relations of trust in medicine built upon a series of scandals, sustained political attacks, and popular critiques of experts and professionals emergent from the 1960s onwards.[18] At the heart of many calls for change in British medicine, however, were medical professionals themselves.[19] In recent years, neither medical scandals nor external criticism of medical care have ceased. Public trust in doctors and healthcare practitioners remains high, but a series of interrelated political, economic, cultural, intellectual, and technical transformations in post-war Britain has also rendered medical professionals subject to previously unthinkable managerial technologies, created in the name of quality.[20] Through its history of diabetes management in post-war Britain, this book explores these transfigurations and asks how British medicine was so extensively subjected to management over the second half of the twentieth century. Who promoted managerial mechanisms, and why? And what connected new forms of clinical management

Introduction

with the rise of chronic disease control as a political and medical concern?

Managing medical professionals

To some extent, these are questions that scholars have previously sought to answer. One body of literature, for example, has cast the creation of systems for professional management as predominantly state-driven.[21] Here, the global economic crises of the 1970s are seen to have undermined the funding assumptions of welfare states the world over.[22] In Britain, state support for clinical guidelines and audit structures supposedly developed as a response to this turmoil, serving, as in the USA, to regulate clinical activity and to remove costly variations in healthcare through standardisation.[23] Such efforts, moreover, are seen to have productively intersected with 'New Right' theories of government and economy that became prominent in British politics during the 1970s.[24] Within this framework, guidelines (and other forms of clinical government) thus formed part of a broader remaking of public services, motivated by an ideological distrust of welfare professionals, and a desire to curtail professional autonomy through private-sector accountability techniques.[25]

Such broad-stroke accounts, however, have often downplayed the role of healthcare professionals in constructing the means for their own management, or have portrayed them as successfully restrained or co-opted by the state. To be sure, competing analyses have contradicted arguments of state success. Here, scholars have suggested that medical professionals responded effectively to political and administrative pressures, moving to maintain control over collective autonomy at the expense of reduced individual clinical freedom.[26] Nonetheless, such interpretations still set professional activity as a rear-guard campaign fought in opposition to the state. 'Managerialism', moreover, is taken to represent an external, state-originated construct that ran counter to ideals of medical professionalism, ideals predicated upon collective control over standard-setting and work content.[27] Thus, much of the extant literature has tended to understate the complicated, often synergistic, relationships between state agencies and professional actors upon which national systems for professional management were built. They have also overlooked connections between care guidelines, audit structures, and a broader history of bureaucratised care stretching back before and across the post-war period.[28]

With a focus on diabetes care in twentieth-century Britain, this book reinstates the active role of practitioners – particularly GPs and specialists – as partners with state and non-state agencies in the development of tools and systems for professional management. In what follows, the opening three chapters position the first managerial care systems as local developments. Hospital clinicians and GPs developed models for integrated and structured care in response to growing disease prevalence, strained NHS resources, and shifting understandings of diabetes on the one hand, and as part of professional projects and longer trends towards bureaucratisation of medicine on the other. The instruments produced subjected the rhythms and processes of care to codification, and the local use of audit introduced elements of review. The subsequent three chapters then chart the political career of new models of care, moving with specialists and advocates in turns between clinic and surgery, and national and international policy fora. In so doing, this work builds on a small number of historical studies that situate tools of clinical management in a context of professional politics and concerns over quality.[29] Whilst positioning the promotion of technologies for professional management in terms of cultural and political anxieties about professional accountability, it suggests that specialists and elite medical bodies were not simply reacting to external pressures; rather, elite doctors and academics actively shared these concerns. Apprehensions about accountability and variation informed the development of new technologies, and motivated specialist agencies (and the Royal Colleges) to reposition themselves as governors of medical quality. Despite being sceptical about neoliberal programmes to remake the NHS, professional bodies forged common ground with government departments and statutory organisations over the managerial principles and practices that sat at the centre of their mutual (though somewhat misaligned) political projects.

Reinstating the active role of healthcare professionals in the history of managed medicine, however, does not mean negating the role of 'the state', conceptualised here as a loose collection of political institutions, statutory agencies, regulatory organisations, local and central government departments, welfare bodies, judicial and police systems, and quangos, funded by public monies.[30] At the end of the twentieth century, the medical profession remained closely entangled with the British state. Parliamentary legislation empowered central medical bodies to set educational and disciplinary standards for registered practitioners, and secured for doctors their monopoly supply of labour to tax-funded institutions.[31] Likewise, government departments sought to use clinical and public health expertise to both devise and legitimate central health policy, and continued to depend upon medical professionals to staff health services.[32] It was through such extended connections, moreover, that the policy of elected governments could be influenced by state officials and professionals alike.[33] Over the post-war period, professionals and their organisations interacted with civil servants, health authorities, ministers, and Parliament to construct elements of managed medicine, and elite practitioners worked through statutory agencies to give guidelines and audits greater authority.

The history that follows, therefore, remains a political history as much as a story of technical developments or professional manoeuvrings. Indeed, any history of managed medicine within the British health services must include politics in both its broadest and most traditional historiographical senses. On the one hand, like the scientific medicine of the late nineteenth and early twentieth centuries, managed medicine was promoted by certain segments of the medical profession and associated academic institutions.[34] It required a reordering of resources, institutions, practices, and relations of labour. Healthcare practitioners seemingly accepted some of its forms and practices as uncontroversial, even useful. Yet debates about how clinical guidelines might produce unfeeling and unthinking 'cookbook medicine', removing skill and individuality from practice, also highlight how professionals regarded the reworking of their quotidian lives as inherently political.[35]

On the other hand, managed medicine developed through the pressure and support of more formal political actors, such as government ministers, the civil service, Parliament, and political parties, as well as more dispersed state institutions. Like other parts of the post-war welfare state, the NHS owed its existence to the centralising and collectivising political impulses of Britain's post-war reconstruction, and British medicine continued to be influenced by shifting political and economic tides. Traditionally, historians have debated these currents in terms of 'consensus', the extent to which the three decades after 1945 were characterised by broad policy agreement between elite figures in Whitehall and the major political parties, with all sides supporting a mixed economy, a predominantly Keynesian fiscal policy (to maintain full employment), and a generous welfare state, comprising tax-funded education, social security, and healthcare free at the point of use.[36] It was a framework of policy-making that supposedly ended with the radicalism of Margaret Thatcher's Conservative governments (1979–90).[37]

The existence of consensus, however, is of less importance here than the economic trajectories and changes in frames of policy-making that characterised the five decades after the Second World War.[38] In more recent work, scholars have traced the shifting sands of British politics, providing deep analyses of social and economic planning under the Clement Attlee (Labour) governments of the 1940s;[39] the return to market-oriented policies pursued by the Conservative governments of the 1950s;[40] the conflicts embedded within revived planning of the 1960s, beginning with Harold Macmillan's Conservative government (1959–64) and accelerating under Harold Wilson's Labour premiership (1964–70);[41] the shifts between denationalisation, corporatism, and spending restraints noted within the governments of the 1970s led by Edward Heath (Conservative, 1970–74), Wilson (1974–76), and James Callaghan (Labour, 1976–79);[42] and the complex, contested policy-making around markets and statecraft of the 1980s and 1990s.[43] Moreover, historians of the welfare state have situated policy in relation to government spending and Britain's post-war economic fortunes. The twenty-five years after 1945 have been described as an economic 'golden age', during which strong underlying growth funded an expansion of welfare services.[44] Yet a focus on average rates of Gross Domestic Product (GDP) conceals Britain's turbulent post-war experience.[45] Periodic bouts of stop-start growth, inflation, international credit concern, and instabilities in currency and balances of trade strongly influenced government policy, and British welfare services were often under severe pressure to limit spending across the whole post-war period.[46]

These economic and political trends influenced the development of managed medicine in Britain in two key ways. Firstly, Britain's erratic economy produced a financial environment within which the growing population with diabetes outstripped the available resources for care. To shift or reduce the expense of patient management, pioneering healthcare practitioners developed innovative forms of service delivery, and multiple disciplines and institutions – especially those related to health economics and service research – were forged to assess medical practice and to ensure that public monies were spent effectively.[47] Secondly, as in the case of patient consumerism, managerial reforms considered characteristic of a later period emerged from longer-term political trajectories and medical innovations.[48] From the 1950s onwards, government departments and health authorities – supported by patient bodies, international organisations, and think-tanks – expressed a desire to use data from service monitoring to influence professional decision-making.[49] In the context of scientific innovation and undesired increases in expenditure, it was hoped that the provision of information would guide medical practitioners to more effective and resource-minded care. Furthermore, as political parties came to emphasise the importance of technocratic planning during the 1960s, health departments experimented with expanded information systems, new advisory bodies, and multi-disciplinary management structures, believing that the incorporation of experts and clinicians into formal structures would provide the knowledge and legitimacy for more effective activity.[50] Innovations even stretched to Whitehall during the 1970s, as ministers and civil servants developed various techniques of objective-setting, programme review, and resource management.[51] Although not effective in the ways envisaged, these developments facilitated academic interest in evaluating medicine, and provided political capital for discussions of integrated, multi-sited treatment schemes from which initial technologies for professional management emerged.

Within this context, the growing influence of neoliberal political rationality in British governance after the 1970s can be read anew. Successive British governments during the 1980s and 1990s believed that exposing the central state to the practices and institutions of the so-called private sector provided the key to transforming public services, making them more efficient, less costly, more enterprising, and able to be managed more effectively at a distance.[52] Putting these convictions into practice, Conservative administrations introduced new contracting and performance management arrangements into the NHS, and supported professional efforts to set standards and review practice as a means to benchmark commissioning and enhance accountability. In so doing, however, these governments not only found a platform to cajole, and co-operate with, professional bodies over managerial technologies. They also built on earlier political and medical innovations, with the reforms of the 1980s reorienting tools and subjects developed for planning in the 1960s.[53] The Thatcher governments demonstrated a greater drive to build managed medicine into policy, but they did not originate it.

Where this work departs from the extant literature is in its focus on diabetes care.[54] Although this is a fascinating topic in its own right, much of the historical literature on diabetes and its management has used the condition to examine essential features of modern medicine, from changing models and social relations of knowledge production to the role of new technologies and economic practices in redefining disease and patient experiences.[55] Examining the ways in which British doctors – together with civil servants, government departments, international health organisations, patient associations, and academics – sought to control diabetes illuminates hitherto hidden connections between chronic disease and the creation of systems designed to discipline professional labour.[56]

In essence, this work argues that long-term disease posed challenges to a health system initially organised to treat acute cases.[57] Over the post-war period, the number of NHS patients with diabetes (and other long-term conditions) grew considerably. In 1951, for instance, the eminent physician R. D. Lawrence estimated 0.3 per cent of the population had diabetes, with another 0.3 per cent with asymptomatic forms.[58] By 1991, British Diabetic Association (BDA, a mixed lay and professional organisation established in the 1930s) estimated total prevalence to be near 2 per cent, or around 1 million people with diabetes in England and Wales alone.[59] Without the capacity for cure, or resources to cope with rising demands, doctors had to devise new ways to treat increasing numbers of ambulant patients with long-term disease, and bureaucratic observation became central to tracking patients not directly under hospital observation. Healthcare teams combined existing tools in new ways to ensure that novel forms of organisation – particularly dispersed elements and institutions of community care – were able to function effectively.[60] Appointment systems, recall mechanisms, and patient registers tracked patients and proactively regulated the temporality of oversight; mobile records inscribed and communicated longitudinal data to inform long-term treatment decisions; and letters and records communicated what action had been taken so that concentration in one location was unnecessary. As teams grew, care protocol also formally allocated responsibility and guided practitioners on appropriate clinical activity, organising care along the lines of bureaucracy in the hope that treatment would be integrated and standards maintained.[61] Operating at the intersection between primary and secondary care, doctors, managers, and health service planners believed diabetes to be at the forefront of these developments, casting it as a model chronic disease whose management strategies might be generalised to other conditions.[62]

At national level, political interest in diabetes intensified during the final two decades of the century. As government explicitly designed policy to confront 'chronic disease' during the 1980s and 1990s, conditions and risk factors central to the concept were subject to renewed efforts at cost-control.[63] Diabetes became a condition of rising concern. Specialist practitioners, health economists, civil servants, and the BDA all lobbied ministers, and policy networks produced quantified measures of the costs of the disease and its complications.[64] With the government interested in new forms of professional management, chronic diseases like diabetes provided promising subjects for piloting new programmes. Healthcare teams were already using many of the tools required for implementation, whilst elite professional bodies and international organisations were creating standards documents, clinical guidelines, and model audit systems. There were alternative routes to promoting managed medicine. Some surgical teams, for example, pioneered new forms of management.[65] Yet chronic disease control proved pivotal, not just because of its cost implications and broad policy appeal, but because of how common managerial technologies were already in clinical practice, and how care penetrated both the hospital and the GP surgery.

Managing medicine before 1945

These longer-term influences, however, stretch back before the Second World War. Between the mid-nineteenth and early twentieth centuries, for instance, a recognisable 'profession' of medicine emerged. During this period, practitioners began to more effectively organise themselves on a national basis, and they made sustained ideological claims to professional status, expertise, and authority, successfully converting esoteric knowledge into market control and self-regulation.[66] Discourses of autonomy derived from specialist knowledge outside the purview of the lay person, moreover, had a substantive impact on doctors' identities and work patterns into the 1900s, buttressed by social networks and training.[67] In Britain, the 1858 Medical Act laid the foundations for professional identity and status.[68] With the creation of the General Medical Council, the state charged a small committee of elite doctors with maintaining a register of licensed practitioners, disciplining those found guilty of 'infamous' behaviour, and overseeing formal medical education in approved institutions. Practitioners themselves were thus placed in control of training and regulating their fellow members, positioning standard-setting and professional freedom as principles to be fiercely defended.[69]

Whilst this history means that examining the actions of 'medical professionals' in the post-war period makes analytic sense, serious professional divisions persisted after 1858. The intensification of specialisation, for instance, generated heated disputes over the second half of the nineteenth century. As Granshaw has highlighted, in the absence of a co-ordinated system, the development of specialist institutions siphoned patients away from GPs, as well as from general hospital consultants engaged in medical education.[70] With their livelihoods and status challenged, generalists attacked specialisation as a dangerous innovation of little medical value.[71] Such criticism, moreover, carried an ideological edge. Opponents condemned specialists for focusing on specific diseases and isolated parts of the body. Localised perspectives conflicted with a prevailing holistic medical culture, and generalists continued to argue that the effective understanding and treatment of illness required disease to be placed in the context of the whole patient.[72]

Into the twentieth century, concerted opposition to specialisation faded as administrative pressures within an emergent healthcare system, and a drive for professional unity, saw referral mechanisms, systems of integrated care, and specialist departments in general hospitals develop.[73] However, though these compromises smoothed tensions, they were not a panacea. Even as specialisation became common amongst consultants, professional conflict continued to occur.[74] Links between universities, medical schools, teaching hospitals, and state bodies deepened over the inter-war years, reinforcing divisions between hospital practitioners and rank-and-file GPs. Such interconnections also created new tensions between gentlemanly, individualist consultants and a cadre of specialist academic practitioners dedicated to research.[75] Gradual educational changes ensured that qualified professionals shared a broad outlook and occupational experience by the post-war period, and over time more robust group identities formed. Nonetheless, internal divisions persisted, and splits were most visible during times of great institutional and political change.[76]

Since the mid-nineteenth century, then, medical professionals in Britain have rarely acted with one voice, and have been dependent upon the state for much of their authority. Indeed, rather than working in opposition to the state (as doctors frequently claimed), medical professionals and the state have consistently been partners. Though the 1858

Medical Act was intended, at least in part, to raise standards and protect the public, nineteenth-century doctors also hoped it would harness state authority to limit competition and protect the economic interests of an overcrowded profession.[77] The initial legislation disappointed many registered practitioners, but political developments since 1858 increasingly folded the profession within state apparatus.[78] Through the 1911 National Insurance Act a significant proportion of GPs were contracted into state-funded care.[79] The Local Government Act of 1929 extended state capacity for hospital work, and before this municipal schemes had sought to co-ordinate private, charitable, and local state services.[80] Finally, the creation of the NHS in 1948 consolidated the central role of the British state in funding medical practice, establishing doctors as welfare professionals whose autonomy of decision-making was guaranteed in exchange for working within fixed budgets.[81]

These changing relations of medicine before 1948 had considerable implications for medical professionals and service management. In a landmark article, Steve Sturdy and Roger Cooter suggested that the remaking of financial arrangements in British medicine – and particularly the expansion of state funding – drove the creation of new corporate hierarchies and divisions of labour between 1870 and 1950.[82] Along with charitable investment and burgeoning international connections, these arrangements provided support to laboratory-oriented scientific medicine, and to the standardised views of physical bodies and disease common to scientific and administrative systems.[83] Crucially, the pursuit of institutional efficiency during these decades also reinforced a managerial ethos in health service organisation, with work divided and re-integrated in order to maximise output within available resources.[84] Faced with the accumulating bodies of nationalised structures, medicine during this period gradually embodied the bureaucratic forms and rationalities characteristic of post-Enlightenment 'modernity'.[85] Techniques of abstraction, classification, mapping, grouping, and division had been central to a host of administrative, commercial, and scientific enterprises across Europe and its colonies.[86] Through the remaking of medicine's institutional and social relations, the individualistic tendencies of British practitioners were slowly overcome, and administrative practices were more intensively applied to construct new subjects, 'chart' bodily and organisational domains, and pursue efficiency.[87]

It is important not to exaggerate the extent of change experienced before 1950. In outpatient clinics, claims to efficiency seemingly outstripped practical achievements.[88] Elsewhere, individualistic diagnostic categories and prescribing habits persisted into the mid-century.[89] Yet the forms of organisation and practice introduced during this period left a legacy for the post-war decades. The creation of the NHS reinforced the dominance of an academic elite over British hospital practice, and some British-trained doctors found working relationships in the service, as well as rules governing employment and practice ownership, rigid enough to warrant emigration.[90] The basic units of medical work, moreover, were standardised by the spread of standard tests, drugs, diagnostic labels, and bodies, thus providing the foundation for more tightly defined and managed care.[91] Indeed, with the creation of multi-sited, multi-disciplinary clinical trials, the inter-war period also produced material and intellectual precedents to managed work.[92] Once trials were integrated into the fabric of the health services, they offered doctors experience with protocol, statistical assessment, and models of teamwork that could be drawn upon when designing new systems of structured care and professional management. These technologies also placed knowledge about efficacious treatment outside the individual, to be determined through systematic research, and thus rendered practitioners more open to regulation.[93] Previously embodied and inexplicable knowledge became communicable.[94]

As the 1950s came into view, though, more closely managed medical work was not inevitable. The transformations of the late nineteenth and early twentieth centuries produced values, projects, instruments, and organisational forms that fed into managed medicine as it emerged during the 1980s and 1990s, but earlier developments did not determine end results. Managed medicine had to be created through the determined action of a range of professional, state, and lay actors, within the shifting political, social, and cultural circumstances of the post-war period. As expensive concerns that linked primary and secondary care, chronic diseases provided important testing grounds for new approaches to medicine.

Diabetes, chronic disease, and managed medicine

Diabetes' historical status as a model chronic disease offers it analytical power for the study of the emergence of professional management. During the late 1950s and the 1960s, clinicians, epidemiologists, and social medicine researchers began to discuss 'chronic diseases' as a coherent category. Key figures often used what was then known as 'maturity onset' or later 'non-insulin-dependent' (now type 2) diabetes to discuss some core characteristics of chronic diseases: gradual and asymptomatic onsets; long-term or incurable natures; and profound social and economic repercussions for individuals, communities, and nations.[95] Equally, doctors and nurses often saw diabetes management as a model for pioneering efforts at co-ordinated shared care between hospitals and GPs, one from which practitioners engaged in other forms of long-term disease management might learn.

However, diabetes and its management also have histories that distinguish the condition from others that contemporaries included within discussions of 'chronic disease', such as cancer or hypertension.[96] The medical and political understanding of the disease has changed significantly over time, in ways that have often made its management rather idiosyncratic. Three features are worth highlighting and considering at length. Firstly, doctors developed a quantified and bureaucratic culture of management earlier than in other chronic conditions. Secondly, clinicians, epidemiologists, and public health doctors remained divided over causative factors for diabetes, and rarely promoted primary preventive approaches. Thirdly, medical and nursing professionals provided the leading edge to the BDA, possibly the first patient-advocacy group in Britain. Through the Association, specialists created networks and connections with state agencies and other elite professional bodies. Each of these factors influenced the ways in which diabetes related to managed medicine, and to a broader concept of chronic disease.

Quantifying diabetes in the nineteenth and twentieth centuries
Typically, both academic histories and clinical texts trace the existence of diabetes at least as far back as ancient Greece, where the term 'diabetes' originated.[97] For the present work, though, the most significant developments in the definition and management of the disease occurred in the nineteenth century. Until this point, understandings of the mechanisms and causes of 'diabetes' (or differently labelled states with similar symptoms in non-Greek traditions) had varied considerably between times, places, and practitioners. Despite such variations, physicians defined diabetes in symptomatic terms, diagnosing it upon noting unquenchable thirst, excessive urination, wasting, and/or extreme hunger.[98] Though some ancient physicians from the non-Greek world had discussed similar diseases marked by 'honeyed urine', British doctors did not explicitly discuss urinary sweetness until the

seventeenth century, and the term 'diabetes mellitus' was coined only in the later eighteenth century.[99]

During the nineteenth century, diabetes came to be slowly transformed in British medical discourse and practice, in line with broader epistemological and structural changes in 'Western' medicine.[100] As hospitals grew in importance as centres of medical care, training, and research, medical perception became reorganised around new forms of clinical examination. Lesions and clinical signs – observable only to trained practitioners through skilled examination and technology – became more fundamental than symptoms described by patients in diagnosing and managing disease.[101] The meaning of lesions themselves, moreover, was to be found in relation to scientific observation of the dead and, in the later nineteenth century, in relation to experimentation on the living.[102] These broad trends were not totalising. The exact importance of scientific knowledge and clinical experience in deciphering sign and symptom varied between practitioners and cases during the nineteenth century.[103] Patients also continued to exercise some influence over medical thought and practice, with greater 'passivity' having to be learned.[104] Nonetheless, in terms of diabetes, physicians of the nineteenth century extended experiments with glycosuria (sugar passed into the urine) from the previous century.[105] Chemists produced tests to enable easier assessment of urine content, and the clinical sign of glycosuria became as important as symptoms in the diagnosis of disease.[106]

As well as contributing to a change in disease understandings and patient profiles (new tests shifted the boundaries of who might be diagnosed) these innovations fed into management.[107] Whilst quantitative examination of glycosuria began as a research practice during the 1860s, physiologically minded clinicians like Frederick Pavy (Guy's Hospital, London) used new tests to monitor the extent to which a variety of diets reduced bodily glucose.[108] British doctors had prescribed diets to inhibit the body's production of sugar since the early nineteenth century.[109] After the mid-century, though, glycosuria testing allowed diets to be more finely titrated to affect bodily outputs, following a broader trend of turning 'abnormal' diagnostic signs into quantitative markers of therapeutic success.[110] By the early twentieth century, hospital practitioners had added more markers to their clinical assessments (most notably acids (ketonuria) and nitrogen passed in urine), buoyed by the elevation of basic laboratory practices in pre-clinical training and by the international and imperial expansion of physiological research into diabetes and nutrition.[111] Inter-war innovations even made routine assessment of blood glucose practicable.[112] Though some GPs and specialists disagreed about the necessity of blood testing in ongoing management, by the 1920s authoritative writers had cast diabetes as a disease of the general metabolism, with hyperglycaemia (elevated levels of glucose in the blood) as its diagnostic sign, and glycosuria and ketonuria (acids passed in urine) as markers of therapeutic performance.[113]

Unlike many other conditions later conceived as chronic diseases, diabetes thus had quantified, biochemical management programmes by the early twentieth century. Initial 'stabilisation' involved fasting, careful calculation of carbohydrate, fat, and protein in test diets, and monitoring of physiological changes to assess efficacy.[114] This emergent system of biochemical review and therapeutic adjustment was further strengthened with the spread of insulin therapy in Britain, after early trials with the drug in 1923.[115] Insulin facilitated some changes in approach. As a powerful therapeutic agent (enabling cells to take up glucose circulating in the blood), insulin offered hope to patients who did not take well to planned diets. With insulin, doctors could afford greater leeway on dietary constraints, and they came to emphasise psychological and social factors, as well as biochemical measurements, in devising and assessing treatment.[116] Nonetheless, change had limits. Despite a growing consideration of subjective wellbeing in treatment, clinicians continued to insist on the importance of laboratory-based surveillance and quantified cultures of care. Ensuring a balance of diet and insulin – as measured through biochemical indices – remained central to therapy, as did achieving acceptable metabolic control.[117] Doctors thus sought to maintain a central role in long-term disease management. Patients were charged with daily acts of self-care, but clinical teams retained responsibility for establishing balance in the parameters of individual therapy.[118] Being too lenient might result in hyperglycaemia and ketonuria, risking symptoms and acute complications; being too austere might have iatrogenic consequences, with injections rendering blood glucose levels too low, triggering the novel danger of hypoglycaemia.

In light of these challenges, between the 1890s and 1920s doctors developed a range of tables, graphs, and calculations to assist assessment of diets, insulin requirements, and therapeutic success.[119] They also created new records to monitor biochemical trends and record ongoing treatment. In fact, by the mid-twentieth century, some hospital wards had developed a considerable documentary culture around diabetes management, and records for treatment and laboratory results provided important resources for guiding medical and nursing practice.[120] Creators of new integrated care programmes later developed similar instruments to co-ordinate activity between practitioners. Although some post-war clinicians expressed doubts about the relationship between hyperglycaemia and the development of long-term complications, the close links between diabetes care and laboratory practices thus provided diabetes management with well-developed cultures of quantification and standardisation. Such features made setting and auditing process and outcome standards simpler than for other conditions after the 1970s, and by the 1990s made diabetes care an attractive area for pioneering new target-oriented managerial frameworks.[121]

Diabetes, chronic disease, and risk

Although quantified management programmes were a common feature of diabetes treatment during the post-war period, the exact content of care varied between patients. Before the twentieth century, physicians had made rough divisions between 'types' of patient to provide indicators for diagnosis, therapy, and prognosis. On the one hand, they discussed diabetes with an onset early in life, marked by acute wasting and death following coma. On the other, they wrote of diabetes with later onset, often seen in overweight patients, who tended to live longer but in whom certain ocular, nervous, and kidney complications could occur.[122] Soon after insulin became widely available, clinicians modified their discussions, dividing patients who needed insulin to stave off significant hyperglycaemia, ketonuria, and death from those who did not. Until the 1960s, these criteria roughly equated to classifications of 'moderate' or 'severe' diabetes (generally affecting thinner patients, with acute onset at young age, treated on diet and insulin) and a supposedly 'mild' form of the disease (generally appearing in overweight patients manageable on diet, with onset in middle age).[123] Into the 1960s, doctors began to refer to 'juvenile' and 'maturity onset' diabetes respectively, with these terms replaced during the late 1970s and 1980s by insulin dependent diabetes (now type 1) and non-insulin dependent (now type 2).[124] Researchers from diverse disciplinary backgrounds suggested different forms of classification, proclaiming new types and sub-types, over the century.[125] However, clinicians predominantly classified patients on the basis of liability to coma and response to treatment, with the latter determining therapeutic trajectory and patient experience.

Many of the difficulties in sub-classifying diabetes emerged from uncertainty about its cause. Historically, the condition has been defined and diagnosed by an intermediate effect of pathology – elevated blood glucose – and its potential symptoms or risks, rather than by any specific lesion or trigger. During the 1940s, Harold Himsworth, Professor of Medicine at University College Hospital (London), even suggested that the diversity of disease trajectories in diabetes may have resulted from how the label functioned as an umbrella term, grouping together different problems connected by common pathophysiological processes, biomarkers, and management programmes.[126]

This is not to suggest that doctors before the mid-twentieth century lacked theories about causation. During the second half of nineteenth century, physicians redeveloped older models of disease that equated illness with imbalance, suggesting stress, exposure, alcoholic excess, and 'violent mental emotion' as potential triggers in older patients.[127] Such ideas persisted into the early decades of the twentieth century, and clinicians like R. D. Lawrence considered 'worry' and 'overstrain' alongside heredity, over-eating, obesity, accidents, infections, and other diseases as potential 'immediate cause[s]'.[128] Lawrence admitted, however, that the causes of many 'acute' cases remained 'complete mysteries', and no clear consensus emerged on the precise aetiology of diabetes even after 1945.[129]

Doctors were somewhat uncertain about the aetiology of many chronic diseases in the second half of the twentieth century. After the mid-1950s, the novel application of epidemiological methods to chronic diseases meant that discussions of causation frequently centred upon multifactorial models of onset and statistical assessment of risk.[130] Except for the case of smoking and lung cancer, it was rare for clinicians, epidemiologists, and public health doctors to implicate a single factor as triggering disease.[131] Instead, medical debates about prevention came to focus on the relative contribution of numerous so-called 'modifiable' risk factors (such as diet, exercise, or physiological abnormalities), and preventive programmes were oriented around three levels of intervention: primary prevention (stopping the onset of disease, by either promoting healthy practices or encouraging cessation of 'risky' ones), secondary prevention (instituting early treatment and arresting serious progression of particular conditions), and tertiary prevention (managing long-term complications to prevent further physical deterioration).[132] Although not disappearing completely in Britain, analyses of economic and social determinants of health moved to a minor key.[133] New approaches to causation and prevention took time to become established, and not all parties agreed about the importance of specific risk factors for specific diseases.[134] Nevertheless, doctors still instituted primary preventive programmes for many chronic diseases. Despite strong disagreements over the possible causes of heart disease, for instance, national advisory bodies of the 1970s and 1980s offered preventive advice on smoking and dietary intake. Equally, hospital doctors and GPs proposed targeted, routine blood pressure assessment, and control of patients diagnosed with hypertension.[135] Even private companies turned debates about cholesterol and dietary fats into profit-making opportunities.[136]

As will be noted in Chapter 1, doctors, state agencies, and international organisations spent much less time discussing primary preventive strategies for diabetes than those for other conditions. Between the 1940s and 1960s, some theories about causation were advanced. Several public health doctors implicated sedentary lifestyles and over-eating in the causation of non-insulin-dependent diabetes, whilst a small group of epidemiologists and clinical researchers debated the relative aetiological importance of sugar and other refined carbohydrates. A minority of GPs and hospital doctors also suggested that lifestyle advice could be beneficial to those 'at risk', with risk calculated in relation to characteristics (age, weight, sex, parity, family history) seen most commonly in people with diabetes. However, no part of the profession suggested national primary preventive strategies until the late 1990s. Before this, prevention focused upon secondary and tertiary interventions – on preventing or arresting diabetes' various microvascular and macrovascular complications. Here, dietary composition, blood glucose control, and new therapeutic technologies assumed centre stage, and diabetes itself was conceptualised as a risk factor for myriad acute problems.[137] In other words, with causative factors disputed, clinical activity proved central to prevention, and specialists and the state promoted improved disease management (and, therefore, more intense professional management) as a public health activity during the later 1980s and early 1990s. Whilst this alignment of clinic and prevention was present in the history of other chronic conditions, it was particularly pronounced in diabetes. Doctors in the post-war period thus tended to portray diabetes as a model chronic disease primarily because of features related to its management – long-term surveillance, therapeutic titration, the involvement of primary and secondary health services – or its onset and effects, rather than for its aetiology. Moreover, the alignment of prevention with professional management provided policy-makers with another reason for seeing diabetes as a test site: intervention met public health, as well as clinical and service, interests.

Promoting diabetes services

One final distinctive feature of diabetes that shaped how its professionals became subject to management was the existence of an influential patients' organisation throughout the post-war period. The Diabetic Association (later BDA, and subsequently Diabetes UK) was a mixed lay and professional group established in 1934.[138] The Association itself emerged from attempts by R. D. Lawrence – the pre-eminent British diabetes specialist before the Second World War, and himself a person with diabetes – to gain financial and political support for his Diabetic Department at King's College Hospital (London). In brief, Lawrence turned to his high-profile colleagues and patients to raise capital for the department, and H. G. Wells (a private patient) penned an appeal letter in *The Times* on Lawrence's behalf.[139] From this letter, interest in an association gained ground, and Lawrence pulled together support for the organisation, which was founded in Wells's flat by thirty-two people, including clinicians, nurses, dieticians, industry representatives, and prominent patients.[140]

Membership of the Association grew slowly, but seemingly accelerated over the 1970s and 1980s, and local 'branches' (in which patients might meet and arrange events for their own support) developed in the early post-war decades.[141] However, although the Association was dedicated to work 'for diabetics', healthcare professionals provided the central body with much of its impetus and interests for most of the century. Lawrence was a dominant figure until the later 1950s, and professionals used the Association to form connections, design research programmes, develop their specialism, and influence government policy.[142]

The content and direction of the Association's activity altered over time. As will be noted in Chapter 1, as well as publishing journals and leaflets to support patient self-care, a major early interest of the Association was in promoting the creation and accessibility of specialist outpatient clinics. The development of insulin therapy had intensified patient self-management after the 1920s, introducing painful daily injections and new forms of laborious self-surveillance; where a patient could afford it, doctors encouraged home testing of urine for glucose and ketones (which initially involved boiling urine and applying a reagent in the kitchen) and noting results in record books.[143] This self-monitoring, though, formed part of a larger pattern of patient surveillance grounded in new forms of hospital organisation. The Association held a belief common until the 1950s that clinics were essential to effective diabetes care, providing a space for expertise, high-technology surveillance, and (in a minority of institutions) a growing multi-disciplinary care team. Its leadership thus spent much of the 1940s, 1950s, and 1960s surveying existing facilities and lobbying for better clinic organisation.[144] Its interests, however, did not remain static. Along with investigations into a range of welfare concerns over the post-war period, the Association increasingly co-operated with major professional bodies such as the Royal College of Physicians of London (RCP) during the 1970s and 1980s, producing guidance on service provision and clinical care.[145] During these decades, leading figures reconceived of the BDA as a body for setting and reviewing standards, and lobbied government for support in its efforts.[146]

The existence of such a body distinguished diabetes from many other chronic diseases. Patient-supported organisations had existed a few years before the creation of the BDA, though bodies like the Asthma Research Council focused on basic and clinical research funding.[147] The Association, therefore, remained unique in its work and composition for many years after the Second World War, and attained a position of moral and scientific authority seemingly unrivalled by other disease-specific organisations.[148] Crucially, it influenced the way in which diabetes care became subject to innovative forms of management. Its members developed new models of structured and shared care, spreading them through networks developed within the BDA until they formed something of an accepted 'common sense'. These models were then promoted nationally, and the Association actively engaged in the creation of guidelines and audits, including joint ventures with the Department of Health. Relations were not always cordial, and successive governments were wary of activities that might increase short-term costs. Nonetheless, the tireless work of the Association was a key feature of promoting diabetes as a subject for political interest.

Introduction 23

Managing diabetes and medical professionals in post-war Britain

Through the following chapters, then, this work tells a particular history of diabetes management in Britain. It is one that offers new perspective on the development of instruments for managing professional labour, and which explores a broader history of managed medicine after 1945. Before providing an overview of the following chapters, it is worth briefly pausing to reflect upon the work's silences and parameters.

Given the interests of the study, patients will be seen only fleetingly.[149] Patient testimonies are used to explore how certain systems functioned, or to examine how patients' concerns promoted professional management, whilst the figure of 'the patient' appears when the ways in which medical and political discourse used such a construct are traced, perhaps to justify stasis or encourage change.[150] Similarly, although references will be made to other healthcare professionals (notably managers, nurses, and technical staff), the primary focus remains on doctors and how their work became subject to codification, division, temporal regulation, and review. This is not to diminish the importance of other healthcare professionals in the management or history of diabetes care. Indeed, nurses played a considerable role both in patient management and in designing and promoting schemes for integrated care.[151] Nonetheless, doctors – specialists, academics, and GPs alike – sat at the heart of managed medical practice in Britain. They were the most influential actors promoting new forms of oversight and guidance, and it was their labour and status which was most radically reworked during the twentieth century. Therefore to fully appreciate how managed medicine emerged in post-war Britain, it is crucial to place medical professionals at the centre of the forthcoming analysis.

With regard to the chosen geographical frame for the study, it might well be asked whether it makes sense to focus on 'Britain'.[152] This question can be tackled on three levels. Firstly in terms of whether differences in medical culture, society, and politics undermines the implied unity of England, Wales, and Scotland.[153] It was certainly the case, for instance, that medical culture and politics in Scotland made the development of integrated care schemes much simpler than in England and Wales, and Scottish elites appeared slightly ahead of their southern counterparts in constructing guideline systems.[154] Yet, as this work shows, diabetes management (and the development of professional management) was a very 'British' affair. Specialists, evidence, and models of care moved freely across internal borders during the decades discussed. Major reviews of, and guidelines for, diabetes care often covered the whole of Britain or, if taking place within individual countries, were closely connected to counterparts elsewhere.[155] Developments in one country, in other words, informed developments in others. Similarly, in political terms, major actors and organisations – such as Parliament, the NHS, or the BDA – had British coverage. Undoubtedly, examinations of specific institutions or practices might reveal local peculiarities. But in a broad study such as this, a focus on Britain makes considerable analytical sense.

Secondly, there may be a case for adopting a wider geographical focus. For instance, as recent scholarly work has pointed out, the creation of clinical guidelines and audit was a transnational phenomenon, something perhaps characteristic of 'modern' medicine, with its emphasis on scientific rationalities and administrative pressures for standardisation and efficiency.[156] Indeed, the organisations and actors that promoted the management of professional labour often moved across borders, operating in global institutions and promoting international programmes for reform.[157] Yet the history told here is also one shaped by British peculiarities. As Day, Klein, and Miller point out, the generation and imposition of guidelines were linked far more closely to financial concerns in the USA than in Britain. In the USA, market structures and a disaggregated profession left doctors less able to institute their own vision of professional management.[158] In Britain, different conditions prevailed. Popular appreciation of the NHS curtailed attempts to fully privatise health service provision, and elite specialists and local doctors were more like partners in creating managerial instruments.[159] Likewise, in terms of diabetes management, British clinicians, epidemiologists, and researchers were prime movers within international agencies. They promoted models of structured, managed medical practice within these institutions, and used their organisational prestige to influence domestic practice. Once again, the peculiarities of the British political and medical context influenced the way in which international trends were received, and even informed those trends directly.

It is thus worth noting the productive power of focusing on Britain itself. With the creation of the NHS, Britain possessed a redistributive health service funded from central taxation that was of great interest to countries around the world.[160] By studying its history we can examine how disease and professional management developed in a collectivised (non-insurance-based) system with a mature medical profession. We are also able to tease out the possible contributions of significant political and cultural change to such developments, with Britain experiencing the loss of empire and constant shifts in governance strategies between 1945 and 2000. In other words, by ensuring that 'Britain' is situated within local and international scales this work can provide an illuminating study of modern medicine in the post-war period, but one which does not reduce British history to a variation on a theme. It is therefore hoped that the findings offered here can contribute to a broader literature on diabetes care and managed medicine, providing empirically grounded scholarship that facilitates comparative perspectives.

British distinctiveness can be seen almost immediately in Chapter 1. This chapter examines the ways in which diabetes care came to be remade with the creation of the NHS, and highlights the complex relationships connecting diabetes with a reconstructed concept of chronic disease. The new service accelerated the growth of hospital-based care, with a minority of clinicians developing rudimentary bureaucratic tools for managing the disease and a growing care team. At the same time, doctors, epidemiologists, and public health practitioners interested in 'chronic disease' also began to reframe diabetes as an exemplar of disease management, equating prevention with good clinical care.

These developments are taken up in Chapters 2 and 3, which discuss further expansions of the care team. As patient numbers grew and resources became constrained, clinicians tried to expand the role of GPs, both in formal shared care schemes and more informally in special clinics. GPs themselves were interested in assuming greater responsibility for their diabetic patients during this period, and they actively cultivated multi-disciplinary, cross-institutional ventures to bring diabetes management into primary care. This transition, however, provoked concerns about standards of care and the ability to co-ordinate clinical activity. To solve these problems, clinicians and GPs deployed tools developed from research – and instruments created to facilitate new forms of chronic disease management – to manage care more effectively. Reflecting on what made 'good practice', clinical teams set new standards for undertaking patient management, against which care could be measured and reviewed.

Early schemes did not spread beyond the local institutions in which they were first mobilised. This situation changed for later initiatives. Chapter 4 outlines how diabetes re-emerged as a concern of central government during the late 1970s, setting the scene for the move of managed care from clinical to policy arenas. Specifically, this interest in diabetes arose in relation to diabetic retinopathy, a major cause of blindness nationally. Reflecting changed understandings of prevention in chronic disease, as well as the shifting connections between medical organisations and government, the BDA and elite professionals promoted the cause of retinopathy prevention in government circles. Although these efforts found a supportive ear amongst medical civil servants, finance departments demanded new forms of health-economic evidence before they would consider funding pilot studies of early detection and treatment. Ministers, moreover, picked up schemes for trialling new modes of organisation during the mid-1980s only because of the party politics surrounding public health.

In contrast, the Department of Health (and its predecessor) quickly supported and adopted new standards documents, guidelines, and audit systems during the later 1980s. As Chapter 5 shows, interest in standards and auditing was much broader than their application to diabetes, being closely related to new political rationalities regarding public services, and to anxieties about professional culpability and accountability. In medicine, the creation and use of standards had a long heritage. During the mid-1980s, however, various professional, charitable, and international agencies converged on diabetes to produce their own standards of care process (and intermediate outcomes), which mapped neatly onto managerial principles and practices developed over the previous century. These standards provided a new layer of management in medicine, adding national guidelines for practice and audit to the local systems which had emerged in previous years, and on which such guidance had often been based.

Between the late 1980s and early 1990s, the principles of managed care, if not the content of these new standards documents, made their way into policy circles. Chapter 6 examines how this occurred. It begins by situating government interest in guidelines and audit systems within the influence of neoliberal ideas about competition, professional accountability, and the role of regulated market systems in social and economic life. A new consensus was forged in this period, in part because political and medical projects for management had clear synergies. However, the movement of prominent diabetologists and experts across policy fora to forge such conceptual and practical connections was also critical. Personnel continuities across different levels of governance ensured rough agreement over managed diabetes medicine, a vision of care which dovetailed neatly with political desires to curb costs and make healthcare operate more like a market. More than this, the public health aspect of managed care attracted successive governments to new guideline and audit structures, with little thought given to the growing interest in social determinants of health that had characterised public health during the end of the twentieth century.

Since the year 2000, public health policy for diabetes has changed direction somewhat. In recent decades, governments have sought to emphasise primary prevention of type 2 diabetes through exercise and dietary strategies, and Diabetes UK (previously the BDA) has also created new risk self-assessment tools.[161] And yet the managerial approach remains. The National Service Framework (NSF) and Quality and Outcomes Framework (QOF) continue to provide the financial and standards structures central to managed care, even where GPs have been brought into primary preventive strategies.[162] Similarly, the new approach of risk identification and early intervention has its heritage in mid-twentieth-century discussions of chronic disease and screening, and is designed to target NHS resources and medical attention more efficiently.

Probably reflecting a mixture of improved case-finding, an ageing society, and changing social and economic structures, rates of diabetes mellitus have increased substantially over the past two decades, and are projected to increase at a faster rate in the coming years.[163] As British health policy gravitates ever closer to managerial approaches to, and market commissioning of, health services, it is likely that bureaucratised clinical care will continue to play a central role in the NHS. In such a context, it will be more important than ever to see the historical trends that shape our approach to both of these major features of British life. This book provides something of a starting place for such an important undertaking. I hope it will also offer scholars a basis to extend conversations about chronic disease and managed care in different types of healthcare systems.

Notes

1 J. Lewis, 'The medical profession and the state: GPs and the GP contract in the 1960s and 1990s', *Social Policy and* Administration, 32:2 (1998), 132–50.
2 Secretaries of State for Social Services, Wales, Northern Ireland, and Scotland, *Promoting Better Health: The Government's Programme for*

Improving Primary Health Care, Cm 249 (London: HMSO, 1987), pp. 12–16; M. D. Moore, 'Reorganising chronic disease management: diabetes and bureaucratic technologies in post-war British general practice', in M. Jackson (ed.), *The Routledge History of Disease* (London: Routledge, 2017), pp. 453–4.

3 'The management of diabetic out-patients', *The Lancet*, 231:5974 (1938), 509; 'Detection of diabetes', *BMJ*, 2:5151 (1959), 555–6.

4 On a growing pool of patients and consultations: J. Walker, *Chronicle of a Diabetic Service* (London: British Diabetic Association (BDA), 1989), p. 91. Cf. J. Fry, *Common Diseases: Their Nature, Incidence, and Care*, 2nd edition (Lancaster: MTP Press Limited, 1979), p. 363; J. Fry and G. Sandler, *Common Diseases: Their Nature, Presentation, and Care*, 5th edition (London: Kluwer Academic, 1993), p. 395, table 41.3. The mutable, contested, often inferential, and culturally informed nature of medical and historical knowledge means that it is impossible to definitively untangle exact causes here: R. A. Aronowitz, *Making Sense of Illness: Science, Society, and Disease* (Cambridge: Cambridge University Press, 1998). For instance, leaving aside philosophical discussions about classification, what 'counted' as diabetes altered over the twentieth century, with symptoms giving way to statistical thresholds of blood glucose in diagnosis: J. A. Greene, *Prescribing by Numbers: Drugs and the Definition of Disease* (Baltimore: Johns Hopkins University Press, 2007). Thus increases in patient populations could be underpinned by changes in diagnosis – including enhanced rates of detection resulting from improved technologies and awareness – rather than increases in prevalence. Indeed, variations in cause of death certification mean that even assessing the contribution of longevity becomes difficult. Cf. M. D. Warren and A. Corfield, 'Mortality from diabetes', *The Lancet*, 301:7818 (1973), 1511–12; J. M. Malins, 'Food and death rates from diabetes', *The Lancet*, 304:7890 (1974), 1201. Nonetheless, given the scale of increase over the post-war period and the developments covered in this book, it appears likely that increases in prevalence and workload resulted from a mixture of factors, including secular increases in the number of cases of diabetes per year. In terms of the latter, alongside age, recent research on weight-loss and 'remission' supports long-held associations between obesity and some forms of diabetes: M. Uusitupa, 'Remission of type 2 diabetes: mission not impossible', *The Lancet*, 391:10120 (2018), 515–16; L. H. Newburgh and J. W. Conn, 'A new interpretation of hyperglycaemia in obese middle-aged persons', *Journal of the American Medical Association*, 112:1 (1939), 7–11. These findings inform the suggestion that transformations in structures of employment, leisure, and diet drove a post-war increase in disease incidence. In brief, it seems that Britain's workforce became more

sedentary after 1945, with a general transition from manual labour and manufacturing to office-based service work probably reducing average daily energy expenditure: P. Addison, *No Turning Back: The Peacetime Revolutions of Post-War Britain* (Oxford: Oxford University Press, 2010), pp. 336-7. The reduction was probably compounded by the demands of 'commuting', and the spread of motor vehicles: J. Obelkevich, 'Consumption', in J. Obelkevich and P. Catterall (eds.), *Understanding Post-War British Society* (London: Routledge, 1994), p. 144. Equally, growing wages, shifts in household time economies, and developments in food production and storage saw an increase in sales of 'convenience' foods and sugared foodstuffs: ibid., p. 143; A. Murcott, 'Food and nutrition in post-war Britain', in Obelkevich and Catterall (eds.), *Understanding Post-War British Society*, pp. 155-64. Finally, diabetes has consistently been found to be more prevalent in older age groups than in younger ones, and the proportion of people living until at least sixty-five increased over the post-war period: A. Tinker, 'Old age and gerontology', in Obelkevich and Catterall (eds.), *Understanding Post-War British Society*, pp. 73-5. This is to say nothing about other demographic and cultural changes related to class, gender, and ethnicity. This argument, however, is only intended to suggest that alterations in incidence and distribution are the result of complex webs of structures, practices, and inheritances, and cannot be reduced to simple explanations.

5 T. Scott and A. Maynard, 'Will the new GP contract lead to cost effective medical practice?', Discussion Paper 82, University of York, 1991, pp. ii, 14-35.

6 The history and definition of neoliberalism is taken up in Chapters 4 and 6. Briefly, neoliberal economic analysis and political philosophy emerged during the 1930s and 1940s in opposition to interventionist liberalism (and totalitarian government). The idea that markets were the most efficient allocator of resources, and political bulwarks sustaining all other freedoms, was central to early analyses: D. Stedman Jones, *Masters of the Universe: Hayek, Friedman, and the Birth of Neoliberal Politics* (Princeton: Princeton University Press, 2014), pp. 2-4, 37-72. Market management, though, was not to be laissez-faire, and the *raison d'être* of the state lay in constituting, monitoring, and regulating market relations to promote competition. M. Foucault, *The Birth of Biopolitics: Lectures at the Collège de France, 1978-79*, trans. G. Burchell, ed. M. Senellart (Basingstoke: Palgrave Macmillan, 2008), pp. 133-4, 138-41, 161. Though changing over time, these ideas gained political purchase during the 1970s and 1980s.

7 P. Selby, 'W(h)ither diabetes care?', *Diabetic Medicine*, 10:9 (1993), 791-2.

8 C. J. C. Earl, 'Treatment of diabetics as hospital out-patients', *BMJ*, 1:3461 (1927), 831–3; 'The management of diabetic out-patients'; R. D. Lawrence, 'Special clinics for diabetics', *BMJ*, 2:4262 (1942), 322; R. D. Lawrence, 'Regional diabetic services', *BMJ*, 2:4828 (1953), 160.
9 Department of Health for Scotland, *Committee on Scottish Health Services*, Cmd 5204 (Edinburgh: HMSO, 1936), p. 304.
10 M. Foucault, *Discipline and Punish: The Birth of the Prison*, trans. A. Sheridan (London: Penguin, 1991 [1975]).
11 R. Flynn, 'Clinical governance and governmentality', *Health, Risk and Society*, 4:2 (2002), 155–73.
12 The popularity of 'governance' frameworks has grown in response to a history of financial crises and an intensifying academic and political concern with transformations in the nature of 'risk': M. van Daelen, C. Van der Elst, and A. van de Ven, 'Risk management interconnections in law, accounting and tax', in M. van Daelen and C. Van der Elst (eds.), *Risk Management and Corporate Government: Interconnections in Law, Accounting and Tax* (Cheltenham: Edward Elgar, 2010), pp. 191–231; E. A. Rosa, O. Renn, and A. M. McCright, *The Risk Society Revisited: Social Theory and Governance* (Philadelphia: Temple University Press, 2013). Despite consistent failures in protection, however, such frameworks continue to legitimate institutions in technical and popular communities.
13 Flynn, 'Clinical governance and governmentality'. Though often unquestioned, this 'common sense' is a form of political justification: S. Rosenfeld, *Common Sense: A Political History* (Cambridge, MA: Harvard University Press, 2011).
14 National Audit Office, *The Management of Adult Diabetes Services in the NHS* (London: The Stationery Office, 2012); J. Daly, *Evidence-Based Medicine and the Search for a Science of Clinical Care* (Berkeley: University of California Press, 2005).
15 N. Triggle, 'Diabetes care depressingly poor, says MPs', *BBC News*, 6 November 2012, available at: www.bbc.co.uk/news/health-20210823 (accessed May 2015).
16 H. Perkins, *The Rise of Professional Society: England since 1880* (London: Routledge, 1990). Trust to deal with complex cases remains, but discretion operates within a broader framework of increased external oversight and regulation: J. Evetts, 'New professionalism and new public management: changes, continuities, and consequences', *Comparative Sociology*, 8:2 (2009), 247–66.
17 Evetts, 'New professionalism and new public management'. On late-century changes: G. Hanlon, 'Professionalism as enterprise: service class politics and the redefinition of professionalism', *Sociology*, 32:1 (1998), 43–63; M. Power, *The Audit Society: Rituals of Verification* (Oxford:

Oxford University Press, 1999). For a case study: G. Hanlon, 'Institutional forms and organizational structures: homology, trust and reputational capital in professional services firms', *Organization*, 11:2 (2004), 187–210.

18 A. M. Brandt and M. Gardner, 'The golden age of medicine?', in R. Cooter and J. Pickstone (eds.), *Companion to Medicine in the Twentieth Century* (Abingdon: Routledge, 2003), pp. 29–34; M. Saks, 'Medicine and the counter culture', in Cooter and Pickstone (eds.), *Companion to Medicine in the Twentieth Century*, pp. 113–24. On financial changes: van Daelen et al., 'Risk management interconnections in law, accounting and tax', pp. 191–231. For welfare professionals: I. Kirkpatrick, S. Ackroyd, and R. Walker, *The New Managerialism and Public Service Professions: Change in Health, Social Services and Housing* (Basingstoke: Palgrave Macmillan, 2005).

19 The extent of professional involvement in other fields has seemingly varied: Hanlon, 'Institutional forms and organizational structures'; Evetts, 'New professionalism and new public management'. See also Perkins, *The Rise of Professional Society*.

20 I. Kirkpatrick and M. M. Lucio (eds.), *The Politics of Quality in the Public Sector: The Management of Change* (London: Routledge, 1995). The British Social Attitudes Survey 2014 asked: 'from what you know or have heard, in general, how much do you trust [professional group] to put the interests of their patients above the convenience of the hospital?'. Over 70 per cent of respondents answered 'just about always' or 'most of the time' for nurses, and 65 per cent of them answered the same for doctors. These findings, and the results from other surveys, certainly compare well with responses gathered about trust in other public figures. An IPSOS Mori poll of 2013 put trust in doctors to tell the truth at around 89 per cent, compared with 18 per cent for politicians: A. Charles, 'Do the public still trust doctors and nurses?', *The King's Fund*, 7 December 2015, available at: https://www.kingsfund.org.uk/blog/2015/12/public-trust-doctors-nurses (accessed January 2018).

21 S. Harrison and C. Pollitt, Controlling *Health Professionals: The Future of Work and Organization in the NHS* (Buckingham: Open University Press, 1994); S. Harrison and B. Wood, 'Scientific-Bureaucratic Medicine and UK health policy', *Policy Studies Review*, 17:4 (2000), 25–42; S. Harrison, M. Moran, and B. Wood, 'Policy emergence and policy convergence: the case of "Scientific-Bureaucratic Medicine" in the United States and United Kingdom', *British Journal of Politics and International Relations*, 4:1 (2002), 1–21; S. Harrison and W. I. U. Ahmad, 'Medical autonomy and the UK state 1975 to 2025', *Sociology*, 34:1 (2000), 129–46; Flynn, 'Clinical governance and governmentality', pp. 155–6, 159–60; Kirkpatrick et al., *The New Managerialism*.

22 R. Klein, 'The crises of the welfare states', in R. Cooter and J. Pickstone (eds.), *Medicine in the Twentieth Century* (Amsterdam: Rodopi, 2000), pp. 155–70.
23 Harrison et al., 'Policy emergence and policy convergence'.
24 Scholars have used the term 'New Right' to refer to a nebulous mixture of thinkers and institutions promoting neoliberal, libertarian, neo-conservative, and traditional liberal political rationalities that flowered after the 1950s: N. Barry, 'Neoclassicism, the New Right and British social welfare', in R. M. Page and R. Silburn (eds.), *British Social Welfare in the Twentieth Century* (Basingstoke: Macmillan, 1999), pp. 55–80. Cf. A. Gamble, *The Free Economy and the Strong State: The Politics of Thatcherism* (Durham, NC: Duke University Press, 1988).
25 Kirkpatrick et al., *The New Managerialism*.
26 P. Day, R. Klein, and F. Miller, *A Comparative US–UK Study of Guidelines* (London: Nuffield Trust, 1998); D. Armstrong, 'Clinical autonomy, individual and collective: the problem of changing doctors' behaviour', *Social Science and Medicine*, 55:10 (2002), 1771–7.
27 Cf. more recent work: J. Evetts, 'A new professionalism? Challenges and opportunities', *Current Sociology*, 59:4 (2011), 406–22.
28 Though, for guidelines, see G. Weisz, A. Cambrosio, P. Keating, L. Knaapen, T. Schlich, and V. J. Tournay, 'The emergence of clinical practice guidelines', *Milbank Quarterly*, 85:4 (2007), 691–727.
29 Ibid.; S. Mars, 'Peer pressure and imposed consensus: the making of the 1984 Guidelines of Good Clinical Practice in the Treatment of Drug Misuse', in V. Berridge (ed.), *Making Health Policy: Networks in Research and Policy after 1945* (Amsterdam: Rodopi, 2005), pp. 149–84.
30 Over the post-war period, the British state experienced considerable shifts in its hinterlands, developing dispersed and fuzzy boundaries: J. Clarke and J. Newman, *The Managerial State: Power, Politics and Ideology in the Remaking of Social Welfare* (London: Sage, 1997). However, as these frontiers themselves have not been crucial to the history of British diabetes care, this book does not trace the state's exact contours throughout, so much as highlight where care has intersected with programmes for change.
31 M. Stacey, *Regulating British Medicine: The General Medical Council* (Chichester: John Wiley & Sons, 1992).
32 S. Sheard and L. Donaldson, *The Nation's Doctor: The Role of the Chief Medical Officer 1855–1998* (Abingdon: Radcliffe, 2005); V. Berridge (ed.), *Making Health Policy: Networks in Research and Policy after 1945* (Amsterdam: Rodopi, 2005).
33 There are probably more definitions of 'the state' than there are scholars who have written about it: A. Sharma and A. Gupta (eds.), *The*

Anthropology of the State: A Reader (Oxford: Blackwell, 2006). This work deploys a common political-scientific model, one that recognises interconnections between government, professionals, and the various local and central arms of the polity, whilst also maintaining distinctions between them.

34 C. Lawrence, *Rockefeller Money, The Laboratory and Medicine in Edinburgh, 1919–1930: New Science in an Old Country* (New York: University of Rochester Press, 2005); S. Sturdy, 'The political economy of scientific medicine: science, education and the transformation of medical practice in Sheffield, 1890–1922', *Medical History*, 36:2 (1992), 125–59.

35 M. Berg, 'Problems and promises of the protocol', *Social Science and Medicine*, 44:8 (1997), 1081–8; G. Weisz, 'From clinical counting to Evidence-Based Medicine', in G. Forland, A. Opinel, and G. Weisz (eds.), *Body Counts: Medical Quantification in Historical and Sociological Perspectives* (Montreal: McGill University Press, 2005), pp. 377–93.

36 P. Addison, *The Road to 1945: British Politics and the Second World War* (London: Pimlico, 1994 [1975]). For sympathetic reviews: R. Lowe, 'The Second World War, consensus and the foundation of the welfare state', *Twentieth Century British History*, 1:2 (1990), 152–82; D. Kavanagh, 'The postwar consensus', *Twentieth Century British History*, 3:2 (1992), 175–90. And for critique: B. Pimlott, 'The myth of consensus', in L. M. Smith (ed.), *The Making of Britain: Echoes of Greatness* (Basingstoke: Macmillan, 1988), pp. 129–42; P. Kerr, *Post-War British Politics: From Conflict to Consensus* (London: Routledge, 2001).

37 D. Kavanagh and P. Morris, *Consensus Politics from Attlee to Major*, 2nd edition (Oxford: Blackwell, 1995).

38 See Chapter 4 for further discussion.

39 J. Tomlinson, 'Planning: debate and policy in the 1940s', *Twentieth Century British History*, 3:2 (1992), 154–74; R. Toye, 'Gosplanners versus thermostatters: Whitehall planning debates and their political consequences, 1945–49', *Contemporary British History*, 14:4 (2000), 81–106.

40 J. Tomlinson, '"Liberty with order": Conservative economic policy, 1951–1964', in M. Francis and I. Zweiniger-Bargielowska (eds.), *The Conservatives and British Society* (Cardiff: University of Wales Press, 1996), pp. 274–88.

41 G. O'Hara, *From Dreams to Disillusionment: Economic and Social Planning in the 1960s* (Basingstoke: Palgrave Macmillan, 2007).

42 S. Ball and A. Seldon (eds.), *The Heath Government, 1970–1974: A Reappraisal* (Longman: London, 1996). And for their international connections: B. Clift and J. Tomlinson, 'Negotiating credibility: Britain and the International Monetary Fund, 1956–1976', *Contemporary European History*, 17:4 (2008), 545–66.

43 P. Pierson, *Dismantling the Welfare State? Thatcher, Reagan and the Politics of Retrenchment* (Cambridge: Cambridge University Press, 1994); Clarke and Newman, *The Managerial State*; Kirkpatrick et al., *The New Managerialism*. For nuanced overviews of the whole period: R. Lowe, *The Welfare State in Britain since 1945*, 3rd edition (Basingstoke: Palgrave Macmillan, 2005); Addison, *No Turning Back*.
44 P. Howlett, 'The "Golden Age", 1955–1973', in P. Johnson (ed.), *Twentieth Century Britain: Economic, Social and Cultural Change* (London: Longman, 1994), pp. 320–39.
45 A. Cairncross, *The British Economy since 1945: Economic Policy and Performance, 1945–1990* (Oxford: Blackwell, 1992).
46 Lowe, *The Welfare State in Britain since 1945*, pp. 80–4; C. Webster, *The Health Services since the War*, vol. I: *Problems of Health Care: The National Health Service before 1957* (London: HMSO, 1988); C. Webster, *The Health Services since the War*, vol. 2: *Government and Health Care: The British National Health Service, 1958–1979* (London: HMSO, 1996).
47 C. Cook, 'Oral history – Walter Holland', *Journal of Public Health*, 26:2 (2004), 121–9; S. Sheard, *The Passionate Economist: How Brian Abel-Smith Shaped Global Health Policy and Social Welfare* (Bristol: Policy Press, 2013); S. Sheard, 'Space, place and (waiting) time: reflections on health policy and politics', *Health Economics, Policy, and Law*, 13:3–4 (2018), 226–50.
48 A. Mold, *Making the Patient-Consumer: Patient Organisations and Health Consumerism in Britain* (Manchester: Manchester University Press, 2015); G. O'Hara, 'The complexities of "consumerism": choice, collectivism and participation within Britain's National Health Service, c.1961–1979', *Social History of Medicine*, 26:2 (2013), 288–304.
49 T. Cutler, 'Managerialism *avant la lettre*? The debate on accounting in the NHS hospitals in the 1950s', in V. Berridge and K. Loughlin (eds.), *Medicine, the Market, and the Mass Media: Producing Health in the Twentieth Century* (London: Routledge, 2005), pp. 124–45.
50 See Chapters 5 and 6 of this volume.
51 A. Gray and B. Jenkins, 'Policy analysis in British central government: the experience of PAR', *Public Administration*, 60:4 (1982), 429–50; O'Hara, *From Dreams to Disillusionment*. From a Foucauldian perspective, this growing use of budgeting and review could be said to form part of the advanced liberal state's focus on governing at a distance: N. Rose, 'Government, authority and expertise in advanced liberalism', *Economy and Society*, 22:3 (1993), 283–99.
52 Clarke and Newman, *The Managerial State*; Kirkpatrick et al., *The New Managerialism*; R. Klein, *The New Politics of the NHS: From Creation to Reinvention*, 5th edition (Oxford: Radcliffe, 2006), pp. 140–86.

53 P. Dunleavy and C. Hood, 'From old public administration to new public management', *Public Money and Management*, 14:3 (1994), 9–16, esp. p. 10.
54 For important histories: R. B. Tattersall, *Diabetes: The Biography* (Oxford: Oxford University Press, 2009); E. L. Furdell, *Fatal Thirst: Diabetes in Britain until Insulin* (Leiden: Brill, 2009); M. Bliss, *The Discovery of Insulin*, 25th Anniversary Edition (Chicago: University of Chicago Press, 2007).
55 C. Sinding, 'Making the unit of insulin: standards, clinical work, and industry', *Bulletin of the History of Medicine*, 76:2 (2002), 231–70; M. Edwards, *Control and the Therapeutic Trial: Rhetoric and Experimentation in Britain, 1918–48* (Amsterdam: Rodopi, 2007); Lawrence, *Rockefeller Money*, pp. 270–304; C. Feudtner, *Bittersweet: Diabetes, Insulin, and the Transformation of Illness* (Chapel Hill: University of North Carolina Press, 2003); Greene, *Prescribing by Numbers*; C. Sinding, 'Flexible norms? From patients' values to physicians' standards', in W. Ernst (ed.), *Histories of the Normal and the Abnormal: Social and Cultural Histories of Norms and Normativity* (London: Routledge, 2006), pp. 225–44. On state–industry relations: J. Liebenau, 'The MRC and the pharmaceutical industry: the model of insulin', in J. Austoker and L. Bryder (eds.), *Historical Perspectives on the Role of the MRC: Essays in the History of the Medical Research Council of the United Kingdom and its Predecessor, the Medical Research Committee, 1913–1953* (Oxford: Oxford University Press, 1989), pp. 163–80.
56 As will be explored further in Chapter 1, social medicine provided a common intellectual ancestor of chronic disease epidemiology and health service assessment: V. Berridge, *Marketing Health: Smoking and the Discourse of Public Health in Britain, 1945–2000* (Oxford: Oxford University Press, 2007), pp. 15–16.
57 This curative and acute-disease orientation can be seen, for instance, in the policy assumptions that 'expenditure on healthcare would tend to be self-liquidating by producing a healthier population': Klein, *The New Politics of the NHS*, p. 26. Britain differed from the USA in its nationalisation of financial risk of ill-health, but British policy-makers shared their US counterparts' focus on scientific knowledge, specialised labour, hospital treatment, and medical technology: D. Fox, *Power and Illness: The Failure of American Health Policy* (Berkeley: University of California Press, 1993). See Conclusion below for further discussion.
58 R. D. Lawrence, 'Regional centres for the treatment of diabetes', *The Lancet*, 257:6668 (1951), 1318.
59 K. G. M. M. Alberti, 'The role of diabetes', *BMJ*, 303:6805 (1991), 769.
60 Moore, 'Reorganising chronic disease management', 453–72. For similar developments in acute care: J. D. Howell, *Technology in the Hospital:*

Transforming Patient Care in the Early Twentieth Century (Baltimore: Johns Hopkins University Press, 1995).

61 By bureaucratic, then, I mean work being performed according to codified rules and within prescribed roles. Action taken is also documented and reviewed, often within a hierarchical organisation. This is a generalised view adapted from M. Weber, *Economy and Society: An Outline of Interpretive Sociology*, G. Roth and C. Wittich (eds.), trans. E. Fischoff et al., vols. 1 and 2 (Berkeley: California University Press, 1978), pp. 217–26, 956–1005, esp. pp. 956–8, 973–5. Medical systems often demonstrated the same 'gaps' between model and practice, and the same reliance on tacit knowledge, as many other bureaucratic organisations: E. Freidson, 'The changing nature of professional control', *Annual Review of Sociology*, 10 (1984), 11–12.

62 J. Hasler, 'The size and nature of the problem', in J. Hasler and T. Schofield (eds.), *Continuing Care: The Management of Chronic Disease*, 2nd edition (Oxford: Oxford University Press, 1984), p. 10.

63 This is a slight revision of G. Weisz, *Chronic Disease in the Twentieth Century: A History* (Baltimore: Johns Hopkins University Press, 2014), pp. 176–203.

64 W. Laing and R. Williams, *Diabetes: A Model for Health Care Management* (London: Office of Health Economics, 1989). On post-war lobbying: Berridge, *Marketing Health*; M. Hilton, N. Crowson, J. McKay, and J.-F. Mouhot, *The Politics of Expertise: How NGOs Shaped Modern Britain* (Oxford: Oxford University Press, 2013).

65 H. Dudley, 'Necessity for surgical audit', *BMJ*, 1:5902 (1974), 275–7. In the USA, surgeons performed the earliest recorded audits during the 1910s: S. Reverby, 'Stealing the golden eggs: Ernest Amory Codman and the science and management of medicine', *Bulletin of the History of Medicine*, 55:2 (1981), 156–71.

66 T. J. Johnson, *Professions and Power* (London: Macmillan, 1972); M. S. Larson, *The Rise of Professionalism: A Sociological Analysis* (Berkeley: University of California Press, 1977).

67 E. Freidson, *Profession of Medicine: A Study of the Sociology of Applied Knowledge* (Chicago: University of Chicago Press, 1988 [1970]); H. S. Becker, B. Geer, E. C. Hughes, and A. L. Strauss, *Boys in White: Student Culture and Medical School* (New Brunswick, NJ: Transaction Books, 1984 [1961]). On the shifting limits of medical autonomy and control in nineteenth-century hospitals: K. Waddington, *Charity and the London Hospitals, 1850–1898* (Woodbridge: Boydell Press, 2000), pp. 159–88.

68 M. J. D. Roberts, 'The politics of professionalization: MPs, medical men, and the 1858 Medical Act', *Medical History*, 53:1 (2009), 37–56.

69 Stacey, *Regulating British Medicine*.

70 L. Granshaw, '"Fame and fortune by means of bricks and mortar": the medical profession and specialist hospitals in Britain, 1800–1948', in L. Granshaw and R. Porter (eds.), *The Hospital in History* (London: Routledge, 1989), pp. 199–220.

71 Critiques of specialisation were wide-ranging, encompassing not just effects on medical education and professional unity, but also, for instance, the reputational damage brought to hospitals, and the disrepute that advertising could inflict on the profession. See also G. Weisz, *Divide and Conquer: A Comparative History of Medical Specialization* (Oxford: Oxford University Press, 2006), pp. 28–35.

72 Ibid., p. 33; C. Lawrence, 'Incommunicable knowledge: science, technology and the clinical art in Britain, 1850–1914', *Journal of Contemporary History*, 20:4 (1985), 503–20. The idea of the 'whole patient' was rather flexible, but it generally incorporated ideas of seeing the patient as an integrated biological whole, treating the patient as an individual, and knowing the patient as a person, one who interacted with complex social and physical environments.

73 Weisz, *Divide and Conquer*, pp. 34–43; M. Gorsky, '"Threshold of a new era": the development of an integrated hospital system in northeast Scotland, 1900–39', *Social History of Medicine*, 17:2 (2004), 247–67.

74 J. V. Pickstone, *Medicine and Industrial Society: A History of Hospital Development in Manchester and its Region, 1752–1946* (Manchester: Manchester University Press, 1985), pp. 184–211; F. Honigsbaum, *The Division in British Medicine: A History of the Separation of General Practice from Hospital Care, 1911–1968* (London: Kogan and Page, 1979).

75 S. Sturdy and R. Cooter, 'Science, scientific management and the transformation of medicine in Britain, c.1870–1950', *History of Science*, 36:4 (1998), 421–66; Lawrence, *Rockefeller Money*.

76 Such as the creation of the NHS: Klein, *The New Politics of the NHS*, pp. 1–21.

77 Roberts, 'The politics of professionalization'; I. Waddington, *The Medical Profession in the Industrial Revolution* (Dublin: Gill and Macmillan, 1984), pp. 135–52.

78 Waddington, *The Medical Profession in the Industrial Revolution*; A. Digby, *Making a Medical Living: Doctors and Patients in the English Market for Medicine, 1720–1911* (Cambridge: Cambridge University Press, 1994), pp. 19–20.

79 A. Digby and N. Bosanquet, 'Doctors and patients in an era of national health insurance and private practice', *Economic History Review*, 41:1 (1988), 74–94.

80 B. M. Doyle, *The Politics of Hospital Provision in Early Twentieth-Century Britain* (London: Pickering and Chatto, 2014); M. Gorsky, 'Local

government health services in interwar England: problems of quantification and interpretation', *Bulletin of the History of Medicine*, 85:3 (2011), 384–412.
81 Klein, *The New Politics of the NHS*, p. 37.
82 Sturdy and Cooter, 'Science, scientific management and the transformation of medicine in Britain'.
83 International connections are stressed in Lawrence, *Rockefeller Money*.
84 R. M. M. Domenech and C. Casañeda, 'Redefining cancer during the interwar period: British Medical Officers of Health, state policy, managerialism and public health', *American Journal of Public Health*, 97:9 (2007), 1563–71. For an earlier development of managerial attitudes and structures in hospitals: Waddington, *Charity and the London Hospitals, 1850–1898*, pp. 135–58.
85 Foucault, *Discipline and Punish*.
86 T. P. Porter, *Trust in Numbers: The Pursuit of Objectivity in Science and Public Life* (Princeton: Princeton University Press, 1995); J. C. Scott, *Seeing Like a State: How Certain Schemes to Improve the Human Condition Have Failed* (New Haven: Yale University Press, 1998); G. C. Bowker and S. Star, *Sorting Things Out* (Cambridge, MA: MIT Press, 1999); N. Dirks, *Castes of Mind: Colonialism and the Making of Modern India* (Princeton: Princeton University Press, 2001); Weisz, *Divide and Conquer*, pp. xix–xx.
87 This is not to suggest that inscription, categorisation, or standardisation had been absent in British medicine. Rather that such practices (and associated concepts of the body and disease) tended to intensify in large-scale provision and third-party payment, being particularly prominent within medical institutions and in public health: G. Mooney, 'Diagnostic spaces: workhouse, hospital, and home in mid-Victorian London', *Social Science History*, 33:3 (2009), 357–90.
88 G. Forsyth and R. Logan, *Gateway or Dividing Line? A Study of Hospital Outpatients in the 1960s* (Oxford: Oxford University Press for the Nuffield Provincial Hospitals Trust, 1968); interview with H. Keen performed by the University of Oxford, 21 November 2006, available at: www.diabetes-stories.com/interview.asp?UID=52 (accessed April 2017).
89 T. Osborne, 'Epidemiology as an investigative paradigm: the College of General Practitioners in the 1950s', *Social Science and Medicine*, 38:2 (1994), 317–26; Webster, *The Health Services since the War*, vol. 1, pp. 223–7.
90 Sturdy and Cooter, 'Science, scientific management and the transformation of medicine in Britain'; D. Wright, S. Mullally, and M. C. Cordukes, '"Worse than being married": the exodus of British doctors from the National Health Service to Canada, c.1955–75', *Journal of the History of Medicine and Allied Sciences*, 65:4 (2010), 546–75.

91 Weisz et al., 'The emergence of clinical practice guidelines'; S. Timmermanns and M. Berg, *The Gold Standard: The Challenge of Evidence-Based Medicine and Standardization in Health Care* (Philadelphia: Temple University Press, 2003).
92 Edwards, *Control and the Therapeutic Trial*; H. Valier and C. Timmermann, 'Clinical trials and the reorganization of medical research in post-Second World War Britain', *Medical History*, 52:4 (2008), 493–510.
93 D. Armstrong, 'Clinical sense and clinical science', *Social Science and Medicine*, 11:11–13 (1977), 599–601.
94 Cf. Lawrence, 'Incommunicable knowledge'.
95 See Chapter 1. Today, diabetes is divided into numerous 'types' and subtypes, aligned with different possible causes, treatments, and prognoses. Broadly, the two most clinically important are types 1 and 2. Type 2 accounts for approximately 90 per cent of cases in Britain. The ultimate cause is still debated, though the immediate mechanism is currently believed to be insufficient endogenous insulin production, or the inability of the body's cells to react to insulin. Type 1 accounts for approximately 10 per cent of cases in Britain. Again, the ultimate cause is unknown, though the immediate mechanism is believed to be the autoimmune destruction of pancreatic cells, eliminating insulin production. Type 2 is treated primarily through dietary management and oral drugs, type 1 by diet and exogenous insulin injections. Both conditions are characterised by blood glucose levels elevated beyond normal statistical ranges, and patients with either type have significantly increased risk of experiencing a range of complications affecting almost every system and organ in the body. The development of this classification is discussed later in this Introduction.
96 D. Cantor, 'Introduction: cancer control and prevention in the twentieth century', *Bulletin of the History of Medicine*, 81:3 (2007), 1–38; C. Timmermann, 'A matter of degree: the normalization of hypertension, c.1940–2000', in Ernst (ed.), *Histories of the Normal and the Abnormal*, pp. 245–61.
97 L. J. Sanders, 'From Thebes to Toronto and the 21st century: an incredible journey', *Diabetes Spectrum*, 15:1 (2002), 56–60; C. Feudtner, *Bittersweet*, pp. 4–6. Others trace the earliest recorded concerns with diabetes to Hindu authors writing as early as 1600 BCE: Furdell, *Fatal Thirst*, p. 13.
98 Furdell, *Fatal Thirst*, pp. 13–37.
99 Ibid., p. 17.
100 M. Foucault, *The Birth of the Clinic: An Archaeology of Medical Perception*, trans. A. M. Sheridan Smith (London: Routledge, 2010 [1973]).
101 N. Jewson, 'Disappearance of the sick man from medical cosmology, 1770–1870', *Sociology*, 10:2 (1976), 225–44; S. J. Reiser, *Medicine and the Reign of Technology* (Cambridge: Cambridge University Press, 1978); M.

E. Fissell, 'The disappearance of the patient's narrative and the invention of hospital medicine', in R. French and A. Wear (eds.), *British Medicine in an Age of Reform* (London: Routledge, 1991), pp. 91–109.
102 W. F. Bynum, *Science and the Practice of Medicine in the Nineteenth Century* (Cambridge: Cambridge University Press, 1994).
103 Lawrence, 'Incommunicable knowledge'.
104 N. M. Theriot, 'Negotiating illness: doctors, patients and families in the nineteenth century', *Journal of the History of Behavioural Sciences*, 37:4 (2001), 349–68.
105 Physicians had evaporated urine from patients with diabetes to examine the substances left behind, and used diabetic urine in fermentation: Feudtner, *Bittersweet*, pp. 5–6; Tattersall, *Diabetes*, p. 15.
106 Tattersall, *Diabetes*, pp. 19–20. There was, however, some debate about the importance of glycosuric test results, particularly between the 1870s and 1890s: Furdell, *Fatal Thirst*, pp. 143–4.
107 H. Keen and S. Ng Tang Fui, 'The definition and classification of diabetes mellitus', *Clinics in Endocrinology and Metabolism*, 11:2 (1982), 283–7.
108 F. W. Pavy, *Researches on the Nature and Treatment of Diabetes* (London: John Churchill & Sons, 1869); Tattersall, *Diabetes*, p. 20.
109 Tattersall, *Diabetes*, pp. 15–17.
110 J. H. Warner, *The Therapeutic Perspective: Medical Practice, Knowledge and Identity in America, 1820–1885* (Cambridge, MA: Harvard University Press, 1986), pp. 83–162.
111 H. MacLean, *Modern Methods in the Diagnosis and Treatment of Glycosuria and Diabetes* (London: Constable Co., 1922), pp. 107–30. On the importance of international research: C. Feudtner, 'Pathway to health: juvenile diabetes and the origins of managerial medicine', in A. M. Stern and H. Markel (eds.), *Formative Years: Children's Health in the United States, 1880–2000* (Ann Arbor: University of Michigan Press, 2002), pp. 208–32. On colonial research and nutritional sciences: D. Arnold, 'British India and the "beri-beri problem", 1798–1942', *Medical History*, 54:3 (2010), 295–314. On pre-clinical sciences in medical education: K. Waddington, *Medical Education at St Bartholomew's Hospital, 1123–1995* (Woodbridge: Boydell Press, 2003), pp. 115–45.
112 Tattersall, *Diabetes*, pp. 19–20.
113 M. D. Moore, 'Food as medicine: diet and diabetes management in twentieth-century Britain', *Journal of the History of Medicine and Allied Sciences*, 73:2 (2018), 150–67. But see Lawrence, *Rockefeller Money*, pp. 270–304. On testing, cf. H. MacLean, *Modern Methods in the Diagnosis and Treatment of Glycosuria and Diabetes*, 5th edition (London: Constable Co., 1932), p. 163; H. P. Himsworth, 'Management of diabetes mellitus, part II', *BMJ*, 2:3942 (1936), 190. Most agreed, however, that blood testing was necessary to commence therapy.

Introduction

114 Furdell, *Fatal Thirst*, pp. 148–9; A. C. Begg, *Insulin in General Practice: A Concise Clinical Guide for Practitioners* (London: William Heinemann, 1924), pp. 44–6.
115 Trials with the drug were central to standardising the unit of insulin. Although doctors recognised that each patient would require a tailored amount of insulin (subject to affordability), the same volume of insulin from different batches initially had varying levels of potency: Sinding, 'Making the unit of insulin', pp. 231–70. The trials also represented the efforts of the Ministry of Health and the MRC to manage British medicine and to develop sites of scientific expertise during supply shortages of 1922–23. Supplies were directed to trusted sources and institutions with required laboratory facilities, centring expertise in hospitals and fostering a physiological approach to patient management: D. Maksimov-Cox, 'The making of the clinical trial in Britain, 1910–1945: expertise, the state and the public' (PhD dissertation, University of Cambridge, 1997), pp. 96–137. By July 1923, the Ministry removed controls, and the drug became widely used both within non-teaching hospitals and in GP practices, often with a compromise between physiological and clinical perspectives on treatment.
116 Moore, 'Food as medicine'.
117 R. D. Lawrence, *The Diabetic Life: Its Control by Diet and Insulin. A Concise Practical Manual for Practitioners and Patients*, 6th edition (London: J. & A. Churchill, 1931), pp. 30–65.
118 For a broader examination of the role of professional and patient in diabetes management: M. D. Moore, 'Balance and the "good diabetic" in Britain, c.1900–60', in M. Jackson and M. D. Moore (eds.), *Balancing the Self: Medicine, Politics, and the Regulation of Health in the Twentieth Century* (forthcoming).
119 Ibid.
120 P. L. Robinson and E. T. Baker-Bates, 'A new diabetic chart', *BMJ*, 2:4790 (1952), 919–21.
121 This was the view expressed by one interviewee, a retired academic epidemiologist and health authority member. They worked within major centres of diabetes care and research between the 1970s and 2000s, as well as undertaking government advisory and university administration work: interview with Professor Davies conducted by the author. All participants in interviews with the author have been given pseudonyms.
122 Tattersall, *Diabetes*, pp. 25–6.
123 Lawrence, *The Diabetic Life*, 6th edition, pp. 48–59. In later years, 'moderate' fell out of use: R. D. Lawrence, *The Diabetic Life: Its Control by Diet and Insulin and Oral Treatment by Sulphonyl-Ureas. A Concise Practical Manual*, 16th edition (London: J. & A. Churchill, 1960), pp. 39–40.

124 J. Malins, *Clinical Diabetes Mellitus* (London: Eyre & Spottiswoode, 1968), pp. 101–2; W. G. Oakley, D. A. Pyke, and K. W. Taylor, *Diabetes and its Management*, 3rd edition (Oxford: Blackwell Scientific Publications, 1978), pp. 61–6.
125 A. M. Hedgecoe, 'Reinventing diabetes: classification, division, and geneticization of disease', *New Genetics and Society*, 21:2 (2002), 7–27. See discussion of the 'J-Type' variety of diabetes in: M. D. Moore, 'Harnessing the power of difference: colonialism and British chronic disease research, 1940–1975', *Social History of Medicine*, 29:2 (2016), p. 390.
126 H. P. Himsworth, 'The syndrome of diabetes mellitus and its causes', *The Lancet*, 253:6551 (1949), 465–73.
127 Furdell, *Fatal Thirst*, p. 135; S. O'Donnell, 'Changing social and scientific discourses on type 2 diabetes between 1800 and 1950: a socio-historical analysis', *Sociology of Health and Illness*, 37:7 (2015), 1108–11.
128 Lawrence, *The Diabetic Life*, 6th edition, pp. 9–10.
129 Ibid., p. 10. But reviews for insulin-dependent diabetes would often involve discussion of specific genes, viruses, and autoantibodies during the 1980s and early 1990s: WHO, *Diabetes Mellitus: Report of a WHO Study Group*, Technical Report Series, 727 (Geneva: WHO, 1985), pp. 32–7; Fry and Sandler, *Common Diseases*, 5th edition, pp. 392–3.
130 G. M. Oppenheimer, 'Profiling risk: the emergence of coronary heart disease epidemiology in the United States (1947–70)', *International Journal of Epidemiology*, 35:3 (2006), 720–30; D. Porter, *Health Citizenship: Essays in Social Medicine and Biomedical Politics* (Berkeley: University of California Press, 2011), pp. 154–81. For the reception in different territories: C. Timmermann, 'Appropriating risk factors: the reception of an American approach to chronic disease in the two German states, c.1950–1990', *Social History of Medicine*, 25:1 (2012), 157–74.
131 Berridge, *Marketing Health*; Oppenheimer, 'Profiling risk', pp. 720–1.
132 Weisz, *Chronic Disease in the Twentieth Century*.
133 Ibid., pp. 196–7; D. Porter, 'From social structure to social behaviour in Britain after the Second World War', *Contemporary British History*, 16:3 (2002), 58–80.
134 L. Berlivet, '"Association or causation?" The debate on the scientific status of risk factor epidemiology, 1947–c.1965', in Berridge (ed.), *Making Health Policy*, pp. 39–74.
135 On the fractious debate over heart disease: M. Bufton and V. Berridge, 'Post-war nutrition science and policy making in Britain c.1945–1994: the case of diet and heart disease', in D. Smith and J. Phillips (eds.), *Food, Science, Policy and Regulation in the Twentieth Century: International and Comparative Perspectives* (London: Routledge, 2000), pp. 207–22.

136 J. Hand, 'Marketing health education: advertising margarine and visualising health in Britain from 1964–c.2000', *Contemporary British History*, 31:4 (2017), 477–500.
137 D. Armstrong, 'The rise of surveillance medicine', *Sociology of Health and Illness*, 17:3 (1995), 393–404.
138 J. G. L. Jackson, 'R. D. Lawrence and the formation of the Diabetic Association', *Diabetic Medicine*, 13:1 (1996), 17–21.
139 H. G. Wells, 'Diabetics in sympathy', *The Times*, 15 February 1934, p. 10.
140 R. D. Lawrence, 'The beginning of the Diabetic Association in England', in D. von Engelhardt (ed.), *Diabetes: Its Medical and Cultural History. Outlines, Texts, Bibliography* (New York: Springer-Verlag, c.1989 [1951], pp. 451–3; Jackson, 'R. D. Lawrence and the formation of the Diabetic Association', pp. 18–19.
141 In 1957, the Association estimated membership at 22,000, reaching over 100,000 by 1988: J. G. L. Jackson, *Employment Survey* (London: BDA, 1961), p. 2; BDA, *Helping People Live with Diabetes* (London: BDA, 1988), pp. 1–2.
142 Jackson, 'R. D. Lawrence and the formation of the Diabetic Association', p.19; J. G. L. Jackson, 'The formation of the Medical and Scientific Section of the British Diabetic Association', *Diabetic Medicine*, 14:10 (1997), 886–91.
143 R. D. Lawrence, *The Diabetic Life: Its Control by Diet and Insulin. A Concise Practical Manual for Practitioners and Patients* (London: J. & A. Churchill, 1925), p. 54; F. C. Eve, 'Diabetic treatment simplified', *BMJ*, 1:3362 (1925), 1033–5.
144 C. M. Fletcher, 'Inquiry into diabetic care', *BMJ*, 2:4357 (1944), 58; The National Archives, London (TNA), BD 18/793, 4621, letter by H. Bristow (BDA), untitled, 8 March 1966.
145 During the period under discussion, there were two Royal Colleges of Physicians in Britain, the Royal College of Physicians of London and Royal College of Physicians of Edinburgh. Both feature in the following history, but the Royal College of Physicians of London is discussed most heavily because of that College's political importance and relationship to the British Diabetic Association. All references to the Royal College of Physicians, and abbreviation RCP, will therefore be to the Royal College of Physicians of London, unless specified otherwise. Citations will reflect the self-identification of the authorial body, and as such will vary.
146 J. Nabarro, 'BDA present and future', *Diabetic Medicine*, 7:6 (1990), 476.
147 M. Jackson, *Asthma: The Biography* (Oxford: Oxford University Press, 2009), p. 21.
148 See Chapter 4.
149 For excellent scholarship in this regard: Feudtner, *Bittersweet*.

150 On how patients negotiated medical discourses: Sinding, 'Flexible norms?'; Moore, 'Food as medicine'.
151 H. Valier and R. Bivins, 'Organization, ethnicity and the British National Health Service', in J. Stanton (ed.), *Innovations in Health and Medicine: Diffusion and Resistance in the Twentieth Century* (London: Routledge, 2002), pp. 37–64.
152 The history of Northern Ireland and its own health services is connected to, but very distinct from, that of the rest of Britain. It is an area of history that deserves far greater attention than could be covered here, and demands further research.
153 J. Stewart, 'The National Health Service in Scotland, 1947–74: Scottish or British', *Historical Research*, 76:193 (2003), 389–410; P. Michael and C. Webster (eds.), *Health and Society in Twentieth-Century Wales* (Cardiff: University of Wales Press, 2006).
154 Gorsky, '"Threshold of a new era"'.
155 In this respect, committees considering diabetes acted like health commissions reviewing the NHS within individual countries, which tended to operate simultaneously and with close connection to each other.
156 Weisz et al., 'The emergence of clinical practice guidelines'; Harrison et al., 'Policy emergence and policy convergence'.
157 A. Hardy, 'Beriberi, Vitamin B1 and world food policy, 1925–1970', *Medical History*, 39:1 (1995), 61–77. Historically, such movements were also tied with colonial medicine: R. Bivins, 'Coming "home" to (post) colonial medicine: treating tropical bodies in post-war Britain', *Social History of Medicine*, 26:1 (2013), 1–20. See also Sheard, *The Passionate Economist*.
158 Day et al., *A Comparative US–UK Study of Guidelines*.
159 Private, direct-pay healthcare in Britain was not eliminated with the NHS: C. Williamson, 'The quiet time? Pay-beds and private practice in the National Health Service, 1948–1970', *Social History of Medicine*, 28:3 (2015), 576–95. The Thatcher governments introduced some small incentives for individuals and employers to take up private insurance, but, despite think-tanks like the Institute for Economic Affairs suggesting more extensive forms of privatisation, policy alternatives to the NHS quickly dissipated upon public exposure. On Thatcher and the complex issue of 'privatisation': C. Webster, *The National Health Service: A Political History* (Oxford: Oxford University Press, 1998), pp. 142–58; Klein, *The New Politics of the NHS*, pp. 123–30.
160 Webster, *The National Health Service*, p. 1.
161 Department of Health, *National Service Framework for Diabetes: Delivery Strategy* (London: Department of Health, 2002); Diabetes UK, 'Risk Score', *Diabetes UK*, 2015, available at: https://riskscore.diabetes.org.uk/start (accessed June 2015).

162 A. Dixon, A. Khachatryan, A. Wallace, S. Peckham, T. Boyce, and S. Gillam, *Impact of Quality and Outcomes Framework on Health Inequalities* (London: King's Fund, 2011).
163 Diabetes UK, *Diabetes: Facts and Figures*, version 4, *Diabetes UK*, May 2015, p. 3, available at: https://www.diabetes.org.uk/Documents/Position%20statements/Facts%20and%20stats%20June%202015.pdf (accessed June 2015).

1

Chronicity and the care team in Britain's New Jerusalem

Speaking to the Society of Medical Officers of Health in February 1965, J. J. A. Reid – a well-known public health practitioner – addressed a familiar theme. 'In this country', Reid began, 'the problems with which all branches of our profession are faced are very different from those of the past, when poverty, ignorance and infectious diseases were the main enemies of health.' 'Nowadays', Reid continued, 'it is towards cardiovascular disease, cancer, bronchitis, accidents, mental disorder, and such chronic conditions as diabetes mellitus and arthritis that we must look for the principal sources of mortality and morbidity.' For Reid, medical advances, increased education, and economic growth might have conquered the diseases of the past, and they were probably the sources of progress in the future. In the present, however, this combination had also provided the conditions for 'smoking … overeating, and … [lack of] exercise' that caused 'maladies of plenty'.[1]

For Reid, and other Medical Officers of Health (MOHs), doctors, and lay persons involved in public health activity, this changed profile of morbidity and mortality required new approaches. On the one hand, these practitioners spoke of a 'New Public Health', based on persuasive health education campaigns that would help individuals to manage the imbalanced lifestyles supposedly underpinning novel burdens of disease.[2] On the other hand, they recognised that such campaigns could form only one component of efforts to confront chronic disease. For conditions like diabetes, even contributory factors to onset were unknown, and complete disease prevention was not considered possible. Moreover, patients managing such illnesses were believed to encounter psychological challenges, discrimination, and often painful long-term complications. For these problems, it was argued, early diagnosis and treatment by a multi-disciplinary team of medical, nursing, and technical staff offered the best solutions.

Unfortunately for visionaries like Reid, the tripartite division of the NHS into general practice, hospital, and local government provision made multi-disciplinary and cross-institutional disease management difficult to realise. Reid had, for instance, placed local government health visitors, district nurses, and public health doctors at the heart of his plans to manage the rising toll of chronic disease. In diabetes, public health workers would promote early diagnosis by educating the public about symptoms and screening local populations. Equally, they would contribute to multi-disciplinary disease management by providing aftercare assistance to specialist hospital clinics and GPs responsible for long-term patient surveillance.[3] Ultimately, though, compromises built into the health system meant that promises of rationally planned and integrated care raised during post-war reconstruction were not realised in the ways envisaged by policy-makers.

Taking the gap between vision and practice as its starting point, this chapter analyses the ways in which diabetes management intersected with changing healthcare structures and emergent notions of chronicity during the two decades after 1945. Beginning with an overview of disease management strategies in the 1940s, it traces how the creation of the NHS confirmed diabetes as a hospital condition, one closely connected with specialist labour, a growing care team, and laboratory technologies. The concessions and divisions on which the NHS had been initially built, however, meant that regional organisation of clinic services, whilst much prized by doctors and the leading diabetes patient association, failed to take place. Furthermore, hospital care began to face serious challenges during the 1950s and 1960s. Shifting understandings of diabetes, rising patient loads, and resource constraints within the NHS encouraged clinicians to look beyond hospital management. Early innovations in cross-institutional care provided models for managing other conditions, but new forms of working were again frustrated by the limitations woven into the fabric of the health services.

Changing understandings of disease were related to shifting ideas of chronicity. During the 1940s, discussions of chronic patients generally referred to the large hospital populations deemed 'incurable' and admitted to old municipal and Poor Law institutions.[4] These patients were generally elderly and infirm, or diagnosed with long-term physical impairments and mental health problems. The creation of the NHS and post-war welfare state brought political attention to these populations, just as new techniques for assessing mortality and morbidity drew medical interest to long-term conditions of the middle-aged.[5] Although government departments were absorbed with how the health and social services could care for 'the chronic sick' during the 1950s and early 1960s, epidemiologists, public health agencies, clinicians, laboratory researchers, and social medicine academics all began to consider the problems posed by 'chronic disease' in the general population. Within discussions of chronic disease, diabetes assumed something of a symbolic position, providing a medium through which to discuss pathology and disease management. It was a position diabetes would retain, in various ways, for the rest of the century.

The transformations of the health service, diabetes management, and concepts of chronicity over the first decades of the post-war period, therefore, had ramifications lasting into the new millennium. Within the fluid political contexts of post-war Britain, the initial institutional arrangements of the NHS created dynamics that proved increasingly problematic for politicians and service staff. For professional and state bodies, improved integration and service information became solutions to rising expenditure and cross-institutional challenges of 'chronic disease'. As a prominent chronic condition, diabetes was managed in a way that provided a pioneering example of how to undertake integrated care. The transformations noted here (and in the next chapter) reframed clinical management itself into a preventive act, alleviating pressures to find potential social aetiological factors. For now, this chapter traces the origins of these transformations, the effects of which are considered throughout the book.

Diabetes and reconstruction of the health services

On the eve of the NHS's creation, British clinicians managed diabetes according to many of the same principles and strategies that prevailed in the 1920s. Controlling a patient's metabolism within certain limits (as measured through blood sugar levels, and sugar (glycosuria) and acid bodies (ketonuria) expelled in the urine) remained a key aim of intervention. For patients deemed to be overweight, weight reduction accompanied the pursuit of control in the hope that metabolic dysfunction might be subsequently relieved. Practitioners thus sought to balance dietary schemes and – where required – insulin regimes as well as possible with a patient's metabolic capacities and work demands.[6] Laboratory surveillance and monitoring for signs of long-term complications also remained central to management programmes. Most hospital doctors encouraged patients to test their own urine and to record the results. These clinicians also required patients to attend outpatient clinics at regular intervals, primarily for blood sugar examinations, urinalysis, and, in some instances, tests for skin and chest problems.[7] Of course, aims and practices varied between institutions and practitioners. For instance, the content of dietary plans often differed considerably, and not all patients were expected to undertake self-monitoring.[8] Equally, GPs retaining sole responsibility for their patients might lack access to the hospital's surveillance equipment and have to rely solely on urinary tests to assess treatment efficacy as a result.[9]

Perhaps the major area of contention in disease management during the 1940s was 'free diets'. 'Free dieting' was pioneered by American and European paediatricians who believed that dietary restrictions and the pursuit of normal glycaemia stunted healthy physical and psycho-social development in young patients.[10] Though loosely defined, 'free diets' found a minority of advocates in Britain, with practitioners extending the scheme to adults and seeking to adapt insulin intake to diet. These doctors told patients to disregard glycosuria and instead prioritise health, vigour, and remaining ketone-free in the belief that this allowed a more 'normal' life, free from dangerous reactions to low blood sugar.[11]

Intertwined with this discussion was another about the relationship between persistent hyperglycaemia and the onset of long-term complications in diabetes. As noted in the Introduction, some nineteenth-century physicians and pathologists had recorded the appearance of certain lesions and problems in older patients with diabetes. During the 1930s and 1940s these observations multiplied. Clinicians and researchers increasingly noted distinct patterns of complications in patients with diabetes of long duration, regardless of the age of onset, and they expressed consternation at the development of kidney disease, ocular changes, nerve damage, and other vascular problems.[12] Although British doctors became uncertain about the relationship between metabolic imbalance and the onset of complications during the mid-century, it seems that many adopted a middle-ground position in practice. Here, they combined a desire to 'do no harm' – striving for near-normal glycaemia levels where possible – with a pragmatic acknowledgement that any regimen had to be simple enough to be reasonably followed, and generous enough not to generate resentment or provoke hypoglycaemia.[13] Patients, moreover, approached their prescriptions in similar ways, adjusting diets according to different priorities and structural constraints.[14]

The continued emphasis on laboratory oversight into the 1940s meant that elite hospital doctors (and many GPs) believed the ongoing supervision of patients was best provided through specialist outpatient clinics.[15] These institutions combined the laboratory equipment and expertise considered necessary for high standards of care in a complex condition.[16] In line with a general stasis in views about treatment and institutional efficiency, the organisation of clinic work remained deeply hierarchical.[17] Patients congregated in large waiting areas before moving through the stages of the management process: from seat to testing areas, and from testing to consultation.[18] Where available, ancillary staff – such as nurses and laboratory technicians – might offer advice or undertake the various tests involved (including blood tests, feet checks, and x-rays).[19] Once results were available, doctors then consulted using an accumulation of longitudinal notes, with the most senior clinician organising and overseeing the system itself.[20] Though subject to rising demand, clinics retained high esteem, and the Diabetic Association (later BDA) – one of Britain's first patient-oriented bodies – promoted their creation and advertised their availability to patients.[21]

The key political concern during the 1940s, therefore – and one that it was hoped a national health service would resolve – was access. Before the 1940s, diabetes care operated under the same rules of provision as all other forms of care in Britain's mixed economy of services. Although some clinics had appeared in municipal institutions, in general they remained the province of teaching hospitals and larger voluntary institutions, which by the twentieth century were increasingly centres of paid care.[22] This shift in funding methods reflected the changing role of voluntary institutions; rising demand, novel employment arrangements, and the transformation into important sites for teaching, research, and technologically oriented practice increased expenditure.[23] Access to the diabetic clinics in these hospitals remained free, even if inpatient care often did not, but patients were generally accepted only through referral from GPs or inpatient wards.[24] Furthermore, patients needed to pay for prescriptions of insulin and self-testing equipment. Poorer patients who were members of a contributory scheme might find relief through their plan, and National Insurance patients could consult and receive prescriptions from GPs without charge. By contrast, poorer patients without such access (usually women and children) were reliant upon some form of public assistance.[25]

Along with economic status, geographical location could also structure patient access to oversight and treatment before 1948. Clinics tended to be formed in the largest urban centres, in part a response to larger patient populations.[26] Sometimes this response was positive, with clinicians forming clinics because they sought to develop specialist knowledge. On other occasions, doctors were motivated negatively: diabetes patients were seen to clog up general medical outpatient clinics, and clinicians argued that it would be more efficient to concentrate this work in special sessions.[27]

The creation of the NHS was supposed to rectify this inequitable and unequal geography of expertise, primarily by providing comprehensive health services for the entire population, free at the point of use. As will be noted below, however, compromises built into the service during its formation thwarted the realisation of such ideals.

The NHS was the outcome of a long history of innovation in, and debate about, health service organisation.[28] The first half of the twentieth century was marked by a growing political interest in the moral and physical health of the national population (though particularly of workers, mothers, and children), and was matched by a growing state responsibility for service provision.[29] Political concern with population health was closely connected to imperial and wartime politics, as well as discourses of health rights, responsibilities, and citizenship in liberal and socialist traditions.[30] At the same time, clinical medicine was also organising itself around technologies and concepts of the collective. By the 1940s, experiments had been undertaken with multi-sited clinical trials and community-focused epidemiological research, both of which were later geared towards determining clinical and public health practice.[31]

When launched in July 1948, the NHS was, in theory at least, to form part of Britain's newly planned modernity: a vision for the nation in which rational experts guided state intervention into a vast array of social and economic activity, freeing citizens from 'the five giants' of want, disease, squalor, ignorance, and idleness.[32] Yet, despite high hopes for, and long-term interest in, reformed health services, the creation of the NHS was riven with political compromises that posed problems for diabetes management into the second half of the century. An eclectic mix of actors took part in the formation of policy, and whilst some policy experiments with mass provision and integrated services existed, consensus over broad principles masked sharp divisions about the aims, structures, and mechanisms to be employed.[33]

Ultimately, these disputes became embodied in the final shape of the NHS. Against advice from senior civil servants, Cabinet colleagues, and the Labour Party, the Minister of Health, Aneurin Bevan, promoted a scheme for nationalising almost all Britain's hospitals.[34] The reform, however, did not place the Ministry of Health (or the Department of Health in the Scottish Office) in direct control of hospitals. Rather, several layers of administrative bodies existed between government departments and healthcare providers. Unit committees organised day-to-day provision. These committees reported to hospital management committees (or boards of management in Scotland), which allocated responsibilities between institutions and co-ordinated services. Finally, overseeing these agencies and allocating funds were nineteen Regional Hospital Boards (RHBs) and thirty-six boards of governors of the major teaching hospitals.[35] The exact duties of, and relationships between, these agencies shifted over time, and in England and Wales – though less so in Scotland – ambiguity often impaired their functioning.[36] Regardless of future changes, the lack of clear lines of influence frustrated ministers and doctors in the long term, and had considerable influence on the provision of diabetes care in the short term.

That the hospitals were the only elements of the NHS to be nationalised also caused political and clinical challenges. Voluntary hospitals and consultant staff accepted enrolment in a nationalised sector in exchange for favourable administrative arrangements, generous pay settlements, and some continuation of private practice.[37] By contrast, through the British Medical Association, GPs fervently defended their position as independent contractors, free from state salary and direct employment by local authorities. Building on arrangements developed under the previous National Insurance scheme, GPs contracted their work (now covering the whole population) via executive councils, paid broadly on a capitation basis.[38] The result was that GPs continued to operate without central oversight or involvement in integrated planning. A central Medical Practices Committee retained some ability to limit list sizes, and to direct GPs through positive and negative inducements to new appointments.[39] Equally, some professional advisory and statistical services existed, with statutory bodies mildly regulating prescribing through systems of classification (ruling certain products as ineligible for NHS prescription), and monitoring (sending GPs 'analyses of their prescribing costs compared with the average for the area in which they practised').[40] However, such mechanisms were limited. Attempts to strengthen management in the 1950s were easily rejected, and attempts to co-ordinate care across sites had to take place without connective institutional tissue.

Finally, compounding these managerial and administrative problems, responsibility for a diverse and somewhat incoherent range of preventive and clinical public health responsibilities was assigned to local government health departments under the direction of the MOHs. Some of these activities had fallen under their jurisdiction before 1948 (for instance, sanitation and maternity and child welfare services), whilst others – such as medical social work – were new responsibilities.[41] Crucially, the removal of hospital administration from local government cut short attempts to fully integrate hospital and community services, just as concessions to GPs over local government employment made co-ordinating local services considerably more difficult.[42]

In some respects, the new NHS was a great boon for diabetes care. The adoption of a tax-funded service removed most direct financial obstacles to accessing pharmaceuticals, self-care equipment, and clinic services. In fact, as will be noted in the next chapter, GPs were almost incentivised to refer patients diagnosed with diabetes to hospital. Clinics also became more accessible as the number of clinics grew (from 40 in 1940 to over 190 in 1955), and the regional machinery of the NHS provided a possible means for planning clinic placement.[43]

This regional focus was, in many ways, the result of the Diabetic Association's championing of specialist services. Discussions of reconstruction first provided the Association with an opportunity to campaign for equitable clinic distribution. As R. D. Lawrence wrote to *The Lancet* in 1942, the Association had asked the 'Planning Commission to take steps to establish clinics on a regional basis throughout the country'. Such clinics, he went on, were 'essential for the welfare of … diabetics in general', and regionalisation would enhance accessibility.[44] These efforts intensified following the creation of the NHS. Negotiations between the profession and government during the 1940s secured professional advisory mechanisms throughout the NHS's structures. Through conferences and publications, Lawrence successfully promoted the cause of regional planning for clinics amongst his colleagues.[45] These efforts resulted in support from major medical journals and a review in the early 1950s by the Central Health Services Council (CHSC), an advisory body established with the NHS to advise ministers on service questions.[46] The Council offered its advice to the Ministry of Health in 1953 – based on testimony from Lawrence – and the Ministry issued loosely prescriptive guidance to hospital authorities in

1953.[47] Here, it was recommended that facilities should be planned to prevent patients travelling further than thirty miles for care. The Ministry also recommended bed numbers per population size, offered general guidance on the scale of facilities and staffing for centres of different sizes, and requested that regional plans be created.[48]

Although this political interest in diabetes marked something of a coup for the BDA, success was ultimately hollow because of the concessions made to form the NHS. Already in the 1950s, central departments wanted to exercise some control over service expenditure, even if this infringed upon clinical decision-making.[49] Considerations of costs were shared by some elite GPs and emergent health service researchers, who progressively problematised variations in prescribing and speculated about accountability for resource use.[50] Nonetheless, the NHS had been founded on an informal agreement that doctors would have considerable autonomy of action within set budgets.[51] Appeals to 'clinical freedom' held considerable sway within the profession, and even sceptical politicians and civil servants feared the potential backlash to the nascent NHS that might follow attempts to proscribe clinical autonomy.[52] Thus, as was common at this time, the Ministry's guidance for RHBs focused on facilities and staffing, and left considerable room for interpretation.[53] Furthermore, even had more expansive standards been set, there would have been no guarantee that practitioners, administrators, or health authorities would follow any plan produced. The Ministry's only recourse to implementation was exhortation to RHBs, whilst the muddled relationships between RHBs and hospital units meant that regional plans rarely had a direct relationship with the service delivered.[54] Efforts to 'generalise the best' in diabetes care, to paraphrase Bevan, were difficult to achieve in a system which sought to guarantee the maximum possible devolution of decision-making.[55]

The creation of the NHS, therefore, confirmed diabetes' status as a hospital disease, but dashed hopes for effective regional organisation. Where planning did take place, this was largely the result of efforts from unevenly distributed interested parties. The spread of clinics in Britain compensated for some of this service disorganisation in terms of access, and certain regions managed to co-ordinate their services.[56] More significant problems, though, arose in terms of co-ordinating efforts across institutions and different parts of the service. As we will see below, health authorities and clinicians began experimenting with co-ordinated hospital and community care in diabetes during the 1940s and 1950s. Underpinning such efforts were shifting ideas of chronicity, growing clinic workloads, and novel views on how the new NHS should manage such problems.

Remaking chronicity: the chronic sick, social medicine, and chronic disease

During the 1940s, medical and public health discussions of chronicity centred on a very different set of patients from those in similar discussions later in the century. At this time, the most common use of the term 'chronic' was in reference to 'the chronic sick', a rather loose term applied to an amalgam of patients with diverse concerns and needs.[57] Broadly speaking, by the early 1940s institutions housing 'the chronic sick' tended to provide care for elderly and physically frail patients, particularly older people with physical impairments, mental health problems, and long-term and incurable diseases (such as arthritis or epilepsy), and people deemed likely to have terminal illnesses.[58] During the inter-war years, these were patients for whom the majority of doctors believed cure or rehabilitation was impossible, and who required long-term medical, nursing, and domestic care. They were also patients likely to be excluded from voluntary hospitals on these grounds and to be instead admitted to municipal and former Poor Law institutions, where they received little medical or political interest.[59]

How, then, did a different view of chronicity emerge, one concerned with the conditions prevalent amongst the middle-aged? And how did diabetes relate to these new perspectives? The application of various techniques to questions of mortality and morbidity saw clinicians, epidemiologists, and public health practitioners grow increasingly concerned with new problems. Diabetes served as a useful filter for discussing some common elements shared by various conditions, and its management also provided a model for new forms of cross-institutional care. Before 'chronic disease' could become a political issue, however, the existing label of 'chronic sick' had to be dismantled.

The fate of the chronic sick – as a classification and population – was closely intertwined with the creation of the NHS and the post-war welfare state. There had been some interest in chronic patients before the 1940s. Following legislation expanding the role of local government in hospital administration in 1929, a small number of doctors in newly municipalised hospitals began to pay closer attention to the needs and composition of the chronic sick. Faced with a disparate array of patients, these clinicians devised new systems of diagnosis, classification, and treatment.[60] They rejected passive approaches to care, arguing – and often demonstrating – that recovery and discharge were possible for many patients if they received proper, timely treatment.[61]

This work may have raised the profile of the chronic sick during the 1930s, but it was the nationalisation of Britain's hospitals and creation of post-war welfare services that brought many medical practitioners, healthcare administrators, and government officials into contact with chronically ill patients for the first time.[62] Suddenly, a large number of clinicians and civil servants began to see 'the chronic sick' as a problem in need of management, mobilising humanitarian arguments to motivate improved care for marginalised populations.[63] Moreover, the initial professional response – particularly through bodies like the British Medical Association – was to encourage the development of techniques that figures in municipal institutions had pioneered in the 1930s.[64] Discussions even extended to the internal organisation of institutions, and generated an administrative gaze based upon functionality and social criteria. Here medical officers discussed the importance of segregating 'annoying' patients (incontinent patients, 'senile dements', patients with 'sub-normal minds', and the 'mentally confused'), and of nursing '"likes" together' on grounds of efficiency and patient comfort.[65]

Increased visibility and activity also produced tensions. Many hospital practitioners saw chronic, incurable patients as blocking beds that would be better utilised for younger, acute patients, and promoted the application of new techniques only to increase bed turnover.[66] Yet the creation of a new specialty had resource implications, meaning that consultant support for geriatrics was mixed at best.[67] Conflict also occurred between the health and social services. Interested clinicians and health planners consistently identified the home as the ideal location for ongoing care, and moved surveys into the community to assess both the living conditions of chronic patients and their need for domestic help and nursing.[68] The subsequent discharge of patients caused tension with local government social service authorities, however, as the separation of budgets meant that for every patient removed from a hospital setting, a greater burden fell upon a local authority.[69]

In this sense, the management of the chronic sick became closely connected to questions of how best to use the resources of the post-war welfare state – or rather, how to ensure that heavily scrutinised resources were used for certain ends. Hospital care was a high-cost activity, and the first years of the NHS saw initial expenditure estimates greatly exceeded.[70] These disparities startled the Cabinet and the Treasury, especially in light of post-war economic problems and government commitment to other areas, notably rearmament and the Korean War (1950–53). Officials thus consistently targeted the Ministry of Health to control NHS expenditure.[71] In this context, the Ministry came to share clinical views of the chronic sick as unnecessary users of expensive services, and 'bed blocking' became a political problem.[72]

Political concern with the chronic sick stretched into the early 1970s. Gradually, however, the application of ever more refined administrative, political, and medical classifications transformed the subjects of interest. Though it remained an elastic category, discussions of 'chronic sickness' in the 1960s and 1970s increasingly centred on issues of functionality, on people whose physical condition impaired their ability to move, to undertake basic domestic tasks, or to undertake paid employment within existing architectural and social parameters.[73] Whilst the majority of the chronic sick tended to be frail elderly people, this interest in impairment meant that younger patients came into view and that chronic sickness became intertwined with disability.[74] Concern with the health and social service needs of older people continued into later decades, but authorities considered these needs under the rubric of old age more broadly.[75] And in a similar manner, over the 1950s and 1960s people diagnosed with mental health and cognitive problems were progressively classified, discussed, and treated separately from the chronically sick.[76] The administrative and clinical drive for management sparked by the creation of costly health and welfare services – combined with concerted campaigning from individuals and pressure groups – eventually disintegrated the category.[77]

The dismantling of the concept of 'the chronic sick' did not end interest in chronicity, though. Although the chronic sick attracted considerable political attention, into the 1950s and 1960s figures within clinical medicine, epidemiology, laboratory sciences, and public health became interested in the concept and challenges of 'chronic disease'. In contrast to discussions of chronic sickness, discussions of chronic disease predominantly concerned how best to prevent and manage non-infectious conditions in order to delay impairment and death. Very broadly, that is, whereas discussions about – and management of – chronic sickness sought to ameliorate loss of physical and social functions, in the context of chronic disease such discussions and practices sought to prevent loss of function occurring.[78]

Nonetheless, medical interest in non-infectious conditions emerged from the same concerns that drove political focus on the chronic sick. The collectivising concern with population health that underpinned the NHS continued into the post-war period, and growing state expenditure on health and welfare services intensified interest in improving health and ameliorating financial burdens. Thus, during the 1950s, reviews of changing patterns of morbidity and mortality sparked concern over trends found amongst 'the middle-aged', and especially amongst middle-aged males. Public health doctors and epidemiologists noted how 'female mortality [had] maintained its downward course [since the 1920s]; but the reduction of male mortality [had] slackened and almost stopped'.[79] During the inter-war period, cases of duodenal ulcer, bronchial cancer, and coronary thrombosis increased, and infectious disease deaths proportionally declined.[80] By the 1950s, doctors were less sceptical about possible statistical artificiality, and 'lung cancer, chronic bronchitis, diabetes, arteriosclerosis, heart disease, [and] cirrhosis of the liver' now provided additional concerns.[81]

As George Weisz has argued, however, the findings of novel morbidity surveys perhaps generated the most intense medical concern with chronic disease, with surveillance of illness in local communities revealing a greater prevalence of long-term and degenerative diseases than was expected from mortality figures alone.[82] In Britain, the creation of the post-war welfare state and the transformation of British social medicine provided considerable spurs to such surveys during the 1950s and 1960s. The inter-war social medicine movement had begun as an international project that located the cause and remedy for illness in social and economic structures.[83] Its proponents strived to reorient the thought and practice of clinical medicine along these lines, but efforts to remake medical education largely failed.[84] As a result, post-war social medicine became an academic pursuit associated with epidemiological research and health service assessment.[85] Now motivated by the need to plan services, and using the research opportunities offered by the welfare state, many social medicine researchers conducted extensive morbidity surveys of 'normal' populations in Britain and its colonies during the 1950s and 1960s.[86] They were joined in this pursuit by civil servants and a host of other medical professionals. Government officials used statistical returns from GPs to map general morbidity patterns, whilst hospital clinicians, MOHs, and general practice research communities undertook extensive detection surveys of ostensibly healthy populations in the community.[87] This work produced important studies on the prevalence and causes of heart disease, diabetes, and high blood pressure, alongside now-famous mortality studies on lung cancer.[88] Moreover, the activity generated increasing public health attention.

Research into diabetes prevalence provided an important vehicle for such work, and raised pertinent social and medical questions. Early studies took their cue from similar exercises in North America, and formed part of international and colonial research programmes.[89] In Britain, important community investigations were undertaken in Ibstock, Birmingham, and Bedford during the late 1950s and mid-1960s.[90] These surveys varied in structure, scale, and origin, but all were predicated upon initial screening of post-prandial urine to identify persons suspected of having diabetes, before formal glucose tolerance tests were used to assess their metabolic state.[91] By moving away from hospital populations, this work found surprising levels of diabetes in the community, and claimed that for 'every known case there is another as yet undetected and untreated'.[92] After several studies reported, the projected national prevalence of the disease increased substantially, from between 0.3 and 0.6 per cent of the population in 1953 to around 1.2 per cent in 1959.[93] It was in relation to such research – and work on diabetes in particular – that practitioners began to talk of 'the existence of the clinical "iceberg" of undetected and untreated disease'.[94] Indeed, the Bedford study was so successful that it not only generated follow-up studies and clinical trials, but even provided the basis for surveys into other conditions.[95]

Such findings provoked comment in the medical and lay press, with articles discussing disease prevalence and the possibility of living with a 'hidden' disease.[96] Culturally, the idea of a submerged enemy surreptitiously eroding the integrity of the physical and social body resonated with imagery of espionage and subversion slowly pervading British popular culture.[97] Medical journals and doctors discussed the consequences of unaddressed, silent, diseases for the individual.[98] Yet references to 'impaired efficiency' in their reflections indicate how the sick body was also a political concern for the nation, presenting a challenge to economic activity.[99] Productivity was a key index of comparison in the ideological contest of the Cold War, and relative economic growth rates provided a measure by which cultural critics, politicians, and journalists discussed Britain's post-war industrial and imperial decline.[100] Moreover, Britain's welfare state was funded through tax receipts, and was thus dependent upon the fiscal yield from productive work. It was amid such concerns that doctors and health economic agencies produced assessments of the financial and productivity implications of long-term illness.[101] Specifically, they built on work undertaken in the 1930s to estimate 'working days lost' and social security money paid out.[102] That the highest rates of death and morbidity for many conditions occurred amongst those who dominated Britain's political, cultural, and economic institutions possibly compounded existing anxieties.

It was in relation to such findings, as well as transatlantic influences and exchange, that epidemiologists, clinical practitioners, and public health doctors came to discuss the unique challenges of 'chronic disease'. As the renowned epidemiologist and social medicine academic Jerry Morris put it, many found 'chronic diseases' a 'useful term for the miscellany of degenerative, metabolic, malignant and mental conditions that increasingly dominate the practice of medicine and public health'. 'The term', he went on, 'had some value because it emphasises certain common features: the life-time or very long process of development, the often insidious onset, the usual impossibility of cure, the tendency to relapse and to remit; and often their profound economic and social repercussions, particularly on the family.'[103] The term did not provide the basis for service reform movements, as in the USA.[104] It did, nonetheless, provide a useful shorthand for integrating seemingly diverse diseases into broad discussion and, as we will see below, for drawing out models of local service provision that might be adapted in different sites.

Diabetes fitted quite neatly within this framework during the 1960s. As noted, clinicians had long recognised the social and financial difficulties that patients with diabetes faced, and regularly discussed the psychological and physical challenges that patients might experience as a result of privations of diet. From the 1930s onwards, doctors admitted the need to make dietary and pharmacological concessions to ease these burdens, whilst into the post-war decades the BDA explored employment discrimination and welfare issues affecting specific patient groups.[105] Finally, as well as mentioning its incurability, doctors frequently referred to diabetes' long onset (outside childhood), with easily mistaken early symptoms.[106] Indeed, diabetes often provided an example of hidden disease.[107]

At this time, though, diabetes became most widely discussed in relation to pre-symptomatic detection and diagnosis of disease. Research into prevalence, and studies of what was termed the 'natural history' of several chronic conditions, raised questions about when disease was said to begin.[108] The relationship between asymptomatic physiological abnormalities (such as elevated blood pressure), symptoms, and the development of functional disease and long-term complications was often uncertain. For instance, surveys of diabetes revealed that glycaemia levels in the population were continuously distributed, with no strict cut-off point at which symptoms manifested (a threshold that traditionally divided healthy from pathological). Moreover, such initial research could not reveal whether borderline cases closest to diagnostic thresholds would become symptomatic in the future, whether such individuals were at risk of diabetic complications, or whether earlier treatment would prevent these outcomes.[109] This interest in borderline cases generated longitudinal community research, as well as clinical trials of early intervention, with researchers and clinicians undertaking similar projects for hypertension.[110] However, when discussing diagnosis and quantitative thresholds of disease, doctors regularly mentioned diabetes as challenging present assumptions. For example, opening a discussion on emergent patterns in community medicine at the annual conference of the Society of Medical Officers of Health in 1966, Reid noted that 'although epidemiological research answered many questions, it also posed many questions: in the field of diabetes for instance, recent studies have made even an acceptable definition of the disease very difficult and have led to the suggestion that all men are diabetic, but some are more diabetic than others!'[111]

As we will see in the next chapter, findings from this research eventually led to a reclassification of diagnostic boundaries and therapeutic practices, with diabetes itself becoming a risk factor for heart disease, stroke, and other conditions. Notably, unlike those for other chronic conditions, the diagnostic thresholds for diabetes were revised upwards rather than downwards.[112] In the meantime, uncertainty meant that many doctors were sceptical about pathologising borderline cases without being able to promise benefits. Approaches to diabetes, therefore, were unlike other those taken to other conditions, though new organisational approaches to its treatment would soon come to influence other forms of chronic disease management.

Diabetes, chronic disease, and the limits of the NHS

According to many doctors and epidemiologists during the 1950s and 1960s, the NHS and British society were confronting new and complex problems. Faced with wide-ranging and prevalent chronic diseases, medical practitioners and public health doctors asked how to prevent tragic loss of labour, social function, and life. Rising expectations of modern medicine during its 'golden age' meant that neither doctors nor lay public necessarily saw the onset or outcome of many chronic conditions as inevitable.[113] Medical discussions of how to respond to new threats bifurcated around two interlinked poles: wholesale prevention and better disease management.

Wholesale prevention efforts were closely tied to new forms of risk-factor thinking.[114] To confront rising tolls of chronic disease, MOHs and medical practitioners sought to use research into disease aetiology to build 'primary' preventive efforts – interventions to completely avoid onset of disease (see Chapter 2). However, studies of many conditions did not reveal simple causative mechanisms. Instead, drawing on complex statistical methods (and recent understandings of multi-factor causation pioneered in studies of epidemics), researchers developed a range of techniques and study designs for teasing out associative, predictive, and possibly contributory factors to specific diseases.[115] These new understandings of causation altered the targets and methods of preventive medical intervention. British experts studying a range of conditions began to shift frequently used explanatory frameworks for patterns of morbidity away from social structures of inequality and towards behaviours and 'accumulated vices'.[116] These perspectives formed the basis for new policy networks and large-scale public health campaigns targeting 'risky' lifestyle choices, with health education programmes designed to cultivate self-managing subjects through the persuasive provision of advice and coded cultural messages.[117] To fine-tune their practices, moreover, state bodies assumed responsibility for undertaking research-based surveillance on public attitudes and behaviours.[118] Individuals, though not overtly coerced, were to be benevolently guided to healthy decisions.

The international adoption of risk-factor approaches to prevention, in socialist as well as capitalist democratic states, was the product of number of political projects.[119] In Britain, the focus on individuals and education dovetailed neatly with the country's recent political history, and with the liberalism which infused the Labour Party's social democratic approach to economic and social management.[120]

Yet, as the NHS itself symbolised, state agencies and medical professionals provided services as well as education. In some rare instances, such as lung cancer, single agents were highlighted as definitively causative, even if such assessments were opposed for some time.[121] However, doctors during the 1950s and 1960s noted that a lack of knowledge about causation in many conditions excluded a reliance on primary preventive health education. In diabetes, for instance, there were a number of theories about contributing factors – genetic predisposition, weight, consumption of sugar or refined carbohydrate, and age – but none were certain.[122] As Reid bluntly put it in a 1963 symposium on diabetes, 'the scope for primary prevention is yet limited'.[123] Thus local government efforts focused upon educating the general population about the symptoms of disease, and (despite scepticism about efficacy and cost-effectiveness) establishing some screening programmes to find undiagnosed cases of the condition.[124] Both methods, in other words, were dedicated to finding unknown symptomatic patients and instituting treatment, in order to, at the very least, remove symptoms and prevent the development of acute diabetic emergencies. To be sure, some medical practitioners used the knowledge gained from surveys of prevalence to construct a list of groups considered most 'at risk' of developing the condition.[125] Others, like Reid, recommended 'the avoidance of obesity in such groups as the relatives of diabetics', thus translating predictive models of risk into theories about causation and practices of intervention.[126] Nonetheless, programmes of primary prevention did not form the backbone of approaches to diabetes during the 1950s and 1960s.

Instead, doctors saw effective disease management in diabetes – and in conditions such as cancers – as the best means to prevent deterioration into symptoms and long-term disability.[127] As noted above, even as doctors grew uncertain about the value of blood glucose control, they adopted pragmatic approaches to metabolic balance as a precaution, and surveillance remained important in order to remove symptoms and avoid certain complications.

Undertaking this work, at least in more elite institutions, was an expanding hospital care team, reflecting the growing complexity of managing patients and their complications. Clinicians, nurses, and technicians, who had been central to diabetes management in the 1930s, were increasingly assisted by dieticians, chiropodists (to monitor feet and prevent injury turning into infection), and obstetricians (for joint care of pregnant patients) during the first two decades of the postwar period.[128] As teams and patient populations expanded, however, doctors acknowledged that clinical labour required co-ordination to be effective.[129] Within ward settings in particular, new tools and bureaucratic cultures of systematic recording developed as a means to maintain standards of practice. Senior doctors in Cheshire, for instance, complained of problems in treating patients 'scattered in numerous non-medical wards throughout a large general hospital', with the result that such patients received care from staff with 'little experience in the practical management of diabetes'.[130] In response, these doctors designed new records, building upon the rich history of form-creation and techniques for tabulating and visualising data in diabetes research and care.[131] The new records contained pre-formatted boxes and graphic arrangements for the most important treatment and monitoring measures, as well as designated areas for recording the timings of actions undertaken (where the temporal gap between tests would offer important clinical information). The new forms were thus clearly laid out 'so that doctors, nursing staff, and patients can see [information] at a glance', and so that practitioners would be guided on what data, tasks, and tests they should prioritise.[132] Clearly targeting nursing staff in their efforts to influence practice, the designers even used moral judgements and institutional pressure to ensure use of the document. 'Any sister', they concluded, 'who is not prepared to keep it accurately is unsuitable to nurse diabetics.'[133]

However, specialist doctors during these post-war decades were beginning to reflect more systematically on the psychological, social, and economic problems that patients with chronic diseases faced, with repercussions for organising services.[134] For instance, Ronald Tunbridge, Professor of Medicine at the University of Leeds, concentrated a considerable part of a prestigious lecture delivered to the BDA answering the question 'why do patients fail to maintain a satisfactory level of control?' In response, he suggested that 'failure is due to three main groups of causes – psychological, social, and educational'.[135] In terms of social causes, he pointed out that doctors before the Second World War regularly prescribed dietary composition in relation to four meals ('breakfast, lunch, dinner, and a supper snack'), ignoring the fact that 'few working-class families had … two cooked meals a day'. Expanding further, he recalled a survey he had conducted with a dietician, finding that the average cost of a diabetic diet exceeded that of normal diets, even when carefully planned by the two researchers. He concluded that 'the failure of many diabetics, particularly the elderly, to maintain a steady diet is undoubtedly [due to] financial stringency'. Likewise, he stressed the educational difficulties faced by ordinary patients, especially older individuals who had already formed strong habits, in adjusting to new demands. Even for a doctor with physiological training, Tunbridge noted, it might take 'at least three months of dietary control before he [sic] can enter a restaurant and order an accurate meal without undue emotional tension'.[136]

Turning to questions of care, Tunbridge supported clinic supervision of patients, but placed considerable emphasis on being conscious of costs, tailoring treatment to individual patients, and using repetition and 'every device possible' with a 'team' of almoners, nurses, and dieticians to educate patients on the essentials.[137] In general, approaches to education varied between practitioners, and it is likely that the size of most clinics, and the distribution of inpatients across wards, made tailored treatment and education difficult to deliver.[138] Yet a minority of clinics did incorporate 'socio-medical' insights into practice, generally where clinical leads had either personal experience of long-term conditions or a strong professional interest in chronic disease management.[139] Moreover, where strong links between hospitals and local health departments existed, the most innovative practitioners were able to extend oversight into the community. Recognising that pressures on clinics prevented care teams from offering patients sufficient support, these doctors designed schemes for health visiting that moved follow-up education and surveillance directly into domestic settings. Such programmes contributed to the gradual expansion of the health visitor's remit beyond infant and child health.[140] More importantly for diabetes care, however, the attachment of health visitors outside local government provided one possible means for integrating care across the NHS's administrative barriers.[141]

Pioneering work in this direction had taken place during the 1940s in Cardiff, where 'specialist health visitors' for diabetes were employed to provide 'aftercare' for patients previously admitted to the Llandough Hospital.[142] This aftercare required health visitors to discuss prescribed regimen with doctors, ward sisters, dieticians, and almoners, and then to visit patients' homes to ensure that 'the regimen recommended in hospital was carried out'. Whilst there, health visitors would also undertake 'sound health education'.[143] Just as with the prevalence research noted earlier, doctors subsequently extended the arrangements created for diabetes management into care for such long-term conditions as gastric diseases, asthma, and tuberculosis.[144] In all such cases, self-care was essential in the absence of daily professional encounters, and by passing into the home health visitors were able to use the disciplinary technology of surveillance to reinforce adherence to the parameters of self-management.

A similar scheme was also established under the Leicester Royal Infirmary in the early 1950s.[145] Here, health visitors undertook an array of domiciliary tasks, focusing on the newly diagnosed as well as children and elderly patients.[146] Co-ordinating with the district nurse, health visitors paid all new patients at least three domiciliary visits. The substance of individual visits varied, but health visitors were generally responsible for delivering educational content (on diet, hypoglycaemia, general principles of self-care, and urine testing); taking notes on social circumstances (social status, work, relatives, accommodation, and hygiene); co-ordinating and advising on other services (from home helps to National Assistance benefits); and even dealing with employment troubles and school demands.[147] Particularly in the case of the aged, visitors could observe competency in self-care, assess the possibilities of keeping patients in their homes, and inspect patients for possible signs of complications (especially in the feet). In addition, health visitors were supposed to subject obese patients to additional scrutiny. For these patients, the Infirmary's clinical lead wanted staff to inspect the kitchen and undertake intense dietary surveillance and education, tightening the disciplinary mesh for patients whose weight had been framed as the result of dietary 'transgression'.[148]

As within the hospital itself, records played an important role in health visitor schemes, with reports sent to the clinic and a patient's GP to ensure therapeutic continuity. However, the reports compiled by health visitors were designed to expand surveillance beyond biochemistry to the patient as subject. Reflecting a systematic interest in the social and psychological world of patients that was common within discussions of chronic disease, health visitor reports turned a person's character, health practices, social relationships, and means of support into objects of interest.

As noted, some clinicians extended the model set up for diabetes management into other chronic conditions. MOHs also saw opportunities to craft new positions for themselves, liaising with clinics and providing educative services for conditions like diabetes. As Dorothy Egan, President of the Society of Medical Officers of Health, suggested in 1965, 'the image of the personal friend and mentor who guides the family from the cradle to the grave is being replaced by one of the team. In this team-work other disciplines have their part to play, but it is essential that the three branches of the NHS should have a common aim and a shared responsibility.'[149]

Ultimately, resources were just as scarce for local authorities as for clinics. Domiciliary and community care staff were already stretched, dedicated primarily to supporting elderly patients in their homes, and innovative schemes did not always last. Crossing the boundaries of the NHS, moreover, depended upon dedicated personnel with an interest in diabetes, meaning that provision was patchy rather than universal. As we will see in the next chapter, MOHs had been politically undermined by the early 1970s, just as financial and political pressures on clinics were intensifying. Such pressures meant that hospital clinicians were still looking for means to ensure cross-institutional disease prevention and management. With the decline of the MOHs and the reframing of clinical activity as preventive work, GPs made claims for diabetes care. Healthcare politics, economics, and philosophy all mutually reinforced a shift away from the hospital, and GPs saw such changes align with their own interests. Once again, diabetes provided something of a pioneer in these efforts, but with the development of cross-institutional care also came calls to ensure management of professional labour.

Conclusion

Although the creation of the NHS brought considerable change to British healthcare, hospitals retained their leadership in, and authority over, diabetes care in the three decades after the Second World War. Hospital practice, however, was not necessarily static over this period. The number of clinics grew considerably under the NHS, with a greater emphasis in policy placed on their staffing, facilities, and organisation. Likewise, diabetes management became closely entwined with medico-political emphasis on managing chronic sickness in the community. Experiments with health visitor schemes marked the beginning of a more socially oriented medical gaze, focusing on the home conditions, attitudes, and practices of young and elderly patients, along with the newly diagnosed. As academics, public health practitioners, and clinicians began to talk more about the challenges of 'chronic disease', doctors even experimented with travelling clinics for continuing care of all adult patients.

The growing healthcare team demanded co-ordination, and new forms of guidance and records emerged in the bureaucratic culture of the hospital. These tools loosely managed labour, but focused primarily upon nursing and ancillary staff, and there was clearly great flexibility in the work undertaken. These dynamics were to play out over a much larger canvas and geographical area during the next two decades, as GPs and other community care actors sought to expand the care of diabetes outside hospital walls. As diagnosis improved and rates of diabetes continued to rise, clinics faced patient loads that they were never designed to handle. At the same time, their resource requirements continued to outstrip the funding available under the NHS. The result was falling standards and unsatisfactory care, and clinicians complained of clinics filled with patients who did not require their skilled labour. Moving care beyond the hospital and into GP practices, however, was not a simple affair. As we will see in the next chapter, this remaking of diabetes management involved numerous innovations, and was driven by complex aims and professional interactions. In the event, these local efforts at spatial innovation brought new forms of bureaucratised practice into the community. When combined with increased drives for surveillance and regulation of quality, they also produced local forms of professional management. It is to the changing role of primary care, and its implications for professional management, that we now turn.

Notes

1 J. J. A. Reid, 'A new public health – the problems and the challenge', *Public Health*, 79:4 (1965), 183–4.
2 V. Berridge, 'Medicine and the public: the 1962 report of the Royal College of Physicians and the new public health', *Bulletin of the History of Medicine*, 81:1 (2007), 286–311.
3 J. J. A. Reid, 'Some public health aspects of diabetes mellitus', *Public Health*, 77:3 (1963), 145–57.
4 G. Weisz, *Chronic Disease in the Twentieth Century: A History* (Baltimore: Johns Hopkins University Press, 2014), p. 181.
5 The social and psychological concerns of middle age were also becoming a familiar part of the cultural and political landscape: M. Jackson, '"Life begins at 40": self-help, marriage guidance, and the making of the midlife crisis in Britain and America', in M. Jackson and M. D. Moore (eds.), *Balancing the Self: Medicine, Politics, and the Regulation of Health in the Twentieth Century* (forthcoming).
6 W. Oakley, 'The treatment of diabetes mellitus', *The Practitioner*, 157:942 (1946), 420–5.

7   F. G. Lescher, 'The modern treatment of diabetes mellitus and the use of zinc protamine insulin', *BMJ*, 1:4017 (1938), 13–14; 'The management of diabetic out-patients', *The Lancet*, 231:5974 (1938), 509.
8   G. F. Walker, 'Reflections on diabetes mellitus: answers to a questionary', *The Lancet*, 262:6800 (1953), 1329–32; '"Calorie control" diabetic diet', *BMJ*, 1:4282 (1943), 143–4.
9   H. P. Himsworth, 'Management of diabetes mellitus, part II', *BMJ*, 2:3942 (1936), 188–90.
10 C. Feudtner, 'The want of control: ideas, innovations, and ideals in the modern management of diabetes mellitus', *Bulletin of the History of Medicine*, 69:1 (1995), 80; R. B. Tattersall, *Diabetes: The Biography* (Oxford: Oxford University Press, 2009), pp. 85–90.
11 R. H. Micks, 'The diet in diabetes', *BMJ*, 1:4297 (1943), 598–600.
12 'Modern views on diabetes', *BMJ*, 2:4568 (1948), 209–10.
13 Walker, 'Reflections on diabetes mellitus', pp. 1330–1.
14 M. D. Moore, 'Food as medicine: diet, diabetes management and the patient in twentieth-century Britain', *Journal of the History of Medicine and Allied Sciences*, 73:2 (2018), 150–67.
15 L. J. Witts, 'Special clinics and planning', *BMJ*, 2:4259 (1942), 226.
16 R. D. Lawrence, 'Special clinics for diabetics', *BMJ*, 2:4262 (1942), 322.
17 S. Sturdy and R. Cooter, 'Science, scientific management and the transformation of medicine in Britain, c.1870–1950', *History of Science*, 36:4 (1998), 421–66.
18 'A diabetic clinic', *BMJ*, 1:3828 (1934), 906; H. Droller, 'An outbreak of hepatitis in a diabetic clinic', *BMJ*, 1:4400 (1945), 624.
19 'The management of diabetic out-patients'.
20 Ibid.
21 See Introduction.
22 B. Abel-Smith, *The Hospitals, 1800–1948: A Study in Social Administration in England and Wales* (Cambridge, MA: Harvard University Press, 1964).
23 S. Cherry, 'Regional comparators in the funding and oranisation of the voluntary hospital system, c.1860–1939', in M. Gorsky and S. Sheard (eds.), *Financing Medicine: The British Experience since 1750* (London: Routledge, 2006), pp. 59–76.
24 'London diabetic clinics, provincial diabetic clinics', *Diabetic Journal*, 3:3 (1940), 32–4. Free inpatient admission might be given for research purposes: C. Lawrence, *Rockefeller Money, The Laboratory and Medicine in Edinburgh, 1919–1930: New Science in an Old Country* (New York: University of Rochester Press, 2005), p. 288.
25 TNA, MH 55/422, 186284/1/13, report by Office Committee of the Ministry of Health, 'Supply of insulin for the treatment of diabetes', 14 January 1924, pp. 4–5.
26 'London diabetic clinics'.

27 TNA, BD 18/793, FLD/G, letter by F. L. Dyson (Neath General Hospital) to Dr A. Trevor Jones (Senior Administrative Medical Officer, Welsh Hospital Board), 'Regional planning of diabetic services', 11 August 1953, p. 1.
28 C. Webster, *The Health Services Since the War*, vol. 1: *Problems of Health Care: The National Health Service before 1957* (London: HMSO, 1988).
29 M. Gorsky, 'Local government health services in interwar England: problems of quantification and interpretation', *Bulletin of the History of Medicine*, 85:3 (2011), 384–412.
30 J. Seymour, 'Not rights but reciprocal responsibility: the rhetoric of state health provision in early-twentieth century Britain', in A. Mold and D. Reubi (eds.), *Assembling Health Rights in Global Context: Genealogies and Anthropologies* (Oxford: Routledge, 2013), pp. 23–41; J. Stewart, 'Ideology and process in the creation of the British National Health Service', *Journal of Policy History*, 14:2 (2002), 115–19.
31 D. Armstrong, *Political Anatomy of the Body: Medical Knowledge in Britain in the Twentieth Century* (Oxford: Oxford University Press, 1983); H. Valier and C. Timmermann, 'Clinical trials and the reorganization of medical research in post-Second World War Britain', *Medical History*, 52:4 (2008), 493–510.
32 M. Francis, 'The Labour Party: modernisaton and the politics of restraint', in B. Conekin, F. Mort, and C. Waters (eds.), *Moments of Modernity: Reconstructing Britain, 1945–1964* (London: Rivers Oram Press, 1999), p. 153. The 'five giants' are from William Beveridge's influential 1942 report into social insurance: N. Timmins, *The Five Giants: A Biography of the Welfare State* (London: Fontana Press, 1996), esp. pp. 11–62.
33 R. Klein, *The New Politics of the NHS: From Creation to Reinvention*, 5th edition (Oxford: Radcliffe, 2006), pp. 1–21; D. Fox, *Health Policies, Health Politics: The British and American Experience, 1911–1965* (Princeton: Princeton University Press, 1986). Cf. C. Webster, 'Conflict and consensus: explaining the British health service', *Twentieth Century British History*, 1:2 (1990), 120–33. On policy experimentations: M. Gorsky, '"Threshold of a new era": the development of an integrated hospital system in northeast Scotland, 1900–39', *Social History of Medicine*, 17:2 (2004), 247–67.
34 Webster, *The Health Services since the War*, vol. 1, pp. 84–8.
35 There were five RHBs in Scotland, one in Wales, and thirteen in England. Teaching hospitals were integrated into regional machinery in Scotland.
36 Webster, *The Health Services since the War*, vol. 1, pp. 274–87, 298–316.
37 Klein, *The New Politics of the NHS*, 15–16.
38 I. Loudon and M. Drury, 'Some aspects of clinical care in general practice', in I. Loudon, J. Horder, and C. Webster (eds.), *General Practice under the*

National Health Service, 1948–1997 (Oxford: Oxford University Press, 1998), p. 103.
39 G. Rivett, *From Cradle to Grave: Fifty Years of the NHS* (London: King's Fund, 1998), p. 81.
40 Ibid., p. 83; see also pp. 50–1, 112; Webster, *The Health Services since the War*, vol. 1, p. 246.
41 Webster, *The Health Services since the War*, vol. 1, pp. 92–3; M. Gorsky, 'Local leadership in public health: the role of the Medical Officer of Health in Britain, 1872–1974', *Journal of Epidemiology and Community Health*, 61:6 (2007), 468–72.
42 On post-war activities of the MOHs: J. Lewis, *What Price Community Medicine? The Philosophy, Practice and Politics of Public Health since 1919* (Brighton: Wheatsheaf, 1986). Cf. J. Welshman, 'The Medical Officer of Health in England and Wales, 1900–1974: watchdog or lapdog?', *Journal of Public Health Medicine*, 19:4 (1997), 443–50; S. McLaurin and D.F. Smith, 'Professional strategies of Medical Officers of Health in the postwar period – 2: "progressive realism": the case of R. J. Donaldson, MOH for Teeside, 1968–1974', *Journal of Public Health Medicine*, 24:2 (2002), 130–5; Gorsky, 'Local leadership in public health', pp. 470–1.
43 'London Diabetic Clinics', pp. 32–4; TNA, BD 18/793, memo, 'Diabetic clinics', 1955.
44 Lawrence, 'Special clinics for diabetics', p. 322.
45 'British Medical Association: scientific sections', *The Lancet*, 254:6567 (1949), 67; R. D. Lawrence, 'Regional centres for the treatment of diabetes', *The Lancet*, 257:6668 (1951), 1318–19.
46 'Diabetes and insulin', *BMJ*, 1:4662 (1950), 1122; CHSC, *Report of the Central Health Services Council for the Year Ended December 31, 1952*, House of Commons Papers, 218 (London: HMSO, 1953), pp. 13–15. On the CHSC: Webster, *The Health Services since the War*, vol. 1, pp. 241–9.
47 CHSC, *Report of the Central Health Services Council for the year Ended December 31, 1953*, House of Commons Papers, 190 (London: HMSO, 1954).
48 TNA, BD 18/793, Ministry of Health circular, 'National Health Service: regional planning of diabetic services', RHB (53) 66, 1953, pp. 1–2. See Chapter 5.
49 Klein, *The New Politics of the NHS*, pp. 23–45. See Chapter 6 below.
50 See Chapter 5.
51 Klein, *The New Politics of the NHS*, p. 37.
52 See the discussions of autonomy in Chapter 5 and of prescribing in Chapter 6. See also Webster, *The Health Services since the War*, vol. 1, pp. 222–7, 246. On languages of freedom: A. Seaton, 'Against the "sacred cow": NHS opposition and the Fellowship for Freedom in Medicine, 1948–72', *Twentieth Century British History*, 26:3 (2015), 424–49.

53 The most specific norms set during this period related to beds, but such explicit standards were unusual: P. Bridgen, 'Hospitals, geriatric medicine, and the long-term care of elderly people, 1946–1976', *Social History of Medicine*, 14:3 (2001), 507–23.
54 M. Gorsky, '"To regulate and confirm inequality"? A regional history of geriatric hospitals under the English National Health Service, c.1948–1975', *Ageing & Society*, 33:4 (2013), 611–12.
55 Klein, *The New Politics of the NHS*. For the Bevan quote: p. 212.
56 Lawrence, 'Regional centres', pp. 1318–19.
57 M. Denham, 'The surveys of the Birmingham chronic sick hospitals, 1948–1960', *Social History of Medicine*, 19:2 (2006), 279–80.
58 M. W. Warren, 'Care of chronic sick: a case for treating chronic sick in blocks in a general hospital', *BMJ*, 2:4329 (1943), 822–3; L. Fairfield, 'Care of the chronic sick', *The Lancet*, 242:6267 (1943), 455–7.
59 A. Levene, 'Between less eligibility and the NHS: the changing place of Poor Law hospitals in England and Wales, 1929–39', *Twentieth Century British History*, 20:3 (2009), 322–45.
60 M. Martin, 'Medical knowledge and medical practice: geriatric medicine in the 1950s', *Social History of Medicine*, 8:3 (1995), 446–7.
61 S. Pickard, 'The role of governmentality in the establishment, maintenance, and demise of professional jurisdictions: the case of geriatric medicine', *Sociology of Health and Illness*, 32:7 (2010), 1077.
62 Weisz, *Chronic Disease in the Twentieth Century*, pp. 180–1; Martin, 'Medical knowledge and medical practice', pp. 445–6. Post-war surveys of hospitals, which provided the basis for reform, were also important precursors.
63 Martin, 'Medical knowledge and medical practice', pp. 445–7; 'Neglect of the chronic sick', *The Lancet*, 248:6416 (1946), 240–1.
64 A. N. Exton-Smith and G. S. Crockett, 'The chronic sick under new management: experiences in starting a geriatric unit', *The Lancet*, 253:6563 (1949), 1016–18; Gorsky, '"To regulate and confirm inequality"?', pp. 609–12.
65 Warren, 'Care of chronic sick'; A. R. Culley, 'The care of the aged and infirm and the chronic sick', *Public Health*, 60:5 (1947), 103–4.
66 Bridgen, 'Hospitals, geriatric medicine, and the long-term care of elderly people'.
67 P. Thane, 'Old age', in R. Cooter and J. Pickstone (eds.), *Companion to Medicine in the Twentieth Century* (Abingdon: Routledge, 2003), pp. 624–8; Martin, 'Medical knowledge and medical practice', pp. 446–53. Support was slightly more forthcoming in Scotland.
68 Martin, 'Medical knowledge and medical practice', pp. 453–61; Denham, 'The surveys of the Birmingham chronic sick hospitals', pp. 284–5.

69 P. Bridgen and J. Lewis, *Elderly People and the Boundary between Health and Social Care, 1946–91: Whose Responsibility?* (London: Nuffield Trust, 1999).
70 T. Cutler, 'Dangerous yardstick? Early cost estimates and the politics of financial management in the first decade of the National Health Service', *Medical History*, 47:2 (2003), 217–38.
71 Webster, *The Health Services since the War*, vol. 1, pp. 133–83.
72 Bridgen, 'Hospitals, geriatric medicine, and long-term care of elderly people'.
73 Chronically Sick and Disabled Persons Act 1970, c. 44; Local Government Operational Research Unit, *Identifying the Chronically Sick and Disabled in Reading* (London: Royal Institute of Public Administration, 1973).
74 'The young chronic sick', *BMJ*, 1:5637 (1969), 134–5. For background: J. Hampton, *Disability and the Welfare State in Britain: Changes in Perception and Policy, 1948–79* (Bristol: Policy Press, 2016).
75 Local Government Operational Research Unit, *Manchester's Old People: A Study for the Social Services Department*, 2nd edition (London: Royal Institute of Public Administration, 1972).
76 Gorsky, '"To regulate and confirm inequality"?', pp. 610–11. In policy terms: J. Welshman and J. Walmers (eds.), *Community Care in Perspective: Care, Control and Citizenship* (Basingstoke: Palgrave Macmillan, 2007).
77 On campaigning: G. Millward, 'Social security policy and the early disability movement – expertise, disability and the government, 1965–77', *Twentieth Century British History*, 26:2 (2015), 274–97.
78 D. Armstrong, 'Chronic illness: a revisionist account', *Sociology of Health and Illness*, 36:1 (2014), pp. 19–26.
79 J. N. Morris, 'Uses of epidemiology', *BMJ*, 2:4936 (1955), 395.
80 Ibid.; Weisz, *Chronic Disease in the Twentieth Century*, pp. 179, 189.
81 R. W. Elliot, 'The prevention of illness in middle age', *Public Health*, 79:6 (1965), 317–25.
82 Surveys played a different role in the USA, emerging from different political and disciplinary contexts. In both countries, however, research indicated that long-term illness was far more prevalent than anticipated: Weisz, *Chronic Disease in the Twentieth Century*, pp. 77–100.
83 D. Porter, 'From social structure to social behaviour in Britain after the Second World War', *Contemporary British History*, 16:3 (2002), 59–63.
84 N. T. A. Oswald, 'A social health service without social doctors', *Social History of Medicine*, 4:2 (1991), 295–315; M. Perry, 'Academic general practice in Manchester under the early National Health Service: a failed social experiment', *Social History of Medicine*, 13:1 (2000), 111–29.
85 Lewis, *What Price Community Medicine?*; S. Murphy, 'The early days of the MRC Social Medicine Research Unit', *Social History of Medicine*, 12:3 (1999), 389–406; V. Berridge, *Marketing Health: Smoking and the*

Discourse of Public Health in Britain, 1945–2000 (Oxford: Oxford University Press, 2007), pp. 15–16.
86 M. D. Moore, 'Harnessing the power of difference: colonialism and British chronic disease research, 1940–1975', *Social History of Medicine*, 29:2 (2016), 384–404.
87 T. Osborne, 'Epidemiology as an investigative paradigm: the College of General Practitioners in the 1950s', *Social Science and Medicine*, 38:2 (1994), 317–26; C. Timmermann, 'A matter of degree: the normalization of hypertension, c.1940–2000', in W. Ernst (ed.), *Histories of the Normal and the Abnormal: Social and Cultural Histories of Norms and Normativity* (London: Routledge, 2006), pp. 245–61.
88 J. N. Morris, J. A. Heady, P. A. B. Raffle, G. C. Roberts, and J. W. Parks, 'Coronary heart disease and physical activity of work', *The Lancet*, 262:6795 (1953), 1053–7; Berridge, *Marketing Health*, pp. 22–51.
89 Working Party of the College of General Practitioners, 'Diabetes survey', *BMJ*, 1:5291 (1962), 1497–503; WHO, *Diabetes Mellitus: Report of a WHO Expert Committee*, Technical Report Series, 310 (Geneva: WHO, 1965).
90 'Detection of diabetes', *BMJ*, 1:5291 (1962), 1535–6; J. B. Walker, 'Diabetes in the community', *Public Health*, 77:3 (1963), 158–64; 'British Diabetic Association', *BMJ*, 2:5315 (1962), 1251.
91 The Birmingham study, for instance, enrolled 20,000 subjects through local GPs, and was run under the auspices of the College of General Practitioners as part of efforts to establish the College as a central figure in epidemiological research. By contrast, the Ibstock and Bedford surveys were overseen by innovative hospital clinicians. The former surveyed a small community of 5,000 persons, the latter – pioneered by the local public health department – emerged from the will of a local inhabitant (whose wife had died of diabetes), and covered a population of 45,000 to become one of the largest surveys in Europe: '350,000 may have diabetes', *The Times*, 17 July 1962, p. 6.
92 'Detection of diabetes', *BMJ*, 2:5151 (1959), 555.
93 Ibid. Cf. Lawrence, 'Regional centres', p. 1318.
94 'Symposium on the practical applications in general practice, public health and industry', *BMJ*, 2:5404 (1964), 306.
95 'Symposium on glaucoma', *BMJ*, 2:5404 (1964), 303; H. Keen, 'Diabetes detection', in G. Teeling-Smith (ed.), *Surveillance and Early Diagnosis in General Practice* (London: Office of Health Economics, 1966), pp. 19–24.
96 '350,000 may have diabetes'.
97 On the complexities and shifts in British anxieties about Communism: M. Jones, *Science Fiction Cinema and 1950s Britain: Recontextualizing Cultural Anxiety* (London: Bloomsbury, 2018).
98 W. Oakley, 'Detection of diabetes', *The Lancet*, 282:7311 (1963), 787.

99 'Diagnosis of diabetes', *The Lancet*, 276:7153 (1960), 745–6.
100 J. Tomlinson, *The Politics of Decline: Understanding Post-War Britain* (Harlow: Pearson Education, 2001).
101 'Continuing care in chronic disease', *BMJ*, 2:5404 (1964), 308; Tomlinson, *The Politics of Decline*.
102 Office of Health Economics, *The Common Illness of Our Time: A Study of the Problem of Ischaemic Heart Disease* (London: Office of Health Economics, 1966), esp. pp. 18–19; Department of Health for Scotland, *Committee on Scottish Health Services*, Cmd 5204 (Edinburgh: HMSO, 1936), pp. 73–9.
103 J. N. Morris, 'The prevention of disease in middle age', *Public Health*, 77:4 (1963), 237.
104 Weisz, *Chronic Disease in the Twentieth Century*, pp. 176–202.
105 M. D. Moore, 'Balance and the "good diabetic" in Britain, c.1900–60', in M. Jackson and M. D. Moore (eds.), *Balancing the Self: Medicine, Politics, and the Regulation of Health in the Twentieth Century* (forthcoming.
106 R. D. Lawrence, *The Diabetic Life: Its Control by Diet and Insulin. A Concise Practical Manual for Practitioners and Patients*, 6th edition (London: J. & A. Churchill, 1931), p. 14; 'Diagnosis of diabetes'.
107 J. Fry, 'General practice to-morrow', *BMJ*, 2:5416 (1964), 1065. Most famously, see the discussion of diabetes in Julian Tudor Hart's 'rule of halves': J. T. Hart, 'A new kind of doctor', *Journal of the Royal Society of Medicine*, 74:12 (1981), 872–5. Hart was a renowned socialist GP and fervent supporter of the NHS.
108 'Natural history' is a problematic term, but by and large it was used to discuss the progress of disease from onset to termination in the absence of medical intervention: J. N. Morris, *Uses of Epidemiology*, 3rd edition (Edinburgh: Churchill Livingstone, 1975), pp. 121–41.
109 J. Malins, *Clinical Diabetes Mellitus* (London: Eyre and Spottiswoode, 1968), pp. 66–82.
110 Keen, 'Diabetes detection'; R. J. Jarrett, H. Keen, J. H. Fuller, and M. McCartney, 'Treatment of borderline diabetes: controlled trial using carbohydrate restriction and phenformin', *BMJ*, 2:6091 (1977), 861–5; Medical Research Council [MRC] Working Party, 'MRC trial of treatment of mild hypertension: principal results', *BMJ*, 291:6488 (1985), 97–104.
111 'Thursday morning: opening remarks', *Public Health*, 81:5 (1966), 207.
112 Cf. Timmermann, 'A matter of degree'.
113 A. M. Brandt and M. Gardner, 'The golden age of medicine?', in Cooter and Pickstone (eds.), *Companion to Medicine in the Twentieth Century*, pp. 21–37.
114 D. Armstrong, 'The rise of surveillance medicine', *Sociology of Health and Illness*, 17:3 (1995), 393–404; W. Rothstein, *Public Health and the Risk*

Factor: A History of An Uneven Medical Revolution (New York: University of Rochester Press, 2003).
115 G. M. Oppenheimer, 'Profiling risk: the emergence of coronary heart disease epidemiology in the United States (1947–70)', *International Journal of Epidemiology*, 35:3 (2006), 720–30.
116 Porter, 'From Social Structure to Social Behaviour'; Elliot, 'The prevention of illness in middle age', p. 318.
117 Berridge, 'Medicine and the public'; J. Hand, '"Tucking your tummy in isn't the answer": visualising obesity as a public health concern in 1970s and 1980s Britain', in Jackson and Moore (eds.), *Balancing the Self*.
118 Berridge, *Marketing Health*, pp. 75–7.
119 C. Timmermann, 'Appropriating risk factors: the reception of an American approach to chronic disease in the two German states, c.1950–1990', *Social History of Medicine*, 25:1 (2012), 157–74; R. A. Aronowitz, *Making Sense of Illness: Science, Society, and Disease* (Cambridge: Cambridge University Press, 1998).
120 P. Addison, *No Turning Back: The Peacetime Revolutions of Post-War Britain* (Oxford: Oxford University Press, 2010). Even under Labour, planning in Britain quickly shed compulsory controls over labour and materials, and governments adopted voluntary agreements as the basis for engaging with private industries: R. Toye, 'Gosplanners versus thermostatters: Whitehall planning debates and their political consequences, 1945–49', *Contemporary British History*, 14:4 (2000), 81–106; G. O'Hara, *From Dreams to Disillusionment: Economic and Social Planning in the 1960s* (Basingstoke: Palgrave Macmillan, 2007).
121 L. Berlivet, '"Association or causation?" The debate on the scientific status of risk factor epidemiology, 1947–c.1965', in V. Berridge (ed.), *Making Health Policy: Networks in Research and Policy after 1945* (Amsterdam: Rodopi, 2005), pp. 39–74.
122 H. P. Himsworth, 'Diet in the aetiology of human diabetes', *Proceedings of the Royal Society of Medicine*, 62 (1949), 323–6; Malins, *Clinical Diabetes Mellitus*, pp. 3–26; T. L. Cleave, G. D. Campbell, and N. S. Painter, *Diabetes, Coronary Thrombosis, and the Saccharine Disease*, 2nd edition (Bristol: John Wright & Sons, 1969).
123 Reid, 'Some public health aspects of diabetes', p. 155.
124 R. J. Donaldson, 'Multiple screening clinics', *Public Health*, 81:5 (1967), 218–21.
125 See Chapter 2.
126 Reid, 'Some public health aspects of diabetes', p. 155; Oppenheimer, 'Profiling risk', pp. 725–7.
127 Morris, 'The prevention of disease in middle age'. It was variously described as secondary or tertiary prevention: see Chapter 2.

128 Although recommended in the 1953 standards, these additions could be difficult to achieve in practice: J. Walker, *Chronicle of a Diabetic Service* (London: BDA, 1989).
129 M. D. Moore, 'Reorganising chronic disease management: diabetes and bureaucratic technologies in post-war British general practice', in M. Jackson (ed.), *The Routledge History of Disease* (London: Routledge, 2017), p. 456.
130 P. L. Robinson and E. T. Baker-Bates, 'A new diabetic chart', *BMJ*, 2:4790 (1952), 919–21, esp. p. 919.
131 See Introduction.
132 Robinson and Baker-Bates, 'A new diabetic chart', p. 919. On how records controlled action through communication: J. D. Howell, *Technology in the Hospital: Transforming Patient Care in the Early Twentieth Century* (Baltimore: Johns Hopkins University Press, 1995). This is taken up more extensively in Chapter 3.
133 Robinson and Baker-Bates, 'A new diabetic chart', p. 921.
134 J. Walker, 'Sociological implications of diabetes', *BMJ*, 2:4934 (1955), 317–19.
135 R. E. Tunbridge, 'Sociomedical aspects of diabetes mellitus', *The Lancet*, 262:6792 (1953), 895.
136 Ibid., p. 896.
137 Ibid., pp. 893–9, quotations at p. 896. Tunbridge's suggestions were supported by other practitioners: J. Lister, *The Clinical Syndrome of Diabetes Mellitus* (London: H. K. Lewis, 1959), pp. 211–19, 221–5.
138 H. Valier and R. Bivins, 'Organization, ethnicity and the British National Health Service', in J. Stanton (ed.), *Innovations in Health and Medicine: Diffusion and Resistance in the Twentieth Century* (London: Routledge, 2002), p. 41.
139 For instance, R. D. Lawrence (King's College Hospital, London) was a person with diabetes as well as a pioneering specialist in diabetes, and he promoted the use of health visitors in clinics within his local NHS region and around the country: Lawrence, 'Regional centres'. Joan Walker had connections with Lawrence, and her visits to the USA informed her thinking around community diabetes care: J. Welshman, 'Growing old in the city: public health and the elderly in Leicester, 1948–74', *Medical History*, 40:1 (1996), 83–4. D. A. Williams suffered asthma and had previously worked closely with the Cardiff MOH, J. Greenwood Wilson, to establish an asthma clinic before again collaborating with the use of health visitors in diabetes care: A. J. Thomas, 'Lives of the Fellows: David Aelwyn Williams', *Royal College of Physicians*, 2009, available at: http://munksroll.rcplondon.ac.uk/Biography/Details/4780 (accessed March 2018).

140 On early schemes and imperial, gender and class politics: H. Marland, 'A pioneer in infant welfare: the Huddersfield scheme, 1903–1920', *Social History of Medicine*, 6:1 (1993), 25–50; R. W. J. Dingwall, 'Collectivism, regionalism and feminism: health visiting and British social policy', *Journal of Social Policy*, 6:3 (1977), 291–315; C. Davis, 'The health visitor as mother's friend: a woman's place in public health, 1900–14', *Social History of Medicine*, 1:1 (1988), 39–59.

141 On attachment: McLaurin and Smith, 'Professional strategies of Medical Officers of Health', pp. 130–5.

142 'One hundred and eighteenth annual meeting of the British Medical Association: aftercare by health visitors', *BMJ*, 2:4673 (1950), p. 291.

143 Ibid.; 'British Medical Association annual meeting, Cardiff, 1953: health visitor and the family doctor', *BMJ*, 2:4830 (1953), 276.

144 'British Medical Association annual meeting, Cardiff, 1953', p. 276.

145 Welshman, 'Growing old in the city', p. 84.

146 J. B. Walker, 'Field work of a diabetic clinic', *The Lancet*, 262:6783 (1953), 445.

147 Ibid., pp. 445–6; interview with J. Wilson conducted by the University of Oxford, 11 December 2006, available at: www.diabetes-stories.com/interview.asp?UID=53 (accessed April 2017).

148 Walker, 'Field work of a diabetic clinic', p. 447; Walker, *Chronicle of a Diabetic Service*, p. 31. For attitudes to overweight patients: Lawrence, *The Diabetic Life*, 6th edition, p. 48.

149 D. F. Egan, 'Towards a new public health', *Public Health*, 79:4 (1965), 181.

2

Diabetes, risk management, and the birth of modern primary care

Although the creation of the NHS had strengthened the role of hospitals in diabetes management, a minority of innovative practitioners began to experiment with more community-oriented care schemes in the 1950s. Clinics and local government health departments co-operated to extend the surveillance and educative reach of clinicians, with nursing and health visiting staff forming part of expanded care teams. With their growing mix of skills, the new teams sought to confront the myriad social and medical problems facing patients with a common chronic disease.

These arrangements had generally marginalised GPs. Many GPs either lacked confidence with the condition (referring sole responsibility for diabetic problems to clinics) or, reflecting wider tensions within the profession, did not have patients returned to them by hospital colleagues, who lacked faith in GPs' capabilities. Moreover, whilst some GPs undoubtedly assumed a significant amount of responsibility for diabetes care, divisions of labour with hospitals were rarely systematised. Responding to a Ministry of Health questionnaire issued in 1963, one consultant physician from Caerphilly summarised a situation common across Britain: 'on the whole, G.P.'s [sic] prefer to leave the care of diabetics to the clinic and none has expressed special interest [in patients with the condition]'.[1]

Despite such trends, within ten years of this assessment a host of systems and research programmes emerged around general practice and shared care in diabetes. Into the 1980s, many hospital practitioners remained sceptical about the abilities of GPs, and evaluations of new organisational arrangements highlighted numerous problems. Yet innovations spread in face of such difficulties, with novel patterns of GP-led and community-based care reaching from Stirling to Poole and from Powys to King's Lynn.[2]

This chapter explores how GPs became enrolled in novel diabetes management programmes, and why schemes for integrated care spread across the country. At its heart, the chapter positions the changing organisation of diabetes care within professional political projects. For hospital consultants, the attractions of co-operating with GPs were clear. Patient numbers were outstripping hospital resources, with the result that clinicians felt standards of care were falling. Moreover, the politicisation of hospital costs and waiting times during the 1960s and 1970s meant that conditions in clinics could no longer be tolerated. With local government health departments atrophying, the greater incorporation of GPs in systematic diabetes care offered a way to alleviate pressures on clinics, spreading the cost of care and freeing consultants to focus on the patients who they believed were in most need of skilled oversight.[3] Consultants also suggested that GPs would be able to provide more attentive care than clinics to patients whose management was deemed more 'routine'. These were patients who were generally not on insulin regimes, who had no long-term complications, and who did not regularly experience hypoglycaemia or significant hyperglycaemia. As such, they were also patients whose straightforward oversight proved less clinically challenging or interesting.

By contrast, the motivations of GPs to involve themselves in diabetes care are less obvious on first sight. Diabetes management increased their clinical work, with no compensatory increase in resources, and there were more prevalent 'chronic illnesses' that could have drawn GPs' attention.[4] Of course, many GPs became involved in diabetes care because they believed standards could be improved. Diabetes management, however, also tied neatly into the shifting politics of general practice following the 1950s, and became incorporated into broader efforts to improve the status of GPs within the profession and British health services. The first appeals for greater GP involvement, for instance, emerged in relation to pre-symptomatic disease and prevention, areas of considerable interest to some GPs, especially those connected with academic institutions. By the early 1970s, poor-quality evidence and cost concerns had seen such claims superseded, with GP care entangled in long-held discussions about the unique social, psychological, and clinical skills of GPs. Finally, appeals to preventive risk management returned alongside the themes of practice organisation in the 1980s and 1990s, as bodies like the Royal College of General Practitioners (RCGP) incorporated diabetes care into projects of quality assurance and public health practice. Diabetes, in other words, became a disease more feasibly managed in general practice because of changes in the institutional environment, but it was also a disease around which general practice could be remade in ways consonant with broader professional projects.

Such endeavours cannot be divorced from post-war political and economic developments. The spectre of cost-control – and related calls for greater service integration and efficiency – haunted debates. New schemes for diabetes were part of wider NHS readjustments, particularly in chronic disease care, and diabetes management provided something of a 'model' for other chronic conditions.[5] Similarly, this chapter suggests that ground-breaking schemes would not have been possible without determined pioneers and important technological innovations. Particularly in the 1960s and 1970s, structured GP care for diabetes was rare, and integrated schemes tended to emerge where local clinicians and GPs either were especially interested in the condition or were convinced by persuasive colleagues.

Bringing these factors into a single analysis will articulate the rich political, professional, and technological histories underpinning important shifts in British diabetes management. The reorganisation of responsibilities for diabetes could involve conflict or even founder upon passive resistance, and in the short term GP involvement in structured care schemes was geographically uneven. However, the extent of occupational and institutional change involved in new arrangements was significant enough to raise awkward questions. GPs and hospital practitioners alike became concerned about standards of care and the possibility of dividing and integrating labour across time and space. As will be explored in Chapter 3, the answers that doctors produced to these challenges had repercussions for medical professionals and for the status of diabetes as a 'model' chronic disease. Likewise, the ways in which managed labour become aligned with public health policy is taken up in the rest of the volume. To understand the magnitude of these changes, however, it is important to first have a sense of the landscape of care in the 1950s.

GPs and diabetes management in the first decade of the NHS

Although the referral system had a long lineage, the creation of the NHS confirmed and generalised the role of the GP as part personal doctor, part gatekeeper.[6] Most GPs lost or dropped private practice work after 1948, instead serving registered populations of up to 4,000 patients in the new service.[7] Registered patients could access a GP for consultation whenever they felt it necessary – generally upon experiencing symptoms – either by making an appointment (though this was rare before the 1960s), receiving a home visit, or simply waiting at the practitioners' surgery. Upon attendance, GPs would diagnose problems and prescribe treatment for patients who they thought were within their competence and means (with wide variation), referring on to hospital those who they felt required special investigations or therapy.[8] In principle, any test results, diagnoses, or treatment plans made at hospital would be explained to the GP via a letter on discharge, thereby ensuring that the GP had a complete medical history of the patient for future contact. Although ideals were only patchily realised, patient access to costly hospital services were mediated through these mechanisms of registration and referral, and the GP became the primary medical contact for patients over their lifetime.

In diabetes care, the introduction of the NHS also accelerated inter-war trends. Despite specialist diabetes outpatient clinics growing after the 1920s, the financial arrangements of the inter-war medical system were complex. Patients could avoid direct charges for diagnostic tests, medical consultation, and therapeutic agents under certain conditions, but not under others. Access to clinics (and even GP care) thus varied across the country. The NHS, however, removed most financial barriers to hospital care for patients. Moreover, its generalisation of capitation payments for general practice meant that GPs would also have no monetary incentive to keep hold of patients making heavy demands on their time, as was the case with patients with diabetes.[9] In general, therefore, patients with diabetes were the perfect candidates for referral, and a significant proportion of GPs passed all diabetes care on to specialists.[10]

Financial factors in referral were buttressed by intra-professional aversions and anxieties. On a local level, consultant staff and GPs could maintain good relations, but the existence of private medicine often helped to facilitate friendly co-operation.[11] In terms of diabetes, some GPs even served as 'clinical assistants' in specialist outpatient clinics, undertaking clinical assessments and consultation under direction of senior hospital doctors.[12]

Broadly speaking, though, hospital doctors did not hold general practice in high regard during the 1950s. Despite the fact that general practice provided the most likely employment after qualification, one survey undertaken in 1961 indicated that only one quarter of 'senior medical students and newly-qualified doctors' made general practice their first-choice occupation.[13] The views of junior practitioners seemed to dovetail with, and be shaped by, the values expressed by senior doctors. Taking one frequently cited example, Lord Moran, the President of the RCP, suggested to a Royal Commission on pay in 1958 that GPs were generally doctors who had 'fallen off' the professional 'ladder'.[14] These opinions generated considerable backlash, and Lord Moran later attempted to modify his statement. By contrast with hospital specialties, entrance into general practice required no vocational training during the late 1950s, with a pre-registration year in hospital practice considered sufficient for a graduate to be appropriately qualified.[15] Referring to this difference, Lord Moran claimed that his initial statement was meant only to support the rewarding of lengthy specialist training.[16] Nonetheless, the underpinning sentiment was telling, and seemingly common within diabetes care. Surveys of doctors from the late 1950s indicated that clinicians did not always trust GPs to be skilled or confident enough to look after patients with diabetes, and specialist liaison after referral could be poor.[17] During the 1960s, hospital doctors complained that 'few general practitioners are prepared to treat their diabetic patients', the consequence of which was retention of clinic attenders 'indefinitely'.[18]

However, a minority of GPs did retain almost complete responsibility for their patients with diabetes during the 1950s and 1960s.[19] One well-known practitioner suggested that he referred only sixteen of eighty maturity-onset patients under his care over twenty years.[20] Furthermore, during the 1950s at least, most GPs retained some contact with their diabetes patients. Though highlighting a significant rate of attrition from formal care, one review conducted between 1952 and 1954 estimated that GPs saw approximately 68 per cent of their patients with diabetes annually.[21] Such findings were supported by an earlier study, which recorded an average of around eight consultations with these patients per year, albeit with a wide range across locations (between two and fourteen consultations per year) and age (higher rates for patients aged sixty-five and above).[22]

Yet, whilst regular contact was not uncommon, most consultations were not for management of diabetes *per se*. GPs may have been responsible for initial disease detection, but, following referral, clinics often assumed the lead in diabetes care, and patients contacted community care staff for more quotidian issues, such as daily drug administration or treatment of unrelated illness.[23] In fact, reflecting on her contact with GPs over twenty years between 1960 and 1980, one patient recalled that 'apart from perhaps mentioning it [her diabetes] if I went to him with any other problem, it never seemed to be brought forward at all'.[24] It was a common arrangement, and not just for diabetes. Once patients had been referred or admitted to hospital, specialist services often retained managerial responsibility for patients with supposedly complicated long-term illness.[25] One prominent report from the 1960s even referred to these outpatients as 'detainees'.[26] As such a critical assessment suggests, this division of labour between hospital specialist and GP was soon to be placed under question.

Early challenges in the 1960s: co-ordinating care, risk, and pre-symptomatic disease

The earliest calls for a reorganisation of responsibility and labour in diabetes management came from a handful of GPs, hospital clinicians, and public health practitioners during the 1960s. All these doctors recognised the importance and advantages of specialist outpatient clinics in their usual respects: laboratory facilities, experienced physicians, cutting-edge research, and availability of ancillary services.[27] Yet, for this tiny minority of critics from across the medical spectrum, overwhelming support for specialist outpatient clinics masked important problems. The first, according to clinicians like John Nabarro at the Middlesex Hospital, was that once a patient was referred, there was 'a tendency for the entire treatment to pass to the clinic'. Problems could arise, he concluded, 'when the practitioner is called in, in an emergency', as 'he [sic] is without up-to-date knowledge of the patient's condition and treatment'.[28] The second common concern amongst critics was the ever-growing size of clinic populations. Busy conditions made comprehensive care very difficult. 'The crowded diabetic clinic', wrote the well-known academic clinician, researcher, and diabetologist Harry Keen, 'is not the place where the deeper or more confidential of the diabetics' problems may be easily unfolded.' Rather, he suggested, diet and insulin were the 'chief preoccupations' of the 'busy clinic', despite being 'only the beginning of the diabetic life'.[29]

Indeed, the causes and results of the clinic's problems were summarised succinctly by one GP from the Birmingham region (L. A. Pike) at a joint meeting of MOHs and GPs in the early 1960s:

> At the present time, it seems to be the rule that a patient with suspected diabetes is referred to hospital where the diagnosis is confirmed. The

diabetic clinic then takes the patient under its wing and never lets him [sic] go. Rarely are patients discharged to their family doctor, and of course many family doctors are prepared to delegate this care. The general practitioner copes with illnesses other than diabetes and advises the patient between hospital visits. Clinics serve a valuable function in the assessment of new cases, the management of severe diabetes, and as centres for research and teaching. In my area, however, I feel that these functions are hampered by the deluge of diabetics who turn up to keep their routine appointments but who could well be supervised by their family doctor. In most places the diabetic clinics are working to capacity with a shortage of staff and premises.

With the estimated prevalence of diabetes rising, the author concluded, 'resources are going to be further stretched by the increasing number of diabetics particularly in the older age groups.'[30]

These criticisms would be heavily repeated into the 1970s, and they drove many of the initial experiments with more formal programmes for shared care. During the 1960s, however, hospital clinicians, GPs, and MOHs suggested several solutions to the issue of overcrowding. Harry Keen, for instance, sought to promote roles for GPs as surveillance officers: 'It is a common experience for the diabetic', Keen wrote, 'noting the approach of his [sic] visit to the clinic, to tighten up his control.' As doctors relied on short-term measurements of urine and blood glucose, this meant that when the patient arrived at the clinic, they 'present[ed] an excellent and thoroughly atypical picture of it [their diabetic control]'. Being able to check on patients between visits to the hospital, Keen suggested, GPs could circumvent such strategies, proposing that 'no-one is better situated to assess the degree of control of the diabetic than the family doctor'.[31] Moreover, unburdened by the busy strictures of the clinic, the GP, Keen also implied, might be better placed to deal with the social, psychological, and emotional concerns of patients – with the patient's 'employment problem, his fears about blindness, his sexual impotence, or the veil of prejudice he has met at work.'[32] Whilst the hospital dealt with the 'technical' matters of therapy, GPs could take up responsibility for the broader challenges of chronic disease.[33] No formal programme was forthcoming, however.

GPs who were critical of existing arrangements often sought a more substantive role, primarily for those 'well-controlled' patients who did not require specialist attention or technologies.[34] 'There is no reason why', wrote Pike, 'in a partnership practice the control of diabetes should not be undertaken by one of the partners in the way that maternity work is sometimes undertaken.'[35] In addition to managing already diagnosed patients, Pike also envisioned a greater role in case-finding and preventive medicine. Drawing on the Birmingham detection survey, he ruled out mass screening on grounds of expense. Instead, 'greater results will be obtained with less effort' if practitioners focused on those considered 'at-risk'.[36] In this case, vigilance would be applied to individuals who had relatives with diabetes, who were over fifty years old (especially women over this age), who were obese (or, owing to higher prevalence at different weights, 'lighter' if 'West Indian'), who were multiparous or had a history of giving birth to babies over 10 lb, or who had classic symptoms of diabetes. Such characteristics, according to Pike, might be predictive of diabetes either because population research revealed these groups to contain a disproportionate number of people with diabetes than in control groups (e.g. the under-fifties or the non-obese), or because retrospective study revealed that such characteristics were preponderant amongst people who developed diabetes.[37] Moreover, transitioning from statistical prediction to causative concepts of risk, Pike viewed targeted case-finding as necessary because intervention before symptoms became 'marked' offered the best hope of preventing complications.[38]

For more radical interlocutors, such work would form part of an expanded GP role in chronic disease surveillance more broadly. For instance, according to R. F. L. Logan of the innovative Darbishire House research team at the University of Manchester, screening studies had unlocked new areas of research and practice activity.[39] 'Where 300 persons in an average practice', he argued, 'may have a glucose tolerance test so abnormal that classically it would be considered diabetic, it makes us ask the questions: What is diabetes? When does the disease begin?' The part played by GPs in such investigations meant that 'general practice is now at the front line of these fundamental questions about the nature of non-infectious disease itself and the point of its onset'.[40] Moving on to practicalities, Logan suggested that as many conditions were multi-causal 'you cannot have primary prevention of them'.[41] Instead, intervention would focus on secondary and tertiary prevention. Thus, in the 'medical care of the chronic non-infectious pattern of disease today', Logan suggested, 'the poles of curative medicine on the one side and prevention on the other no longer apply'. Rather, 'what do apply are, early presymptomatic recognition, surveillance of high risks, postponing the onset or reducing its impact, bringing in of adequate care, delaying of handicap, and training residual abilities'.[42]

For conditions like diabetes, hypertension, glaucoma, rheumatoid arthritis, cancers, and mental illnesses, Logan felt that 'something directly effective, often life-saving can be done in general practice'.[43] And even though undertaking care and 'surveillance in the control of chronic disease' could 'swamp' the GP – especially in the context of population growth and rising 'expectations of the lower social classes' – organisational solutions could ensure success. Primarily, change would involve drastic reductions in home visiting, and the GP becoming a 'community doctor' with a large list, 'a team of nurses', and 'a centre equipped with modern facilities'.[44] To use David Armstrong's terms, Logan sought to turn the GP into the embodiment of dispensary medicine: ever watchful of the whole population, not just locating 'submerged' clinical disease but redrawing the boundaries between health and illness in the process.[45]

That academics like Logan were key figures in promoting new understandings of disease and service provision is indicative of the way the NHS provided a productive environment for research and scholarly activity. As Valier and Timmermann have argued, the regional structure of the NHS, based on 'major teaching hospitals and their affiliated universities', provided post-war academics with abundant research opportunities and considerable intellectual influence within the profession.[46] Research and education were initially less integral to establishing authority in general practice, but the situation slowly changed over the 1950s and 1960s.[47]

Nonetheless, unfortunately for Logan, his vision was far removed from the experience of most GPs, and problems of workload, finances, and prominent understandings of disease worked against the creation of new roles for general practice. Some recent service changes may have facilitated novel forms of care. A new GP contract had been agreed in the mid-1960s which extended allowances for administrative, nursing, and other staff.[48] Similarly, some innovative MOHs were keen to attach their staff to GP surgeries, conceptualising the future of public health activity in relation to so-called 'lifestyle diseases' and health service management.[49] Yet, as one respondent to Logan's paper put it, 'medical time, manpower and finance are limited'.[50] 'Although regular effective screening of the community may be a theoretical ideal', the author went on, 'there is a very real danger of forgetting the amount of disease that is and can be prevented by the conventional methods which depend on nature's early warning system [of symptoms] and which are the keystone of good general practice.'[51] Furthermore, not only did many doctors still take symptoms (rather than asymptomatic, quantitative deviations) as the starting point of disease, but clinicians and researchers across the health services also felt that evidence was insufficient to categorically support screening and pre-symptomatic intervention.[52]

In terms of clinical diabetes, there were further obstacles to remaking the role of GPs along preventive lines. The power of metabolic control to protect against longer-term complications was still a matter of dispute during the 1960s, and one tempered by the very practical fear of hypoglycaemia, the inconveniences of testing, and desires for a normal life.[53] With uncertainty about the effects of glycaemic control even for the symptomatic, surveillance and opportunistic lifestyle advice represented the furthest practitioners would go for 'at risk' or 'borderline' patients whilst further research was ongoing.[54] Similarly, whilst medical civil servants were intrigued by the implications of community surveys for screening and diagnostic criteria, they made little movement beyond committee discussions.[55]

In short, economies of time and finance, combined with persistently high opinions of specialist practice, curtailed more systematic general practice interventions into diabetes management during the 1960s. Such arguments did not disappear. Rather they became background to further discussion until changes in knowledge, ideology, and health service conditions made them more persuasive.

Expanding GP care: integration and deputation in the 1970s

At the heart of discussions about GPs and diabetes care during the 1960s were questions about the nature of disease and general practice, about the use of resources, and – as will be noted later in this chapter – about the very structure of the NHS itself. Critically, such discussions were taking place within a context of shifting political and financial circumstances of the health service. As noted in Chapter 1, since its inception, the health service had been under severe pressures to control costs. Negotiations between the Ministry of Health and the Treasury did secure significant capital investment for the NHS during the 1960s as part of the political renewal of central planning.[56] Furthermore, supported by the findings of the now-famous Guillebaud Report in 1956, the NHS also received a real-terms increase in current expenditure over the 1960s, funded in part by an erratically expanding economy.[57] Nonetheless, central pressures to use resources efficiently and to cap current expenditure remained in place. They were even formally agreed in exchange for increased capital investment in the nation's ageing hospital stock.[58]

State drives to control NHS expenditure also extended to encouraging greater professional engagement with questions of resource use. In 1966, the Ministry of Health and Joint Consultants Committee of the British Medical Association established the Joint Working Party on the Organisation of Medical Work in Hospitals.[59] Its reports sought to provide the basis for collective professional governance of hospitals prior to possible service restructuring. Linking individual decision-making to collective resources, the first report suggested that 'practically every clinical decision affects the administrative running of the hospital'. Effective management – 'the smooth and economic running of the procedures concerned with diagnosis, treatment and care' – would thus depend upon 'mobilising the full consciousness of clinicians about the effect of their individual actions on others than the patient'.[60] In 1953, the Ministry had encouraged local medical advisory committees to 'undertake periodic ... systematic review and statistical analysis of the clinical work of all departments in the hospital', but without great success.[61] Now the Working Party suggested improving routine data collection and organising consultant staff in 'clinical divisions' to carry out 'constant appraisal of the services it provides, [to] deploy clinical resources as effectively as possible and [to] cope with the problems of management that arise in its clinical field'.[62] Divisions would be linked via a small medical executive committee, with a senior clinician as chair, to ensure cross-institutional co-ordination. Though not compelling codification of work and performance management review, such reforms did facilitate greater professional oversight of work, and even saw institutions develop clearer guidelines for 'routine' hospital procedures.[63]

Such pressures intensified into the 1970s. Industrial unrest, rising inflation, growing unemployment, and confused policy responses brought down the Conservative administration of 1970–74.[64] The incoming Labour government also had to cope with global economic turbulence, and the persistent mistrust of subsequent Labour administrations (1974–79) on the part of international capital markets resulted in a now infamous International Monetary Fund loan in 1976.[65] These political and economic circumstances provided fertile ground for the spread of neoliberal ideas into British politics.[66] During the 1970s, however, continued frustration with a lack of central control over NHS spending drove interest in increased service planning and management, and underlined persistent structural reforms that began in 1974.[67] Labour administrations even developed a new planning and priorities system for the NHS in 1976, within which central government detailed the money available for specific objectives, and the hierarchy of health authorities then produced plans for resource allocation. 'Superior' authorities provided 'priorities and an indication of the resources available', and 'the 'inferior' authorities produc[ed] plans after consultation', with subsequent review up the chain of command.[68]

Central government departments were not the only policy actors to raise concerns about the use of NHS finances. Driven by older concerns about efficiency and new interests in health economics and patient consumerism, think-tanks and organised consumer groups like the King's Fund, the Nuffield Provincial Hospitals Trust, the Office of Health Economics, and the Patients' Association also raised public concerns about outpatient waiting times and hospital inefficiencies.[69] In particular, they called attention to the large number of chronic patients – like those with diabetes – who they felt were unnecessarily attached to specialist clinics.[70]

Under such circumstances, criticisms of clinics grew louder during the 1970s. For some GPs, the problems of clinics resulted in unsatisfactory care for doctor and patient. As one GP wrote in 1974, once a patient was referred, they were 'doomed to take time off work, travel and wait to see a fresh houseman at almost every attendance … His [sic] notes get thicker and thicker so that both [the patient] and the young doctor find the fleeting consultations more and more unrewarding.'[71] The very *raison d'être* of the clinic – continuous specialist care for individual patients – had become undermined, and specialists themselves complained about compromised management and worsening experiences of care. As one commentator put it, this was an ironic consequence, whereby the 'desire by hospital doctors to look after interesting patients has now backfired'. Instead of improving working conditions, the accumulation of patients had produced 'overcrowding' and the 'aims of treatment were being increasingly frustrated'.[72]

What emerged in the 1970s, therefore, was a synergy of interests between GPs and hospital specialists within a febrile political environment. Building on early critiques, both saw mass outpatient care as costly and as failing patients. The figure causing problems, according to both sides, was the 'well-controlled' patient, with no long-term complications, who was being treated by diet alone (or diet and oral hypoglycaemic agent) and who attended the clinic for 'routine' follow-up.[73]

Their care had become rote for hospital practitioners, based on the periodic repetition of standard tests and, probably, advice to carry on in the same way. They also, according to one prominent clinician, prevented consultants from 'deal[ing] with the difficult problems for which [they had] been trained'.[74]

Such patients sat at the heart of new programmes for more structured diabetes care and a new division of responsibilities for patient management. Incorporating a small, though growing, minority of GPs and consultants, schemes emerged in the first half of the 1970s to integrate GPs into formal diabetes management operations. Broadly speaking, the new arrangements followed from the criticisms of traditional clinic systems. GPs assumed ongoing responsibility for routine surveillance of uncomplicated and well-controlled patients. They monitored physical and biochemical health, watched for signs of complications, and made small adjustments in therapeutic programmes. Clinics were then reserved for most insulin-requiring patients, patients referred for complications, and individuals with 'brittle' diabetes (characterised by wildly fluctuating blood sugars). As will be shown in Chapter 3, the most systematic of these schemes formalised the responsibilities of the GP and clinic in new care protocol, complete with referral criteria, and clinics would see only new and referred patients or undertake yearly reviews.

There were, of course, variations between schemes. For instance, early programmes were predicated on clinic staff visiting general practice surgeries. These arrangements were pioneered during the late 1960s in the Birmingham area, where they were promoted by the nationally renowned diabetologist John Malins in conjunction with a handful of interested GPs. The role of the GP here focused upon involvement in annual review clinics that were now taking place in GP surgeries. Practice and clinic staff would undertake the necessary testing together, and then the patient would have a consultation with the GP and hospital doctor to agree a treatment plan.[75]

These arrangements persisted into later decades but were quickly challenged.[76] Outside annual reviews, it seems that routine oversight continued to be un-organised. Other clinicians and GPs therefore built on these foundations to provide greater involvement and freedom for the GP. A particularly popular alternative emerged in the West Midlands city of Wolverhampton during the early 1970s. This system was created by the consultant P. A. Thorne – who, probably due to geographical proximity or the BDA, was in contact with Malins – and focused on general practice 'mini-clinics'. Here (in line with Pike's suggestion above) one GP in a partnership would take responsibility for surveillance of all of a practice's diet-controlled patients. Special monthly 'mini-clinics' were then organised, in which doctors and nursing staff set aside protected time to review a select number of patients at regular intervals. The usual tests and consultations would take place, and no further contact with the clinic was deemed necessary unless a GP made referrals or organised a yearly visit to the surgery by the clinic team.[77] GPs were given greater responsibility than in alternative plans, but were also more integrated into formal arrangements of care as a result.

One final notable form of systematic care was devised in the southern coastal town of Poole, Dorset. Like most of the early structured care schemes, the Poole system was driven by an influential and determined consultant working in tandem with engaged local GPs. For the consultant clinician R. D. Hill, his 'community care scheme' was more integrated than even the mini-clinic variety. Here, individual GPs kept responsibility for ongoing oversight of their own patients, but also co-ordinated surveillance activities with a range of community care workers – health visitors, opticians, and district nurses. As with mini-clinics, GPs retained responsibilities for routine care adjustments, and hospital laboratory facilities were made open to all scheme members, but hospital staff undertook yearly reviews within the clinic.[78] Although differing slightly, all the above arrangements sought to bring GPs into closer contact with hospitals and facilitate dispersal of duties. Each form, however, afforded slightly different weightings to continuity of care across certain areas of patient management.

Yet, for GPs, the attraction of diabetes care in the 1970s went beyond providing better care for their patients or improving NHS efficiency. Rather, by this decade systematic diabetes management appeared a more feasible proposition, and had become entangled with new visions of general practice itself. On the one hand, the increase in 'open access' arrangements for laboratory services over the 1960s enabled better patient surveillance, whilst familiarity with oral drugs bolstered GPs' confidence about treatment options.[79] Equally, at a local level, good relationships between GPs and charismatic consultants enabled collective ownership of new arrangements. In Poole, for instance, Hill earnestly wrote to all GPs to ensure they were involved in the planning process for his community care system.[80]

On the other hand, pioneers of systematic care schemes discussed diabetes management in ways that harnessed the frustrations of some GPs and envisioned new positions for them in British medicine. During the 1960s, many GPs expressed dissatisfaction with treating high levels of what they saw as minor illness in their practices. In one survey of GPs, for instance, one quarter of the 400 respondents believed that over 50 per cent of their surgery consultations were for 'trivial, unnecessary, and inappropriate reasons'.[81] Anxieties over the status of general practice were thus not uncommon, and proponents of GP-based care framed diabetes management as an absorbing area of clinical medicine. According to Malins and a GP colleague, taking on diabetes patients would prove satisfying, primarily because the GP 'no longer feels that the clinical care of an interesting disease is being taken from him [sic]'.[82] Equally, another GP, promoting systematic care of diabetes by GPs alone, declared how he hoped to 'convey the idea that small numbers of patients suffering from the same disease, as occur in general practice, can provide a wide spectrum of experience in symptomatology, pathology and treatment'.[83] These authors sought to make capital out of dissatisfaction, emphasising how diabetes could keep a doctor's interest and advertising the ways in which diabetes management intersected with highly valued areas of clinical medicine.

By contrast, other GPs drew on languages of personalised and continuous care of individuals and families to promote diabetes care. Although having a long heritage, these ideas gained considerable currency in the decades after the 1950s, as bodies like the College of General Practitioners (later the RCGP) sought to position them at the heart of GPs' professional identities.[84] The College itself had been established in 1952–53, by a group of doctors keen to mould general practice into an independent discipline with its own skills and knowledge.[85] The new body emerged, moreover, at a time when the creation of the NHS, and extensive criticisms of general practice's standards of provision, had damaged the morale of GPs, provoking a period of sustained reflection on the 'essence' and role of general practice in British medicine.[86] Over the early post-war decades, professional bodies and central state agencies alike sought to objectify general practice and to study it in order to understand its nature, and launched formal commissions to plan for its future.[87]

The contrast between the GP and the hospital doctor was a central element in all reflections on general practice. Whereas the clinician dealt with advanced cases of disease in abstract and artificial spaces, the GP treated patients in 'natural' settings of home, community, and surgery.[88] Furthermore, perhaps responding to claims that the NHS was too bureaucratic or impersonal, and hoping to differentiate GPs without detriment to status, some commentators revived a rhetoric that distinguished GPs by their personal knowledge of patients and their ability to build relationships over time.[89] One well-regarded practitioner considered this longitudinal bond to be so strong that, he suggested: 'the GP alone can offer the patient, and his family continuity of medical care over the years. They alone can know the family environment. And they alone can learn what is normal for the individual patient.'[90]

Appeals to personalised practice continued into the 1970s, and medical individualism underpinned claims about general practice diabetes care in that decade.[91] Promoting their scheme for GP-based annual reviews, for instance, Malins and Stuart outlined how patients welcomed the innovation. Not only was review closer to home, they argued, but patients were 'glad to come into an atmosphere which is familiar and to be greeted by staff whom they know. They feel that during the consultations their personal and social circumstances are fully taken into account.' According to Malins and Stuart, GPs would also benefit by gaining new expertise and would be more readily accepted as competent by patients with diabetes.[92] Similarly, Thorn and Russell argued that as a result of GPs taking responsibility for diabetes, general patient care would no longer pass to the clinic, and the care of the 'whole patient' would return to GPs.[93] In fact, being able to take personal and social circumstances into account now made sense for GPs as well. As some articles thus claimed, the combination of 'social and emotional problems' with symptoms, physical, and biochemical changes made diabetes clearly 'of interest' to the GP.[94]

Consolidating new arrangements: prevention and diabetes management

Over the next two decades, appeals for more systematic and integrated diabetes care shifted once again, moving in line with newer visions for general practice. Into the 1980s, discussions of general practice diabetes management returned to themes of prevention, organisation, and anticipatory care, with the psycho-social discourses of the 1960s and 1970s appearing as minor themes. By this decade, moreover, the questions posed in major medical publications were less concerned with whether GPs 'should' have a greater involvement in care, and focused instead on the form that this care could take.

In some respects, doctors in the 1980s revisited questions posed during the 1960s. As noted, a handful of elite and academic practitioners had previously sketched out a vision for GPs as preventive risk managers, but GPs ultimately felt that limitations of evidence and resources made such roles impossible. In terms of diabetes, themes of risk management and prevention reappeared during the 1980s. However, discussions of risk centred on programmes for secondary and tertiary prevention of diabetic complications rather than on primary disease prevention. For instance, during the 1970s several follow-up reports on 'borderline' diabetes appeared that extinguished much interest in these patients for several decades. Firstly, clinical trials found that instituting treatment in borderline patients did not seem to alter their physiological prospects: regardless of intervention, a small minority 'worsened to diabetes', whilst many more either returned to normal or remained the same over five to ten years of study.[95] Secondly, researchers noted that 'borderline' patients were at greater risk of cardiovascular and arterial disease than 'normal' controls. Yet, once again, anti-diabetic treatment appeared to make little impact on clinical outcomes, and statistical analyses suggested that heightened blood pressure was more likely than hyperglycaemia to underpin higher rates of arterial disease.[96] Thus, whilst researchers argued that 'impaired' glucose tolerance could be considered a state of risk – and its physiological abnormalities were worthy of follow-up at the extreme end – they concluded that it was neither a diabetic nor pre-diabetic state, and could not be clinically reversed.[97] Clinicians continued to discuss monitoring individuals with impaired glucose tolerance and those considered at risk for diabetes. But such action was intended to facilitate early diagnosis and treatment for all who required it, rather than to be a means of preventing the onset of disease.[98]

By contrast, over the 1980s, doctors were increasingly convinced that maintaining good blood glucose control might prevent the onset of complications. Much of this support was built on findings from large-scale longitudinal studies of defined populations, combined with clinical research with 'borderline cases'.[99] Specifically, this research suggested that the diagnostic category of diabetes should be restricted to those individuals whose blood sugar levels two hours after glucose intake were over 200 mg per 100 ml.[100] From follow-up investigations of initial prevalence surveys, researchers argued that characteristic pathological changes of the retina could be found almost exclusively in populations with readings above this blood glucose level on initial examination.[101] Not all patients (as they became) with this level of blood glucose developed retinopathy during the study period. Nonetheless, these findings were considered statistically significant, and offered a pathological marker with which to differentiate between populations with gradated variations in blood glucose.

Once doctors applied this knowledge in a clinical setting, they transformed a diagnosis of diabetes into an exercise of risk management and surveillance.[102] Whilst there was no guarantee that any one individual would develop retinopathy, the statistical argument for formalising standard diagnostic criteria at this level proved convincing.[103] Though it was not explicitly stated in publications, the extension of this logic meant that diagnosis was necessary to integrate patients into formal management and surveillance programmes – ones designed to reduce risk via hypoglycaemic interventions, and to deploy new technologies to treat retinal complications upon first indications of their appearance.[104] As we have seen, these arguments were not entirely novel: interviewees suggested that some doctors presumed a link between complications and control before these studies, on 'the balance of probabilities'.[105] However, whereas previously diagnosis may have depended upon the presence of symptoms – or a hypothetical assumption about the relationship between hyperglycaemia and complications – diagnosis now became predicated upon precise statistical calculations of likelihood derived from large-scale datasets, and individual treatment was formally legitimated by this research's predictive possibility.[106]

The relationship between British doctors and international diagnostic standards will be considered further in Chapter 5. However, it is important to note here that discourses of risk management and patient surveillance became a key part of discussions of GP care. For some GPs and hospital clinicians, new epidemiological research confirmed a link between diabetes and long-term complications, corroborated by their clinical experience and some smaller-scale clinical trials.[107] As one GP put it, 'good diabetic control is most important in preventing complications', and though 'extra time is needed to run a clinic', 'diabetics are such a high-risk group tha[t] an average of five minutes per day for prevention and treatment is an efficient use of a doctor's time'.[108]

Indeed, a tighter net of surveillance provided by integrated and systematic care would ensure that this secondary preventive effort could be a complemented by tertiary effort to prevent blindness. As will be seen in Chapter 4, new evidence about the efficacy of photocoagulation therapy in certain types of diabetic retinopathy sparked a push for new treatment programmes. In the words of one widely cited account, this development created a new imperative for tighter surveillance: 'retinopathy is a serious complication which can cause blindness; new treatments are being developed, so early detection is increasingly important'.[109] Such statements found further support amongst proponents of integrating hospital and general practice care. Here, 'regular monitoring of ... glycaemic control, weight, blood pressure' and 'a screening programme for the early detection of the long-term complications of diabetes' were essential activities. Research on defaulting and outcomes in the 1980s indicated that much scope existed for greater organisation and for 'rationalisation of care' and surveillance across the system.[110]

Yet it is important to note that changed discourses around GP diabetes care during the 1980s were not sparked solely by new research evidence unveiling incontestable truths. Instead, motivated by clinical, professional, and political imperatives, doctors and other health policy actors made numerous assumptions that were not strictly supported by available research. Firstly, the clinical interpretation of new evidence was not entirely consistent with what research had demonstrated. Though studies in the 1990s would support efforts to control blood glucose (and other risk factors), the publications of the late 1970s and early 1980s demonstrated only statistically significant, positive correlations between hyperglycaemia and selected end-points over time.[111] They did not, in other words, conclusively exclude the possibility of a hidden factor provoking both raised glucose levels and complications, or prove positive outcomes would result from intervention.[112] Secondly, though it was assumed that more refined disease surveillance would improve outcomes, it took until 1985 for a study to suggest that defaulters had worse physiological markers and complications than clinic attenders, and follow-up work was rare.[113] As with earlier research in coronary heart disease, it seems that clinical imperatives for intervention infused reactions to these observational studies, and medical desire to help transformed risk from a marker of prediction to a causative-but-modifiable variable.[114]

Just as importantly from the perspective of general practice, proactive work in diabetes became of wider interest as GPs made a more concerted effort to move into preventive medicine, and as the RCGP sought to promote better practice organisation.[115] Regardless of the technical validity of their interpretation (from within the bounds of trial-oriented thinking), for a small number of GPs new evidence about complications facilitated professional efforts to reposition diabetes care as a public health endeavour. The lead here was taken by the RCGP itself. Although not pronouncing on diabetes management formally during the 1970s, the College's *Journal* provided significant space for discussion of diabetes care. College support became explicit in the early 1980s, when a working party called for 'routine management of hypertension and non-insulin-dependent diabetes [to] be brought back to general practice'.[116] The justification for this recommendation did not focus solely on clinical experience or benefits that might accrue to patients and practitioners.[117] Rather, the College suggested that people with diabetes were a population 'at exceptional risk for arterial disease', and that the 'control of known diabetics in respect of blood glucose, obesity, smoking, and hypertension' would improve outcomes.[118] The benefits of 'preventive effort', it suggested, would 'flow naturally from improved clinical care'.[119] As will be noted in later chapters, aligning clinical work with preventive medicine in this way would have considerable implications for the political future of managed care.

Diabetes management, therefore, played a symbolic part in broader efforts to incorporate GPs into new public health arrangements. The discussions on diabetes, for instance, came from one of five College working parties considering the role of the GP in health promotion and public health. Their recommendations were unsurprising considering the group's composition. Julian Tudor Hart, a GP working in south Wales, was chair, and was well known for promoting GPs as key figures in the prevention and management of chronic disease on a community basis.[120] Similarly, other members included Laurie Pike (quoted above), and Godfrey Fowler, a GP in Oxford who worked in an academic department of community medicine and general practice and who edited a volume entitled *Preventive Medicine in General Practice* shortly after the publication of the arterial disease report.[121]

The move to establish GPs in preventive medicine situated discussions of diabetes within frameworks of chronic disease management more broadly. Concepts of risk management as a form of secondary and tertiary prevention had first emerged in relation to discussions of 'chronic disease' during the 1960s. Furthermore, the management of conditions like hypertension, though involving different symptomatic patterns from diabetes, experienced similar changes in understanding during the post-war period, whilst pharmacological innovations for other long-term diseases, like asthma, had also made their care more routine.[122] Following such developments and the growth of patient populations, GPs sought to claim responsibility for ongoing care from specialist clinics, or at least to share in management duties. By the 1980s, general practice had been framed as 'ideally suited for the management of chronic disease', and doctors even considered the application of similar models of care to different problems.[123] Discussing group practices, for instance, Hart proposed that 'the expected number of patients may justify concentration in regular mini-clinics for hypertension, diabetes, chronic obstructive airways disease, epilepsy, [and] rheumatic diseases'. Common approaches were possible, Hart suggested, because management of all these conditions had become centred on 'monitoring … a set of variables, support by ancillary staff with at least some special training, the use of equipment not usually used, and giving patients information'.[124] Here a form of care honed in diabetes management was generalised to other conditions, but the flow of influence could also work in the other direction, and doctors outlined how diabetes care in some sites had been altered in light of experience from other conditions.[125] Underpinning such exchanges, however, were a desire to maintain contact with patients and a belief that continuing care of chronic disease in general practice could help prevent mortality, severe morbidity, and disability.[126]

Once again, however, it is important to place professional developments in the context of contemporaneous political and health service change. The 1970s and 1980s were decades in which economic turbulence and global programmes to address disease reinvigorated attitudes to prevention within primary care. Internationally, Marc Lallonde (Minister of National Health and Welfare, Canada) gave his famous set of talks on prevention and responsibility in 1974, and the World Health Organization (WHO) placed prevention at the heart of primary care in the influential Alma-Ata Declaration of 1979. In Britain, economic problems provided grounds for reassessing how prevention might lessen burdens on the state, and Labour's subsequent policy papers on prevention not only drew on Lallonde's work, but also provoked the RCGP's own re-examination.[127]

Equally, these same financial pressures and shifts in thinking had, in part, influenced the reorganisation of the NHS in 1974, which provided

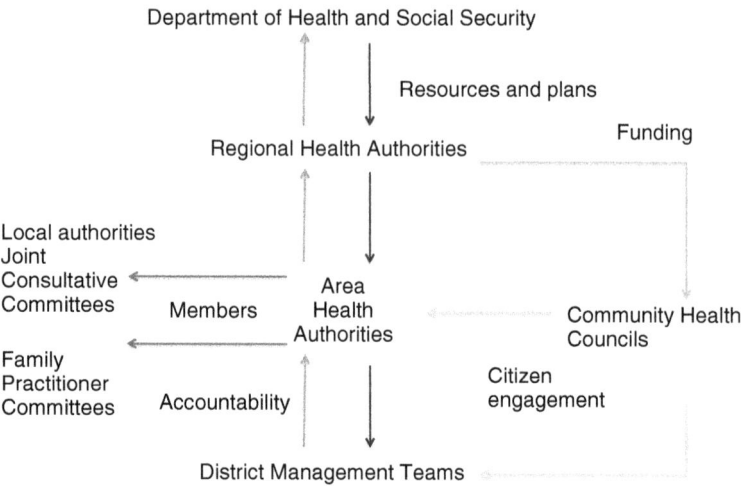

Figure 2.1 Representation of English NHS as envisioned after 1974 reorganisation

the conceptual and institutional space for GPs to move into preventive healthcare.[128] Undoubtedly, the schemes discussed above drew strength from the languages of integrated health and social service planning that characterised debates about reform during the 1960s and 1970s. The working party on medical work discussed above also sought to integrate service planning and management by including GPs in clinical divisions. However, the biggest impact of the 1974 reform on diabetes care came from the abolition of the MOHs as part of broader ambitions for service unification. The reforms played out slightly differently across Britain. In England, new legislation for the NHS eliminated the previous 700 bodies involved in administration, and established in their stead 14 Regional Health Authorities (RHAs), 90 Area Health Authorities, 90 Family Practitioner Committees, and 205 District Management Teams (see Fig. 2.1).

In Scotland, the development of a new settlement ran faster and more smoothly than south of the border, with a less overt emphasis on management and greater stress on political partnership with health authorities.[129] The system was considerably more centralised – with common services organisations providing plans and advice to integrated health

Diabetes, risk, and modern primary care

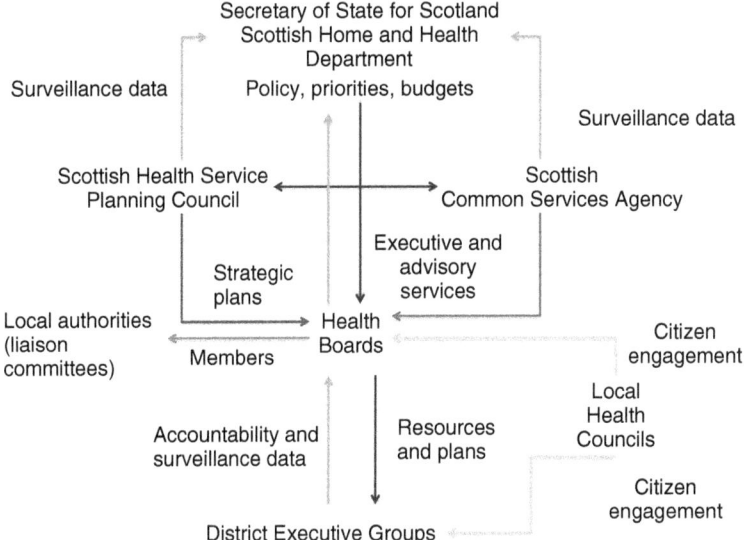

Figure 2.2 Representation of Scottish NHS as envisioned after 1974 reorganisation

boards – and relations between various parts of the service functioned relatively harmoniously (see Fig. 2.2).[130]

Finally, in Wales, the new NHS arrangements appeared as something of a mix of the English and Scottish variants structurally, but the Welsh system leaned much more towards the English version in tensions between central and local institutions (Fig. 2.3).[131]

Although the new structural differences between England, Scotland, and Wales probably had considerable day-to-day effects, the exact relationships of different bodies involved are less important to the story of diabetes care than the fact that, across Britain, the position of the MOH was removed.[132] Eventually, former MOHs were incorporated into the NHS as managers and service analysts, and their earlier clinical service responsibilities fell to GPs and hospitals. Some of the new Community Physicians did play important roles in piloting experiments with GP care in various parts of the country.[133] But the removal of MOHs provided an important space for GPs to claim 'community' practice and service integration as their own field, with visions like that of Reid discussed in the previous chapter now no longer possible.

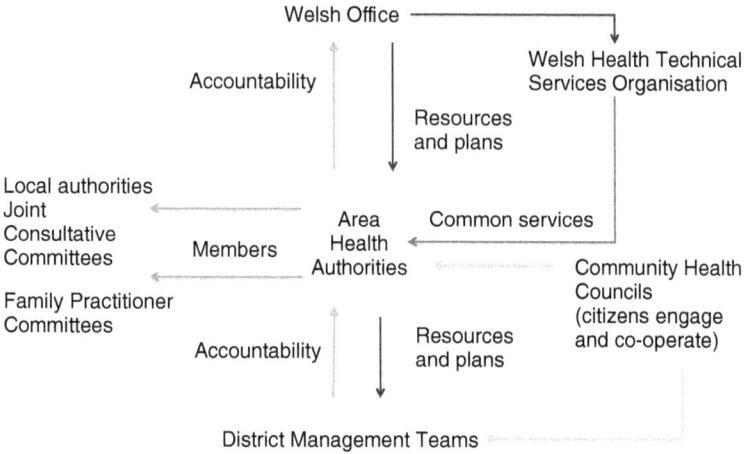

Figure 2.3 Representation of Welsh NHS as envisioned after 1974 reorganisation

Conclusion: political support and questions

Rather than settling issues of NHS structure, the 1974 reorganisation merely marked the beginning of a 'continuous revolution' in service policy and dynamics.[134] Nonetheless, although perhaps considered unsuccessful from this policy perspective, the alterations ushered in by the 1974 reforms had a considerable impact on British medicine. The abolition of the MOH role, for instance, enabled GPs to expand into preventive health work, and – supported by new technologies and new understandings of diabetes management – GPs increasingly considered diabetes as a legitimate responsibility of primary care.

With clinics facing increasing pressures on resources and deteriorating working conditions, specialists were also leading figures in promoting structured programmes of community care for diabetes during the 1970s and 1980s. By the early 1990s, various forms of GP care had spread widely, if not deeply, across Britain as practitioners experimented with forms of systematic and integrated care in major towns and cities. Community schemes, mini-clinics, GP care based on diabetes days or hours, and travelling clinics could be found everywhere from Kirkcaldy to Poole and from Norwich to Cardiff. Schemes spread despite warnings about efficacy. As one exchange of letters to the *British Medical Journal* (*BMJ*) indicated, conflict about the devolution of responsibilities to

GPs could be fierce. In a co-authored letter reviewing the extant literature in 1984, the GP Brian Hurwitz and the renowned epidemiologist John Yudkin proposed that motivated general practice care could match hospital provision, but only when oversight mechanisms were in place. Without these procedures, 'routine general practitioner care … increase[d] the risk of poorer diabetic control and higher overall morbidity and mortality'. Therefore, Hurwitz and Yudkin concluded, 'a global policy of encouraging general practitioners to set up diabetic mini-clinics' was 'unlikely … [to] provide a solution to improving diabetic supervision' and 'reduce the number of patients attending hospital clinics'.[135] Their view formed part of an exchange sparked by an editorial entitled 'Diabetes care: whose responsibility?', in which various forms of GP care were unfavourably compared with one another.[136] In reply to suggestions that GP management in certain locations was 'unacceptable', some correspondents argued that the GP had a duty to ensure follow-up provision regardless of negative assessments, whilst others turned on consultants and declared unsupportive and inattentive hospital staff to be a major block to good general practice care.[137]

Two major points emerge from this exchange. The first is that even by 1984, doctors of all stripes saw GP care as an important innovation. It was one that demanded investigation, but which was to be pursued regardless of results. Conflict had in some areas led to passive resistance and uneven distribution of care, but was not allowed to derail programmes. In places like Sheffield, for instance, whilst the energy and charisma of programme pioneers may have helped launch the scheme, it was the work of mobile specialist nursing staff that sustained such efforts by mediating tensions between GPs and consultants.[138] On a national scale, efforts to promote this form of care received political backing by the late 1980s. As will be discussed in Chapters 4 and 6, the 'cost-effective' realm of primary care proved attractive to the second and third Thatcher administrations (1983–87, 1987–90), which were elected on platforms of public sector reform and reduced central expenditure. Moreover, GP contracts of the early 1990s contained specific financial recompense for running general practice clinics for chronic disease, including diabetes. Such political support for the repositioning of general practice, with diabetes as a major element, undoubtedly underpinned the spread of GP care in spite of medical reservations.[139]

The second point of interest emerges from the conclusions for how to improve general practice care. Hurwitz and Yudkin themselves suggested that the computerisation of schemes – which would prompt GPs when follow-up was needed, and demand results from various tests – might offer one route to improvement, along with further education.[140] This suggestion drew a sharper line around various managerial mechanisms that had medical professionals as their subject.[141] The very earliest GP schemes involved formal referral and care protocol to divide responsibility for patients and to guide decisions about appropriate expertise and decision-making. Recall systems had been in place since the 1970s, and were designed to remind practitioners to proactively make appointments for patient follow-up. Record cards, seemingly inert devices on which to inscribe results, were also intended to prompt clinicians into undertaking certain actions, and moved around the system to facilitate division of labour and clinical review. Structuring diabetes management, in other words, involved structuring the work of the clinician as much as the care received by the patient.

Whilst the drives for managerial technologies that routinised care had been in play for some time, the move to divide responsibility for diabetes management across various sites had thrust them into the centre of diabetological discourse and practice. The repositioning of this work as preventive and public-health-oriented in the 1980s and early 1990s also made national forms of management even more of a priority. It will be these developments – the creation of managerial technologies in structured and shared care schemes, the formalisation of diabetes management as a public health problem, and the politicisation of national structures of healthcare governance – that will now form the interests of Chapters 3, 4, and 5 respectively.

Notes

1 TNA, BD 18/793, questionnaire completed by Dr D. C. Lewin, 'Review of diabetic service', 5 August 1964, p. 4.
2 M. D. Moore, 'Reorganising chronic disease management: diabetes and bureaucratic technologies in post-war British general practice', in M. Jackson (ed.), *The Routledge History of Disease* (London: Routledge, 2017), p. 460.
3 R. D. Hill, 'Community care service for diabetics in the Poole area', *BMJ*, 1:6018 (1976), 1139.
4 Such as asthma or 'chronic rheumatism': J. Fry, *Common Diseases: Their Nature, Incidence and Care*, 2nd edition (Lancaster: MTP Press Limited, 1979), pp. 22–4.

5 See Chapter 3.
6 I. Loudon and M. Drury, 'Some aspects of clinical care in general practice', in I. Loudon, J. Horder, and C. Webster (eds.), *General Practice under the National Health Service, 1948–1997* (Oxford: Oxford University Press, 1998), pp. 103–4.
7 A. Digby, *The Evolution of British General Practice, 1850–1948* (Oxford: Oxford University Press, 1999), pp. 332–7.
8 Loudon and Drury, 'Some aspects of clinical care', pp. 106–8.
9 D. G. French, 'Advances in general practice', *The Practitioner*, 183:1096 (1959), 514. One study estimated that patients with diabetes consulted almost twice as frequently as patients without the condition (once age and sex-matched): C. T. Andrews, 'A survey of diabetes in west Cornwall', *BMJ*, 1:5016 (1957), 431.
10 I. H. Redhead and J. J. A. Reid, 'Diabetic clinics and the general practitioner', *The Lancet*, 281:7273 (1963), 159–60.
11 G. Smith and M. Nicolson, 'Re-expressing the division in British medicine under the NHS: the importance of locality in general practitioners' oral histories', *Social Science and Medicine*, 64:4 (2007), 938–48.
12 'Clinical diabetes mellitus', *Journal of the Royal College of General Practitioners (JRCGP)*, 15:4 (1968), 307. Clinical assistantships were common across different areas of medicine: E. O. Evans and I. McWhinney, 'General practitioner and the general hospital', *BMJ*, 1:5384 (1964), 688–90.
13 J. Horder, 'Conclusion', in Loudon, Horder, and Webster (eds.), *General Practice under the National Health Service*, p. 281.
14 G. Rivett, *From Cradle to Grave: Fifty Years of the NHS* (London: King's Fund, 1998), pp. 163–4.
15 This remained the case until 1982, when voluntary vocational training became mandatory: D. Pereira Gray, 'Postgraduate training and continuing education', in Loudon, Horder, and Webster (eds.), *General Practice under the National Health Service*, pp. 182–204.
16 Rivett, *From Cradle to Grave*, pp. 163–4.
17 Redhead and Reid, 'Diabetic clinics and the general practitioner', p. 160. As this survey indicated, GPs themselves also admitted a lack of confidence.
18 TNA, BD 18/793, questionnaire completed by Dr F. W. Thomas, 'Review of diabetic service', 8 September 1964, p. 3.
19 C. H. Stewart-Hess, 'The management of maturity onset diabetes in general practice', *JRCGP*, 23:137 (1973), 841–60.
20 Royal College of General Practitioners Archives, London, MSS, B Fry C6-1 (i), J. Fry, 'The management of maturity onset diabetes in a general practice (1951–1971)', undated, p. 11.
21 Andrews, 'A survey of diabetes in west Cornwall', p. 431.

22 R. F. L. Logan, *General Register Office Studies on Medical and Population Subjects*, 7 (London: HMSO, 1953). See the consultation and 'patients consulting' numbers in table 2, p. 47.
23 Redhead and Reid, 'Diabetic clinics and the general practitioner', pp. 159–60; Andrews, 'A survey of diabetes in west Cornwall'.
24 Interview with J. Hill conducted by the University of Oxford, 1 October 2004, available at: www.diabetes-stories.com/transcript.asp?UID=19 (accessed April 2017).
25 G. Forsyth and R. Logan, *Gateway or Dividing Line? A Study of Hospital Outpatients in the 1960s* (Oxford: Oxford University Press for the Nuffield Provincial Hospitals Trust, 1968), pp. 59–62.
26 Ibid., p. 61. Diabetes was a prominent example.
27 'Diabetes mellitus – incidence, causation, management', *Proceedings of the Royal Society of Medicine*, 55:3 (1962), 211.
28 Ibid.
29 H. Keen, 'The family doctor and the diabetic', *The Practitioner*, 194:1160 (1965), 244.
30 L. A. Pike, 'A general practitioner looks at diabetes', *Public Health*, 77:3 (1963), 169.
31 Keen, 'The family doctor and the diabetic', p. 246.
32 Ibid., p. 244.
33 See Chapter 1.
34 Especially if GPs were given access to pathological laboratories: 'Annual meeting, Oxford: scientific sections', *BMJ*, 2:5353 (1963), 374.
35 Pike, 'A general practitioner looks at diabetes', p. 169.
36 Ibid., p. 168.
37 Ibid., pp. 167–8.
38 Ibid., p. 165. On associative prediction vs causation: G. M. Oppenheimer, 'Profiling risk: the emergence of coronary heart disease epidemiology in the United States (1947–70)', *International Journal of Epidemiology*, 35:3 (2006), 720–30, esp. pp. 725–7.
39 On Darbishire House: M. Perry, 'Academic general practice in Manchester under the early National Health Service: a failed social medicine experiment', *Social History of Medicine*, 13:1 (2000), 111–29.
40 R. F. L. Logan, 'Control of chronic disease in general practice and industry', *Journal of the College of General Practitioners (JCGP)*, 11:S.1 (1966), 94.
41 Ibid., pp. 94–5.
42 Ibid., p. 95.
43 Ibid., p. 96.
44 Ibid., p. 99.
45 D. Armstrong, *Political Anatomy of the Body: Medical Knowledge in Britain in the Twentieth Century* (Oxford: Oxford University Press, 1983).

46 H. Valier and C. Timmermann, 'Clinical trials and the reorganization of medical research in post-Second World War Britain', *Medical History*, 52:4 (2008), 493–510, esp. p. 498.
47 See the discussion of the College of General Practitioners below.
48 C. Webster, 'The politics of general practice', in Loudon, Horder, and Webster (eds.), *General Practice under the National Health Service*, pp. 28–31.
49 S. McLaurin and D. F. Smith, 'Professional strategies of Medical Officers of Health in the post-war period – 2: "progressive realism": the case of R. J. Donaldson, MOH for Teeside, 1968–1974', *Journal of Public Health Medicine*, 24:2 (2002), 130–5.
50 K. Hodgkin, 'Good general practice without routine screening examinations', *JCGP*, 11:S.1 (1966), 100.
51 Ibid., p. 101.
52 A. L. Cochrane, 'A medical scientist's view of screening', *Public Health*, 81:5 (1967), 207–13; 'Can we prevent it?', *The Lancet*, 288:7474 (1966), 1171–2.
53 J. Malins, *Clinical Diabetes Mellitus* (London: Eyre & Spottiswood, 1968), pp. 138–9, 190–1, 236–7, 447–9.
54 D. L. Crombie, 'Preventive medicine and presymptomatic diagnosis', *JRCGP*, 15:5 (1968), 346; H. Keen, G. Rose, D. A. Pyke, D. Boyns, C. Chlouverakis, and S. Mistry, 'Blood sugar and arterial disease', *The Lancet*, 286:7411 (1965), 505–8.
55 TNA, MH 133/271, internal memo by CHSC staff, 'Diabetic screening', 29–30 November 1961.
56 G. O'Hara, *From Dreams to Disillusionment: Economic and Social Planning in the 1960s* (Basingstoke: Palgrave Macmillan, 2007), pp. 167–204.
57 C. Webster, *The Health Services since the War*, vol. 2: *Government and Health Care: The British National Health Service, 1958–1979* (London: HMSO, 1996), p. 804. See the table 'Appendix 3.5', which outlines current and capital expenditure on the service in real terms according to a special NHS deflationary index. On the economy: P. Howlett, 'The "Golden Age", 1955–1973', in P. Johnson (ed.), *Twentieth Century Britain: Economic, Social and Cultural Change* (London: Longman, 1994), pp. 320–6; see figure 18.3, which outlines GDP deviation from a trend rate of 2.8 per cent per annum.
58 Otherwise known as the Hospital Plan: O'Hara, *From Dreams to Disillusionment*, pp. 184–5.
59 Rivett, *From Cradle to Grave*, pp. 179–80. A separate committee was established in Scotland a year earlier under J. H. F. Brotherston, Chief Medical Officer for the Scottish Home and Health Department (SHHD). The reports were organised differently, the structures suggested for reform varied, and there appeared 'greater suspicion' of new organisational

arrangements in Scotland: 'Cogwheel in Scotland', *BMJ*, 4:5841 (1972), 661–2. Nonetheless, the pressures underpinning the committees were shared. Moreover, the Chief Medical Officers who chaired the respective groups co-operated closely, and the principles and conclusions of the reports were very similar: Webster, *The Health Services since the War*, vol. 2, pp. 312–13.

60 Ministry of Health, *First Report of the Joint Working Party on the Organisation of Medical Work in Hospitals* (London: HMSO, 1967), paras. 27–31.
61 Ibid., para. 24.
62 Ibid., para. 14(b); see also paras. 33–41 and 55–67. Clinical divisions were groups of clinicians linked through specialisms where tools, spaces, and staff were common.
63 J. S. Stewart, 'Cogwheel: a physician's view of a local version', *BMJ*, 4:5680 (1969), 420–3.
64 P. Addison, *No Turning Back: The Peacetime Revolutions of Post-War Britain* (Oxford: Oxford University Press, 2010), pp. 149–56.
65 R. Klein, 'The crises of the welfare states', in R. Cooter and J. Pickstone (eds.), *Medicine in the Twentieth Century* (Amsterdam: Rodopi, 2000), pp. 155–70; B. Clift and J. Tomlinson, 'Negotiating credibility: Britain and the International Monetary Fund, 1956–1976', *Contemporary European History*, 17:4 (2008), 545–66.
66 See Chapters 4 and 6.
67 See discussion later in this chapter.
68 Rivett, *From Cradle to Grave*, pp. 274, 272–5.
69 The Office of Health Economics was founded by the British Pharmaceutical Industry in 1962: W. Laing and R. Williams, *Diabetes: A Model for Health Care Management* (London: Office of Health Economics, 1989), p. 2. The Patients' Association was created by a part-time teacher in 1963: A. Mold, *Making the Patient-Consumer: Patient Organisations and Health Consumerism in Britain* (Manchester: Manchester University Press, 2015), pp. 29–34.
70 'Inquiry is urged into hospital queues', *The Times*, 13 August, 1968, p. 2; Forsyth and Logan, *Gateway or Dividing Line?*, pp. 2–3, 59–62.
71 J. M. Wilks, 'Diabetes – a disease for general practice', *JRCGP*, 23:126 (1973), 46.
72 Hill, 'Community care service for diabetics', p. 1137.
73 P. A. Thorn and R. G. Russell, 'Diabetic clinics today and tomorrow: mini-clinics in general practice', *BMJ*, 5865:2 (1973), 536.
74 Hill, 'Community care service for diabetics', p. 1139.
75 J. M. Malins and J. M. Stuart, 'Diabetic clinic in a general practice', *BMJ*, 5780:4 (1971), 161.
76 I. Benett, 'Diabetes mini-clinic', *JRCGP*, 37:307 (1988), 76–7.
77 Thorn and Russell, 'Diabetic clinics today and tomorrow'.

78 Hill, 'Community care service for diabetics'.
79 Loudon and Drury, 'Some aspects of clinical care', pp. 109–10; Fry, 'The management of maturity onset diabetes', p. 1.
80 C. E. Upton, 'Diabetic community care', *The Practitioner*, 215:1284 (1975), 83.
81 A. Cartwright, *Patients and their Doctors: A Study of General Practice* (London: Routledge and Kegan Paul, 1967), pp. 44–52.
82 Malins and Stuart, 'Diabetic clinic in a general practice'.
83 Stewart-Hess, 'The management of maturity onset diabetes in general practice', p. 859.
84 For a history of familial rhetoric: R. Hayward, *The Transformation of the Psyche in British Primary Care, 1870–1970* (London: Bloomsbury Academic, 2014), pp. 33–6, 57–9.
85 Rivett, *From Cradle to Grave*, pp. 90–1; T. Osborne, 'Epidemiology as an investigative paradigm: the College of General Practitioners in the 1950s', *Social Science and Medicine*, 38:2 (1994), 318.
86 Osborne, 'Epidemiology as an investigative paradigm', p. 318. Histories of general practice have often seen the Collings Report of 1950 as the most damning assessment of general practice, and one connected with the College's creation: J. S. Collings, 'General practice in England today: a reconnaissance', *The Lancet*, 255:6604 (1950), 555–79. C. Webster, *The Health Services since the War*, vol. 1: *Problems of Health Care: The National Health Service before 1957* (London: HMSO, 1988), pp. 356–7.
87 For instance: S. Taylor, *Good General Practice: A Report on a Survey* (London: Oxford University Press, 1954); CHSC, *The Field Work of the Family Doctor: Report of the Sub-Committee* (London: HMSO, 1963); RCGP, *The Future General Practitioner* (London: RCGP, 1972).
88 'Undergraduate education conference, 7th May, 1961', *JCGP*, 5:2 (1962), 290–5. Osborne, 'Epidemiology as an investigative paradigm', pp. 318–19; Armstrong, *Political Anatomy of the Body*, pp. 73–5.
89 J. A. Pridham, 'Future trends in general practice', *JCGP*, 5:4 (1962), 537. For critiques of the NHS as overly bureaucratic: D. Wright, S. Mullally, and M. C. Cordukes, '"Worse than being married": the exodus of British doctors from the National Health Service to Canada, c.1955–75', *Journal of the History of Medicine and Allied Sciences*, 65:4 (2010), 546–75.
90 Taylor, *Good General Practice*, p. 445.
91 RCGP, *The Future General Practitioner*.
92 Malins and Stuart, 'Diabetic clinic in a general practice'.
93 Thorn and Russell, 'Diabetic clinics today and tomorrow', p. 534.
94 A. P. Kratky, 'An audit of the care of diabetics in one general practice', *JRCGP*, 27:182 (1977), 536.

95 R. J. Jarrett, H. Keen, J. H. Fuller, and M. McCartney, 'Worsening to diabetes in men with impaired glucose tolerance ("borderline diabetes")', *Diabetologia*, 16:1 (1979), 25–30.
96 R. J. Jarrett, H. Keen, J. H. Fuller, and M. McCartney, 'Treatment of borderline diabetes: controlled trial using carbohydrate restriction and phenformin', *BMJ*, 2:6091 (1977), 861–5.
97 J. H. Fuller, M. J. Shipley, G. Rose, R. J. Jarrett, and H. Keen, 'Coronary-heart-disease risk and impaired glucose tolerance: the Whitehall study', *The Lancet*, 315:8183 (1980), 1373–6.
98 P. J. Burrows, P. J. Gray, A.-L. Kinmonth, D. J. Payton, G. A. Walpole, R. J. Walton, D. Wilson, and G. Woodbine, 'Who cares for the patient with diabetes? Presentation and follow-up in seven Southampton practices', *JRCGP*, 37:295 (1987), 68.
99 Though animal experiments did feature into some discussions: K. M. West, 'Hyperglycaemia as a cause of long-term complications', in H. Keen and J. Jarrett (eds.), *Diabetic Complications*, 2nd edition (London: Edward Arnold, 1982), pp. 13–18.
100 H. Al Sayegh and R. J. Jarrett, 'Oral glucose-tolerance tests and the diagnosis of diabetes: results of a prospective study based on the Whitehall survey', *The Lancet*, 314:8140 (1979), 431–3.
101 Ibid.
102 D. Armstrong, 'The rise of surveillance medicine', *Sociology of Health and Illness*, 17:3 (1995), 393–404.
103 See the broadly supportive response, with caveats: 'Impaired glucose tolerance and diabetes – WHO criteria', *BMJ*, 281:6254 (1980), 1512–13.
104 J. S. Yudkin, B. J. Boucher, K. E. Schopflin, B. T. Harris, H. R. Claff, N. J. D. Whyte, B. Taylor, D. H. Mellins, A. B. Wootliff, J. G. Safir, and E. J. Jones, 'The quality of diabetic care in a London health district', *Journal of Epidemiology and Community Health*, 34:4 (1980), 277–80.
105 Interview with Professor Whittaker conducted by the author. Professor Whittaker is a retired consultant diabetologist who worked within major centres of diabetes care and research between the 1970s and 2000s.
106 R. J. Jarrett, *Diabetes Mellitus* (London: Croom Helm, 1987), pp. 1–3; J. A. Greene, *Prescribing by Numbers: Drugs and the Definition of Disease* (Baltimore: Johns Hopkins University Press, 2007).
107 Burrows et al., 'Who cares for the patient with diabetes?'; M. T. Wojciechowski, 'Systematic care of diabetic patients in a general practice', *JRCGP*, 32:242 (1982), 531–3.
108 Wojciechowski, 'Systematic care of diabetic patients in a general practice', pp. 531, 533.
109 Kratky, 'An audit of the care of diabetics in one general practice', p. 539.

110 R. D. Hill, *Diabetes Health Care: A Guide to the Provision of Health Care Services* (London: Chapman and Hall, 1987), pp. 91–100, quotations at pp. 91–2.
111 UK Prospective Diabetes Study Group, 'Intensive blood glucose control with sulphonylureas or insulin compared with conventional treatment and risk of complications in patients with type 2 diabetes (UKPDS 33)', *The Lancet*, 352:9131 (1998), 837–53.
112 And questions still abound about the most useful metabolic markers for care and translating trial results into practice: J. S. Yudkin, B. Richter, and E. A. M. Gale, 'Intensified glucose lowering in type 2 diabetes: time for a reappraisal', *Diabetologia*, 53:10 (2010), 2079–85.
113 M. Hammersley, M. Holland, S. Walford, and P. Thorn, 'What happens to defaulters from a diabetic clinic?', *BMJ*, 291:6505 (1985), 1330–2.
114 Oppenheimer, 'Profiling risk'.
115 See Chapter 3.
116 RCGP, *Prevention of Arterial Disease in General Practice: A Report of a Sub-Committee of the Royal College of General Practitioners' Working Party on Prevention*, Report from General Practice, 19 (London: RCGP, 1981), p. 1.
117 Though note C. Waine, *Why Not Care for your Diabetic Patients?*, 2nd edition (London: RCGP, 1988), p. 3.
118 RCGP, *Prevention of Arterial Disease in General Practice*, pp. 7, 1.
119 Ibid., p. 7.
120 J. T. Hart, 'A new kind of doctor', *Journal of the Royal Society of Medicine*, 74:12 (1981), 871–83.
121 Pike, 'A general practitioner looks at diabetes'; M. Gray and G. Fowler (eds.), *Preventive Medicine in General Practice* (Oxford: Oxford University Press, 1983).
122 For instance, hypertension was reframed as a quantitative deviation of physiology after the 1950s, just as diabetes was: C. Timmermann, 'A matter of degree: the normalization of hypertension, c.1940–2000', in W. Ernst (ed.), *Histories of the Normal and the Abnormal: Social and Cultural Histories of Norms and Normativity* (London: Routledge, 2006), pp. 245–61. For asthma: M. Jackson, *Asthma: The Biography* (Oxford: Oxford University Press, 2009), esp. pp. 183–8.
123 M. Lawrence, 'All together now', *JRCGP*, 38:7 (1988), 296–302, esp. p. 297.
124 J. T. Hart, 'Specialization in general practice', *JRCGP*, 30:4 (1980), 218.
125 Such as in computerisation of clinics: G. Brownbridge, A. Evans, M. Fitter, and M. Platts, 'An interactive computerized protocol for the management of hypertension: effects on the general practitioner's clinical behaviour', *JRCGP*, 36:5 (1986), 198–202.

126 J. Gedney, 'Reconstruction of general practice', *BMJ*, 290:6478 (1985), 1350; Lawrence, 'All together now'.
127 Rivett, *From Cradle to Grave*, pp. 209–11; M. Calnan, *Preventing Coronary Heart Disease: Prospects, Policies, and Politics* (London: Routledge, 2002 [1991]).
128 Webster, *The Health Services since the War*, vol. 2, pp. 321–73, 451–579.
129 Ibid., pp. 546–63, esp. p. 551.
130 C. Webster, *The National Health Service: A Political History* (Oxford: Oxford University Press, 1998), p. 92.
131 Webster, *The Health Services since the War*, vol. 2, pp. 572–4.
132 On the decline of MOHs, cf. J. Lewis, *What Price Community Medicine? The Philosophy, Practice and Politics of Public Health since 1919* (Brighton: Wheatsheaf, 1986); J. Welshman, 'The Medical Officer of Health in England and Wales, 1900–1974: watchdog or lapdog?', *Journal of Public Health Medicine*, 19:4 (1997), 443–50; M. Gorsky, 'Local leadership in public health: the role of the Medical Officer of Health in Britain, 1872–1974', *Journal of Epidemiology and Community Health*, 61:6 (2007), 470–1.
133 Interview with Professor Davies conducted by the author. Professor Davies is a retired academic epidemiologist and health authority member.
134 Webster, *The National Health Service*, pp. 140–214.
135 B. Hurwitz and J. Yudkin, 'Diabetes care: whose responsibility?', *BMJ*, 289:6450 (1984), 1000.
136 P. Home and S. Walford, 'Diabetes care: whose responsibility?', *BMJ*, 289:6447 (1984), 713–14.
137 R. Pietroni, 'Diabetes care: whose responsibility?', *BMJ*, 289:6450 (1984), 1001; G. F. Morgan, D. A. Cadman, P. H. Edwards, T. C. O'Dowd, and R. H. Davis, 'Diabetes care: whose responsibility?', *BMJ*, 289:6454 (1984), 1309–10.
138 E. Wilkes and E. E. Lawton, 'The diabetic, the hospital and primary care', *JRCGP*, 30:213 (1980), 199–206; interview with M. MacKinnon conducted by the University of Oxford, 23 April 2007, available at: www.diabetes-stories.com/interview.asp?UID=62 (accessed April 2017).
139 Not that general practice attracted significantly more resources. The current expenditure of general practice in 1976–77 was roughly 6.44 per cent of total NHS current expenditure, compared with 7.08 per cent in 1987–88. These figures were produced by taking the proportion of NHS expenditure allocated to family practitioner services, then calculating the percentage of this allocation spent on general medical services (as opposed to pharmaceutical, general dental, and ophthalmic services). Figures for 1976–77 were 22.6 per cent of NHS current expenditure on family practitioner services, and 28.5 per cent of this allocated to general medical services (22.6 × 0.285 = 6.44): Webster, *The Health Services since*

the War, vol. 2, appendices 3.9 and 3.11. Figures for 1987–88 were 24 per cent and 29.5 per cent respectively (24 × 0.285 = 7.08): Secretaries of State for Social Services, *Promoting Better Health*, p. 7.
140 Hurwitz and Yudkin, 'Diabetes care'.
141 The Poole scheme was already experimenting with computerisation: Home and Walford, 'Diabetes care'.

3
The making of integrated care

Over the four decades that followed the creation of the NHS, British diabetes management slowly spread outside the hospital. During the late 1940s and the 1950s, clinicians first co-operated with local government public health doctors to extend the reach of surveillance and education. From the late 1960s onwards, GPs assumed roles as co-ordinators and providers of care in the community, developing systems of disease management on their own and in collaboration with specialists. Although individual GPs moved into diabetes care for a range of reasons, by the 1980s professional bodies like the RCGP had connected diabetes management to professional projects. The promotion of diabetes management formed part of efforts to enhance GP responsibility for preventive medicine, with understandings of secondary and tertiary prevention recasting GP diabetes care as an innovative form of risk management.

The re-spatialisation of care, together with a growing emphasis on surveillance and blood glucose control, raised questions for clinicians and GPs involved in diabetes management. The first was how doctors involved in new schemes could prevent patients falling through the gaps between different sites of oversight; the second – serving as a mirror image – was how practitioners could avoid unnecessary duplication of labour. In short, how could care be co-ordinated? Furthermore, in the context of political and professional anxiety about professional competence, both specialists and GPs asked how they could ensure that surveillance and treatment would be of sufficient quality. In other words, they asked what counted as good care, and how standards could be maintained within innovative organisational arrangements.

This chapter examines how creators of novel systems for diabetes management sought to answer these questions at a local level. Concentrating on the use of recall systems, patient records, and care protocol, it explores how practitioners drew upon pre-existing bureaucratic cultures of medicine, finding solutions to their concerns in the combination of instruments originally intended for refining patient surveillance. All three devices were initially designed to ensure timely review, to store and provide longitudinal data, to divide responsibility for oversight, and to communicate what tasks had – or had not – been performed. The deployment of such instruments, however, also required the codification of 'good care' (to decide, for instance, when patients should be seen, or what tests should be performed), and inherently regulated the temporality and content of professional work. In fact, over time, the designers of new instruments articulated the politics inherent in these apparently inert 'objects', explicitly framing them as attempts to secure good care through the management of professional labour.[1]

Historically, doctors had perceived almost any formal control over their practice as a threat to professional freedom. Yet in the case of systematic and integrated care, references to instruments' 'built-in reminders' implied a mistrust of unaided professional expertise, and clearly articulated benefits to managed clinical decision-making. To be sure, the 'disciplinary' mesh that regulated the time, space, activity, and visibility of medical practice was far looser than that classically designed in the prison or factory.[2] Similarly, tools like protocols and records could build on routines that already existed, or – once mobilised – might enable practitioners to focus on complex tasks requiring more tacit skill.[3] Nonetheless, the devices discussed here structured and divided medical labour, determined rhythms of activity, recorded work, and subjected professionals to review in ways hitherto unseen. They turned previously implicit and loose clinical norms into explicit guidance. In other words, these new combinations of concepts, instruments, and actors formed what, following historians and sociologists of science, we might call local 'organisational technologies' of quality, ones constructed to subject professionals – not just patients – to management.[4]

It would be easy to assume that the creation of such technologies resulted from Machiavellian politicking on behalf of mistrustful specialists and academics. As noted in Chapter 2, consultants had long been suspicious of GPs' capabilities. Moreover, the instruments used to regulate care emerged from traditional hierarchies of medicine. Indeed, in specific instances specialists pushed for new forms of work out of scepticism about GPs. Nonetheless, the new arrangements also reflected a shared sense within the diabetological community – and, evidently, within elite British medicine more broadly – that quality care depended upon bureaucratising instruments: tools that formally codified work processes and responsibilities and held up actions of team members for review.[5] GPs themselves designed new systems, and once enrolled, all practitioners would find their work patterns reoriented, their responsibilities and actions recorded, and their performance reviewed.

As will be seen in Chapters 5 and 6, the local development of new models for managed, integrated care had implications for, and were tied into, national trends. This chapter, however, looks at the early experiments with professional management on a local level to assess the politics and mechanisms of their spread, and to trace the way in which programmes for diabetes drew upon, and provided a model for, the control of other chronic diseases.

Surveillance, patient-centred care, and managing temporality

As discussed in previous chapters, specialists after the 1960s increasingly emphasised the importance of close surveillance in diabetes management. Shifts in discussions of preventive medicine – triggered by new treatments, NHS reform, and epistemological and evidential change – made oversight more important for all practitioners.

These drives to surveillance found further support from renewed emphases on patient self-management. The 1970s and 1980s saw a marked increase in discussion of patient education and 'patient-centred' care. Textbooks, for instance, professed how 'one of the most important advances in diabetic care has been the recognition that the most important person in the Health Care Team ... is the diabetic'.[6] As discussed at length elsewhere, the drivers for this focus in diabetes management were numerous.[7] Political interest in patient rights, for instance, had grown since the 1960s.[8] Medical scandals, rising costs, and political critiques of medical power also contributed to moves to de-institutionalise patients and increase lay input into healthcare.[9] Medical discourse more broadly had been slowly embracing questions of patient behaviour and social experience since the early 1920s, accelerating in the post-war period as more formal techniques of investigation were imported from sociology, psychology, and economics.[10] In diabetes care itself, technological innovations were also crucial. The development of self-monitoring blood glucose machines and insulin pumps had promised to enhance the ability of patients to manage their own care with greater accuracy.[11] Studies with these machines had delivered positive outcomes, and their use by selected patients found support amongst clinicians.[12]

With patients able to monitor their own physiologies and make relevant therapeutic adjustments to maintain control, it might be thought that clinical teams would relinquish observational duties. However, even the most optimistic doctor felt that pumps and self-monitoring had limits. The growth of patient-centred discourse thus involved a considerable discussion of education, as well as psychological and social support.[13] Technological changes may have enhanced the possibility of self-care, but, handbooks suggested, 'a new responsibility falls upon the Health Care Team' if 'the patient is to accept responsibility for his or her own health care rather than rely on others'.[14] Equally, elite practitioners spoke of the need to offer continued social and psychological support to the patient, innovating with the use of psychologists and lay group therapies.[15] They argued that making effective decisions required more than information, proposing that 'the patient needs someone to whom he or she can turn in order to gain advice'.[16] Moreover, there were concerns that patients could become demotivated by the lifelong grind of self-care and lack of guaranteed results: 'tomorrow never comes', as one leading practitioner put it.[17] Therefore, specialists argued, an increased regularity of follow-up consultations would be beneficial: as well as improving biochemical surveillance, regular follow-up appointments would 'boos[t] the patient's morale and fortif[y] his [sic] determination to continue self-care'.[18]

This emphasis upon the regularity of oversight marked something of a shift from earlier discursive foci. Constant monitoring of disease had been a feature of specialist clinics since the 1920s, but popular handbooks and textbooks rarely discussed the timing of oversight.[19] Even where authors made recommendations about regularity, their deliberations did not extend to active time management.[20] Moreover, whilst hospitals commonly deployed appointment systems by the 1950s, they were not used in a consistent manner, either within or between clinics.[21] Like other outpatient facilities, diabetic clinics block-booked patients for the start of a session, and patients would wait as doctors and nurses worked through their allocation.[22] Such arrangements were predicated upon an economic conception of time as a limited resource, prioritising the efficient flow of medical consultation at the expense of long waits and hurried care for patients.[23] More importantly, although existing temporal systems divided time into minutes, hours, and clinic sessions, they did not track patient attendance or encourage contact with patients who did not appear. Patients might be told to return in three or six months, but before the 1970s providers were seemingly unmotivated or unable to chase patients proactively.

As the frequency and content of patient oversight gained ever greater value, doctors and care teams designed tools to facilitate better tracking of patients. In general practice, the earliest efforts to regulate patient attendance were based upon recall systems, generally in the form of card-index technologies. A Bristol GP, J. M. Wilks, described such a system in a 1973 article for the *Journal of the Royal College of General Practitioners* (*JRCGP*).[24] As for patients with other conditions 'requiring regular surveillance', Wilks kept 'a simple card index system housed in a small box … on the consulting room desk'. Each patient with diabetes had 'a card tagged with a coloured adhesive label', on which Wilks noted the 'significant' details of the patient's condition. These cards were organised in a month and year pattern, with a 'this month' divider separating those to be seen in the current month from those to be seen in the months coming. Cards in each section were then arranged alphabetically for rapid access during consultation. 'At the end of the month', Wilks went on, 'there should be no cards left in [the] "this month" [section]', but if there were, 'these [patients] can be pursued by letter, telephone or health visitor.' Finally, once each patient had been seen, their card was 'put forward to the month in which it is wished to see the patient next', and the process started again.[25]

For Wilks, one of the advantages of the index system was that it reordered the temporality of care for the patient, making it more closely adhere to the rhythms of the health services. Whilst imposing no specific time for consultation, the system still sought to limit patient choice. Moreover, by substituting the body of the patient for an inscription on card index, Wilks also attempted to ensure that absences would be noted and corrected, thereby actively managing the time between visits.[26] Yet, alongside closer management of patients, the index tool also inherently regulated the timing of professional labour. The GP's own work was now inevitably tied more closely to bureaucratic 'clock time' and undertaken within a prescribed schedule.[27] Noting an absence led to telephone calls, with verification rituals undertaken at a specific time at the end of the month. Moreover, as patients returned to the surgery, their reappearance prompted the doctor to undertake review at its scheduled moment. Given the space between visits, and the small number of patients that GPs had on their lists, such effects were undoubtedly small. But they were to form part of a broader complex of instruments and actors directed to surveillance that would inevitably manage professional labour.

Over time, tools for oversight developed and doctors and hospital administrators involved new staff in novel patterns of care. For instance, another article, written approximately eight years after Wilks's, described clerical personnel compiling a separate practice register for diabetes patients, and GPs deputing recall to nursing staff. At this surgery in Wales, an attached diabetic nurse oversaw the card index and used appointment details to record who had missed their pre-arranged consultations. The nurse specialist would subsequently send reminders to those patients who had defaulted, and then visit patients who forgot – or decided not to attend – a second time.[28] Although patients could not be forced into attendance, the system closed the mesh of surveillance around a patient, mapping and regulating time between visits. Likewise, whilst the temporal investment in maintaining follow-up had been deputed, both doctor and nurse still followed the rhythms of the new systems in terms of patient review. Similar changes occurred in the equipment itself. In particular, recall became computerised.[29] Where computers were available, recall packages in general practice had become a standard provision by the late 1980s.[30] Moreover, community care schemes developed systems that proactively assigned patients appointments by letter, and prompted them to attend for laboratory investigations and clinical and optical reviews.[31] Computerisation, therefore, allowed the temporality of practice to be finely calculated for maximum efficiency and oversight.[32]

To be sure, rhetoric did not always match practice. The functioning of systems depended upon the agents involved acting according to predicted patterns. However, as complex individuals enrolled in various relations with competing demands, doctors and patients varied in their commitment to follow-up. For patients, clinics and their doctors could be remote, producing financial and temporal strains.[33] Decisions to attend were also based upon complex physical and psychological assessments. One interviewee with diabetes (diagnosed when aged seven in 1976) reflected on how she often had to wait for over an hour and a half for a consultation as a teenager, only to become 'aggrieved' with the discussion. She felt that consultants (then and since) consistently tried to be her 'headmaster or headmistress', which produced problematic dynamics and contributed to a decision to drop out of medical surveillance for four years as a young adult.[34]

Staff and instruments could also act in ways counter to the roles envisioned. Zest for recall and proactive care could run dry. As one published review of diabetes management in general practice noted, care deteriorated a year or so after more systematic measures had been implemented: 'fewer patients were seen and the intervals at which they were seen had increased'. Upon examination, 'patient notes suggested this deterioration in care was partly due ... to a decrease in the enthusiasm of the staff running the clinic and recall system'.[35] Even computerisation might fail to compensate for such bureaucratic fatigue. Computerised patient registers and recall systems were costly to construct and run, meaning that projects could run out of money.[36] Doctors in the late 1980s also bemoaned how temperamental computer systems could be. 'Relatively minor typographical errors may "lose" a patient in a computer database', one article warned, and 'interruptions of electrical supply or malfunctions in hardware may lose them all.'[37] Across hospital departments, clerical and medical staff often preferred card index systems, and even maintained them alongside computerised lists.[38]

Teething problems with new instruments, their potential costs, and the resistance of some professional and clerical staff to information technologies were not the only obstacles to NHS computerisation. Policy changes and economic disincentives also exacerbated problems within the hospital sector, resulting in unequal adoption of digital technologies across the health service and generating a considerable legacy for later decades.[39] Such problems, though, did not prove harmful to the drive for diabetes surveillance. The major professional groups in favour of computerisation and recall systems (senior diabetologists and GPs, service planners and managers) remained steadfast in their faith, and systems were far easier to organise at a local – as opposed to regional or national – level. Advocates did not regard the technical problems they faced as serious enough to disrupt either the underlying clinical need for more refined long-term patient monitoring or the financial savings and managerial control generated by more efficient oversight and distribution of labour.[40] Instead, with technological change supportive of professional ambitions, these advocates cast disruptions as temporary concerns that could be solved through technical improvements and adjustments in how systems were used. As noted in Chapter 2, some clinicians and GPs confronting problems in community care schemes continued to see a 'centralised computer prompt' as the basis upon which better surveillance could be secured.[41] Similarly, those practitioners highlighting the importance of enthusiasm saw continuous review and contract incentives as potential solutions.[42]

Though clearly diluted in practice, moves to regulate the temporality of patient review nonetheless had clear managerial effects for practitioners. Structured patient care meant structured medical work. In part, such effects were inherent to the instruments used. As will be seen below, however, such outcomes were also an intended part of plans to combine tools to structure the timing and content of care, and to subject both to review.

Records, protocol, and the management of space, teams, and activity

Alongside recall systems, the development of care protocol and the refining of patient records were also crucial to producing the management of professional labour within systematic and integrated care schemes. However, whereas recall registers regulated the timing of surveillance, records and protocol structured the content of care, as well as rendering the actions of care teams visible.

Along with the growing impetus to disease surveillance, doctors were also prompted to create new tools by the expansion of diabetic care teams. The number and types of healthcare worker involved in diabetes management had risen steadily since the 1920s. Within the most sophisticated and dedicated hospitals, patients before the 1950s might have encountered doctors, almoners, nursing staff, dieticians, and technicians, whilst into the post-war period patients had an increased chance of engaging with obstetricians, chiropodists, ophthalmologists, opticians, and new 'primary care' teams of GPs, practice nurses, health visitors, and district nurses.[43] This diverse team was also spreading out across space, taking in clinics, wards, GP surgeries, community settings (such as opticians' practices), and patients' homes. New records and care protocol were thus designed to co-ordinate the activity of multiple workers across diverse sites, beyond single institutions.

To understand why GPs and specialists turned to records and protocol to co-ordinate care, however, it is necessary to trace their emergence, and to note that these tools were objects of broader medical interest over the twentieth century. Crucially, clinical records and protocol were both intertwined with broader changes in health services after 1900. As noted in the Introduction, by the 1930s hospitals had become complex institutions of mass healthcare.[44] Specialisation and the increased sophistication of medical technology often meant that multiple practitioners monitored, treated, and interacted with patients (or at least their samples).[45] Likewise, the emergence of the National Insurance programme introduced notable changes into British general practice after 1913, and state responsibilities for co-ordinated hospital and public health initiatives also expanded dramatically during the early decades of the century.[46]

Such changes transformed administrative and clinical arrangements, especially within hospital settings, and new documentation made further transformations possible.[47] In terms of records, it was during this period that the personal casebook of the physician and the ward notes of the old hospital transformed into the recognisable case file.[48] Under new pressures, clinical notes could no longer be the personal preserve of individual doctors, kept stationary in offices or homes. Instead, clinical documents needed to be mobile, following the patient around the growing spaces of the hospital. They also needed to be collectively compiled, providing a record of test results and clinical opinion and offering a means through which the work of various team members could be noted and co-ordinated. Finally, to handle the flow of patients, and facilitate effective analysis and administration, records were subject to drives for internal standardisation and pre-formatting.[49] Clinical, pathological, and physiological research, just like efficient institutional management, was possible only through the co-ordination of work and the production of focused and comparable records owned by the institution for impersonal analysis.[50]

Equally, as state-funded bodies became involved in cross-institutional research and public health programmes, these agencies used their control of finances and scarce materials to impose new regulations on inter-war medical work.[51] For instance, in pursuit of controlled 'scientific medicine', the UK Medical Research Council (MRC) developed formally codified protocol for its multi-centre clinical trials.[52] Similarly, new public health programmes, especially those involving cancer care, attached norms for organisational patterns and information collection to supplies of materials for operating centres.[53] Indeed, by the mid-century, records and protocol had become objects of overt political interest. Elite practitioners, clinical researchers, service administrators, and Ministry of Health officials all saw the NHS as either an opportunity for research or as an institution in need of significant management. The information that new records might produce was considered of great value to service management, as well as to epidemiological and clinical investigations.[54] Major professional and government bodies introduced centralising pressures – from collective epidemiological research programmes to standard data systems for inpatient analysis – that may have encouraged standardisation.[55] Similarly, during the early 1970s, the Royal College of Physicians of Edinburgh, the Royal College of Surgeons of Glasgow, the RCGP, and the Faculty of Community Medicine formed a joint working party to consider clinical integration. As chronic conditions crossed institutional boundaries the most, the group investigated integration in the care of four common chronic illnesses (dyspepsia, hypertension, stroke, and diabetes). At the heart of their proposals sat the production of clinical protocol to facilitate better specialist–GP interaction.[56]

Such transformations did not always run smoothly. Institutional demands could conflict with cultures of practice in diverse settings. Individualist consultants could ignore protocol, seek control over records, and depute notation to juniors, thus undermining the efforts of reformers.[57] In the individualistic world of general practice, minor efforts to introduce records as part of National Insurance practice faced strong countervailing winds.[58] Records only slowly became part of accepted practice, and were completed erratically into the NHS era.[59] Despite pressures tending towards reform, therefore, a fear of imposing uniform models continued to work against standardisation *per se* into the 1970s.[60] The localism of pre-NHS services ensured both a diversity of practice across Britain and a deep attachment to idiosyncratic forms. Standardisation was even thwarted by basic material differences in storage (such as diverse cabinet sizes).[61]

Nonetheless, by the late 1960s, a wide variety of groups within British medicine were interested in co-ordination and data collection. They saw disorganised care as a problem, and envisaged tools like new records and care protocol as possible solutions. Standardising content of care at this point was less important than the fact that disease management required structure. As suggested, diabetes management, along with the care of other chronic conditions, provided an early testing ground for deploying new instruments, and as noted below some practitioners and researchers were interested in diabetes solely for this reason. At the same time, for doctors who turned to records and protocol to co-ordinate care programmes, this pre-existing bureaucratic culture, albeit with local variations, informed subsequent innovation.

In fact, initial attempts to reform diabetes care records were directly connected to the efforts to standardise hospital medical records noted above, and suffered a similar fate. In 1968, the BDA asked Dr John Bingle, a consultant in York, to review existing clinic documents and to form a panel to consider standardisation.[62] Bingle maintained communication with the Department of Health and Social Security (DHSS, replacing the Ministry of Health from 1968) and its record reforms committee.[63] However, although the BDA subcommittee noted that 50 per cent of the hospitals contacted used their own special charts for routine follow-up (all with similar layout), the proposed standard, composite, form (see Fig. 3.1) did not survive the transition out of committee. Bingle noted that clinic 'requirements ... varied so much' that a

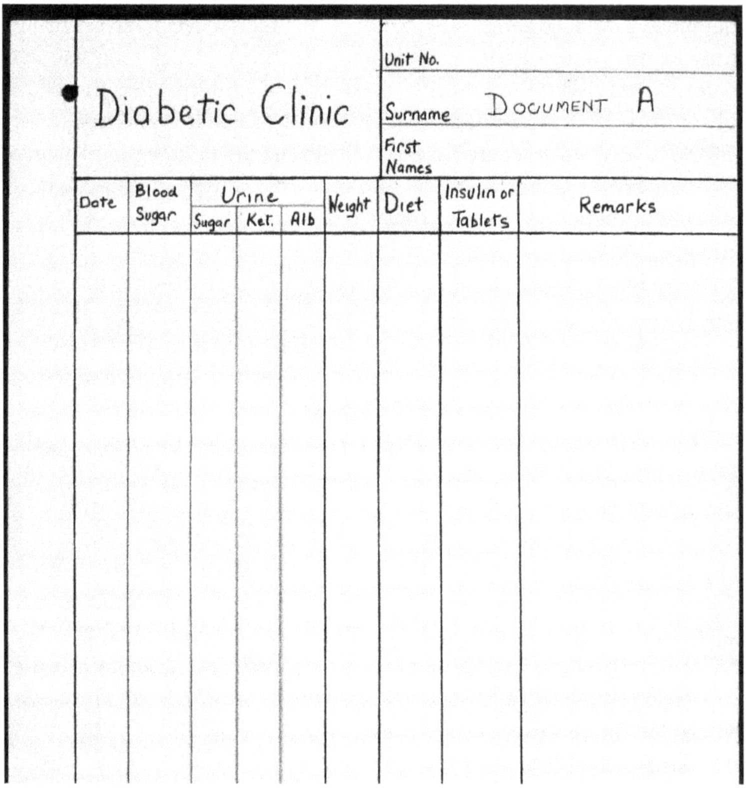
Diabetic Clinic

Unit No.
Surname DOCUMENT A
First Names

Date	Blood Sugar	Urine			Weight	Diet	Insulin or Tablets	Remarks
		Sugar	Ket.	Alb				

Figure 3.1 Standard outpatient clinic review form, c.1968

single form could not suit all purposes, and that 'there is considerable apathy over documentation, each clinic having at some time designed its forms and being somewhat unwilling to change to a new type without a very good reason'.[64]

The record itself, however, was noteworthy for the regulatory and clinical values it embodied. As with earlier innovations in records for inpatient diabetes care, the pre-formatting of the record could be seen as an attempt to influence practice.[65] Lined sections of the form may have restricted the data gathered and passed on, thus ordering the work to be performed.[66] Moreover, the subcommittee had to reflect on what they saw as the most important data to be collected, and members clearly prioritised biochemical markers (blood glucose, glycosuria, ketonuria, and albuminuria), as well as weight and treatment information.[67] They appeared to agree, therefore, that good care involved collecting physiological and clinical information at the very least. At this stage, this control-through-communication may have been somewhat limited, as the record still allowed a large unstructured column for qualitative remarks.[68] Unlike later forms, moreover, this record would have formed part of a range of outpatient observation documentation, with less structured forms perhaps providing additional data.

Although clinic doctors of the 1970s resisted efforts to standardise care nationally, these same practitioners, along with GPs, slowly introduced bureaucratic tools that managed practice at the grassroots level. As with recall, renewed concerns with patient surveillance motivated doctors to introduce new instruments to structure monitoring, often after service reviews revealed deficiencies. For instance, one early and influential study conducted by a trainee GP remarked how the notes in one general practice suggested that 'biochemical investigations relied completely on the patients' own recordings, with no supervised check being carried out'.[69] Some tests were erratically performed. Blood sugar examinations, for example, were seemingly carried out inequitably – 'recorded more often for diet and diet plus oral hypoglycaemic controlled diabetics than in insulin-controlled cases' – and the general conclusion was that 'one could not rely on the last entry in the notes to indicate the biochemical control of the patient's diabetes'. Just as importantly, the recorded information 'was often available only after prolonged searches through sheaves of results and letters from clinics'.[70] The reviewer thus noted three interlinked problems, all of which were a concern given the importance of surveillance and the potential deputation of further responsibility to GPs: key parts of medical work were not being undertaken regularly; when work was performed, doctors had not recorded it; and, when recorded, the results of this work had not been noted clearly.

Within this single site, the reviewer saw the solution to inconsistencies of surveillance in three parts. Firstly, they recommended designing an effective recall system. Secondly, they proposed more systematically dividing the responsibilities of practice nurse (biochemical tests, weighing, dietary advice) and GP (clinical interview, screening for complications, and record completion). Finally, the author stressed the need to create 'an effective follow-up chart' (Fig. 3.2).[71]

The new record card was crucial. The reviewer designed it to solve multiple problems of poor surveillance and recording. The survey section, for example, included a 'simple tick system', enabling easy completion at the front of the form.[72] Through design, the effort required to complete the necessary notes could be reduced and dismantled as an obstacle. Furthermore, this formatting was also intended to structure the practitioner's surveillance of the patient, and correct the problem of work being neglected. On one level, whilst retaining flexibility in its ongoing clinical sections, the record used visibility to encourage adherence, providing clearly marked spaces to note test results, problems, and a 'plan' of action. Of course, notes did not need to be made, and certain actions could easily be forgotten or not undertaken. In such instances, however, the record's spatial zoning would make absences clear to GPs, and would allow them an 'instant review on a yearly basis of [the] routine care and advice offered'. Finally, going beyond visibility, the record itself was created to actively prompt work when in use. The author, for instance, noted that there would be a 'built in reminder' for GPs to screen for complications. The record's minute detailing of the checks to be undertaken within the annual review provided this cue, indicating to the user what tests should be performed as it was being completed.[73] An aide-memoire to previous work was thus transformed into a prompt when the record was in action.

Finally, it is worth noting how the reviewer designed the record to facilitate new kinds of teamwork. Responding to calls for GPs to adopt mini-clinic sessions for efficiency purposes, the author noted that 'with the co-operation of receptionist, practice nurse and doctor' records could be completed adequately, and 'dual appointments to see nurse and doctor could be fitted into a normal surgery session'.[74] The reformulated record, therefore, was intended to be an active part of a broader technology of surveillance, one that facilitated and prompted action

Family history including children	
Initial symptoms	Types of diabetes
Age at onset	Type of control
Problems	Plan

Date	BS	Urine	Wt.	BP	Clinical notes	Treatment

SUGGESTED FOLLOW UP RECORD							
Surname			Forenames				
Sex M/F	Married status S M W D		Date of birth				Age
Occupation			Children				
Height	Weight at diagnosis		Ideal weight target				
Allergies			Seen/not seen hosp. clinic consultant:				
			'76	'77	'78	'79	'80
Diabetic survery and advice							
Join Diabetic Association							
Carry warning card							
Carry sugar							
"Hypo" described							
Urine lest technique shown							
Influenza vaccination							
Regular dental treatment							
Regular ophthalmic check							
Regular chiropody							
Fundi							
Neuropathy							
Nephropathy							
Arteriosclerosis: Coronary							
Peripheral							
Cerebral							
Dietary advice							

Source: A. P. Kratky, 'An audit of the care of diabetics in one general practice', JRCGP, 27:182 (1977), 536–43.

Figure 3.2 Components of a new record card for GP diabetes care, c.1977

and enabled new forms of working and divisions of labour. The record thus played a 'constitutive role' in diabetes care, both inherently and by design.[75]

Over time, more GPs came to adopt such special records. Careful zoning, preformatted priorities, and even 'stamps' for annual reviews became core features of new documents. The RCGP promoted records along these lines as part of its Quality Initiative, including existing models of diabetes records in its 'clinical information pack' for the condition.[76] Indeed, the pack was the second that the College produced, reflecting the importance of diabetes as a gateway to 'the development of … expertise [in] preventive aspects of medical care' and to issues of 'practice organisation and management'.[77]

That early impetus for reform in general practice appeared to come from more junior members of the profession probably indicates that a generational shift contributed to the spread of new approaches to clinical activity. Recent involvement in forms of hospital practice and pioneering vocational GP training may have exposed junior practitioners to cutting-edge concepts of good care centred on surveillance and bureaucracy.[78] Equally, changes in general practice's material and intellectual foundations provided fertile ground for an emphasis on records at this point. Crucially, group practice had slowly become the new norm in primary care, driven by professional interest in peer exchange and financial and organisational imperatives of sharing costs and workload. The result was to undercut 'continuity of care', and doctors could no longer rely on a personal relationship to know their patient's histories.[79] GPs therefore needed records to provide an aide-memoire, as well as to encourage unfamiliar staff to adopt common practices.[80] In a similar vein, the growth of the 'primary care team' within general practice was also influential here, with records facilitated by (and facilitating) the incorporation of specialist clerical staff, practice nurses, and attached health visitors, chiropodists, dieticians, and community nurses following the GP contract of 1965 and NHS reforms of 1974.[81]

A more challenging version of this growing care team, however, appeared in integrated care programmes. Unlike systematic care within general practice, surveillance and therapeutic titration in these schemes occurred in multiple sites (across hospitals, general practice surgeries, and patients' homes), posing several possible problems. Firstly, if schemes were left uncoordinated, patients might fall through gaps in provision, or receive different standards of care based on institutional geography. Secondly, without a clear division of responsibility between practitioners, the system might produce an inefficient repetition of work. And finally, even if lines of communication were established, information could be lost or unintelligible without a formal language shared across services and a changing roster of staff. Within such circumstances, doctors and other 'stakeholders' created tools to clearly allocate, communicate, and review work undertaken across different segments of integrated services.

Records were once again important. In perhaps the most fully realised shared care scheme of all – that in Poole – a working party of GPs and a consultant produced a new form of diabetes record (in collaboration with the local hospital management committee and Hoescht Pharmaceuticals): a 'community care co-operation booklet' that travelled with the patient between practitioners and sites of care (see Fig. 3.3).[82]

The premise of a mobile record itself was not entirely novel. As the designers of the Poole system noted, GPs and hospital practitioners had shared cards for other types of patient, primarily for 'chronic schizophrenics' and antenatal care.[83] However, the community care booklet served multiple functions. It contained advice on diet, 'foot care, illness, insulin reactions, driving, and general instructions about attending the laboratory and general practitioner'. Through its qualitative elements, therefore, it sought to influence the work of its users. Its clinical section also implemented many of the changes in record forms already noted. It contained ruled sections for dates of observation, test results, notes on treatment, and a 'check list to indicate when the patient was last assessed for diseases of the eyes, nervous systems, cardiovascular system, and the feet'.[84]

Perhaps more than when records remained in a single institution, this zoning of the form was crucial to the management of the scheme and its spatially dispersed practitioners. Such techniques, for instance, reduced the possibility of idiosyncratic shorthand, regulating information exchange so that staff across different settings could interpret notes without misunderstanding. Moreover, by clearly boxing specific data, the record could prevent 'wasteful duplication of effort' and allow errors to be checked and corrected.[85] Indeed, the Poole clinical lead hoped that computerisation would provide a 'method of assessing the follow-up and control of patients not regularly seen in the clinic'.[86] Although it was potentially a hospital plan to manage GPs, no punitive measures could be devised in a programme dependent upon co-operation.[87]

Clinical record

Date	WT.	Blood Test		Urine			Check list				Diet	Insulin			Oral therapy	NEXT VISIT
		I.B.S.	HbA1c	S	P	Ac.	Eyes	N.S.	C.V.S.	Feet	G.Cho.	Type	Units	am/pm		

Figure 3.3 The community care co-operation booklet, c.1980s

The designers simply hoped that the record would increase visibility of errors for care teams, with practice review forming the basis for changed behaviour.

During the 1970s and 1980s, hospital hopes for computerised surveillance of professionals were seemingly unrealised. Constrained NHS funding underpinned technical difficulties.[88] Furthermore, doctors using similar records complained that such tools were – in themselves – unable to ensure that professionals always performed 'relevant' disease management.[89] Such problems did not prove fatal for the Poole scheme, or for the record form itself. Hoescht Pharmaceuticals published the booklet as a commercially available product, and GPs and other community care schemes adopted and adapted it.[90] Even the RCGP indirectly recommended it.[91] In this sense, the adoption of the record mirrored the spread of similar forms discussed above.

It was in this form of integrated, structured care that diabetes management appeared as something of a model for other chronic conditions. The interest of the Royal Colleges has already been highlighted, with diabetes appearing as an exemplar of proactive and preventive medicine, existing at the forefront of cross-institutional experiments in integrated chronic disease care. Yet the influence of diabetes care on practices in other conditions did not always derive from success. One article, for instance, detailed how the authors had heard about 'an experiment in shared hospital–GP care of diabetes' which reported 'only limited success, despite careful planning'. They were thus inspired to detail their own experience in the management of hypertension, to address fears that 'shared care of hypertensives would fare no better and that the portable record would be lost, forgotten, badly completed, or illegible.'[92] Despite problems, the use of mobile records and shared care systems nonetheless situated diabetes care at the vanguard of trials in service management, and formed part of a broader discourse around chronic disease and service integration.

However, the power of the record to structure care was truly realised only in combination with care protocols. As noted, protocols for medical practice had numerous origins, and from these sites they seeped into clinical practice after the Second World War. In Britain, the growth of clinical research within the NHS helped to familiarise doctors with using and designing 'protocols', positioning them as a sensible option for co-ordinating action across multiple sites.[93] From the 1970s onwards, several integrated diabetes care programmes used formal protocols to facilitate effective functioning of diverse moving parts. According to early debates, initial agreements may have included 'the circumstances in which patients could or should be kept at home for treatment by the general practitioner, the pattern of investigation of such cases, and the criteria for referral to hospital'.[94] The Poole scheme even supplemented such agreements with extra documentation advising patient and GP about follow-up and 'the standard of control expected'.[95]

Other schemes went further as time passed, tightening the regulatory aims of their protocol. The Ipswich community care scheme, for instance, selected patients for hospital and general practice care using clear criteria, including strict biochemical thresholds of control, age, and various risk and clinical factors. Formal procedures were established for referral and discharge. Furthermore, although GPs were offered freedom of organisation, they agreed to meet 'standards of care, follow-up, and recording', including (1) at least yearly review of 'well-controlled' patients, and either more frequent observation or referral to hospital if control fell outside of agreed parameters; (2) measurement and recording of a minimum agreed set of base surveillance metrics (blood glucose, glycosylated haemoglobin (HbA1c), urine tests, weight); and (3) at least annual assessment of visual acuity, foot condition, and blood pressure, and performance of fundoscopy.[96]

As will be discussed in Chapter 5, by the end of the 1980s, professional organisations were producing model protocols with more finely tuned arrangements, and even GPs outside integrated programmes were promoting their use.[97] The RCGP protocol, for instance, contained a cartographic attachment: the 'diabetes flow-chart', an A1-sized poster which was most likely to be hung on a practitioner's wall for easy consultation.[98] Like other types of mapping, the flow-chart was an exercise in abstraction and legibility.[99] It disaggregated diagnosis and management into certain 'pathways' to be taken if specific conditions were met or not. In so doing, the map embodied an idealised route to care, one that presented it as a simple process of decision-making devoid of contextual factors (about patients and institutions).[100] Crucially, through this decontextualisation and direction, the flow-chart represented a tool to guide patient management, visualising the 'correct' steps to take and highlighting deviations by their absence.

Interestingly, the map also presented a very specific view of care. It contained no 'patient-centred' indicators, such as whether patients were happy with treatment plans. Instead, conditions determining action were clinical and biochemical. It may be that discussions of patient experiences and feelings were informal, the unrecorded product of exchange between practitioner and patient. And this is hinted at in certain protocol that contained points for discussing 'wellbeing'.[101] However, their relative marginality within tools for surveillance is nonetheless notable given how designers used these instruments to prioritise key information and tasks, and to manage professional labour.

Audit, investigatory medicine, and the consolidation of professional management

In each of the tools considered so far, we can trace the emergence and reproduction of a consensus about 'good' diabetes care. Unlike in later years, neither hospital doctors nor GPs defined quality care in terms of outcomes or targets during the 1970s and 1980s. Instead, their records and protocol focused on care process and the same set of physiological markers, checks for complications, and clinically important data on treatment.[102] Moreover, pioneers of GP-based and integrated care all saw a combination of tools as essential to securing good care, coordinating the efforts of care teams, and ensuring regularity and content of oversight. These innovators even slowly articulated the inherently managerial ethos of these new technologies, noting how they prompted activity and recorded performance.

In terms of diabetes, the existence of a professional 'good sense' is perhaps unsurprising. The very creation of the instruments in question forced designers to clarify what they saw as the elements of good care, and the BDA provided a network through which medical professionals could discuss their ideas. As Figure 3.2 above indicates, the organisation exercised considerable influence by the 1970s, and elite bodies like the Royal Colleges also connected interested practitioners and promoted model records and protocol imbued with the emergent consensus.[103]

This articulation of good care, and its connection with regulatory instruments, marked something of a shift in understandings of quality in medicine. During the first half of the twentieth century, doctors (and society more broadly) held that proficiency in medical practice could be guaranteed through effective training and experience. Of course, as noted in this and earlier chapters, professional action would be influenced by any number of other factors. Doctors working in institutions and hospital 'firms' might become socialised into certain approaches, and were constrained by the facilities they had available. Likewise, medical handbooks and journals could provide up-to-date information on trusted or innovative procedures, whilst hospitals might deploy their own documentary aids to help practitioners to tailor observation or therapeutic practices.[104] However, 'the right of private judgement' and clinical individualism were highly prized, and professional action was rarely subject to codified criteria of proper practice, temporal regulation, or recording.[105]

Taken together, therefore, recall systems, specialist records, and care protocol added new local structure to professional action. As discussed in Chapter 5, this structure emerged at a time when professional, public, and political actors had grown concerned about the competence of medical professionals. Professional self-reflection emerged from a cacophony of sources, from media scandals about insensitive care in long-stay institutions to growing critiques of welfare professionals as self-interested bureaucrats (rather than altruistic servants), and from academic studies of variations in care to the rising status of trials as technologies for determining 'best practice'. All contributed to a growing sense that quality care could be secured only through formal regulatory devices.

Devices to structure medical practice could become a 'managerial' technology in a more formal sense, though, only with observation and review. The power of norms derived, in part, from the possibility that adherence, omission, or deviation would be visible to self and others.[106] Thus it was only when recall, records, and protocol were connected to medical audit that their capacity to reshape and manage professional action was fully realised. As noted in the coming chapters, different visions of professionalism and management emerged in relation to protocol and audit. At least within the local systems discussed here, management did not involve formal discipline for deviations, or review being explicitly tied to resource allocation and lay intervention. Rather, doctors saw audit and related tools as educational and as useful for reforming their own practices and systems.[107]

This educational element was perhaps most clearly articulated in the concept of the 'audit cycle'. 'Assessment', noted one influential audit of diabetes care, 'will show in practice if aims are met', quantifying the extent to which this was the case. However, it continued, 'there must be a feedback from "assessment" to "aims", modifying the aims and therefore altering the pattern of care offered'. In this sense, audit was taken to 'represent a continuous process of thought', with 'continuing changes in aims … measured in terms of changing levels of care (assessment)'.[108] Here, protocol could provide a set of standards against which care could be assessed, whilst records and recall systems provided the traces of care upon which analysis would act.[109] Conversely, it was also the case that audit enclosed diabetes care (and medical care more broadly) in a cycle of self-review and management. Without observation, structures could be ineffective and visible actors could deviate. Discipline may have been productive of new forms of working, but it required monitoring.[110]

Audit was a novel practice in British medicine before the 1970s. International influences were important to helping it develop, with American experiences filtering into British discourse.[111] Domestically, doctors themselves were not separated from the society and culture that was making demands for professional regulation. They shared its modes of thought and had knowledge of developments in other professions.[112] Indeed, audit was initially a technology of financial accounting, and British GPs and hospital clinicians had long had connections with private business.[113] In earlier decades, for instance, they had conducted (and been participants in) time-and-motion studies to assess organisational efficiency, hospitals in the late 1960s had drafted in management consultants to improve their administration, and some GPs had even sought to explore general practice in terms of management theory.[114]

Developments within British medical discourse and practice were also of importance. Psychologically oriented theories emerging in the late 1950s emphasised professional fallibility and reflexivity, whilst the NHS's close connection with research saw major figures in British clinical and health services research promote techniques of review as central to efficiency and efficacy.[115] In fact, some doctors saw diabetes as a site for developing audit itself. Chronic disease care developed a rich culture of inscriptions and registers. The supposedly document-heavy nature of diabetes management, therefore, made it a promising target for promoting audit, as did its quantified diagnostic criteria. As one GP put it when justifying their choice of subject for developing audit, diabetes was 'more readily defined than … many of the chronic diseases', and its patients were 'easier to identify'.[116]

Doctors initially audited their diabetes management arrangements, then, as an investigative practice, establishing a co-constructive relationship between talk of standards, structured care, and management. As noted above, early investigators were sometimes concerned that expanding the care team might lower standards, or they sought to demonstrate that improvements in care were possible. As audit occasionally preceded new arrangements, auditors established the very measurements through which it became possible to discuss 'standards' of care.

As one study, cited above, put it, 'one has to set standards against which to measure'.[117] In this instance, the reviewer combined social, clinical, and biochemical factors to classify diabetic care as 'good', 'moderate', or 'poor'. Ultimately, the author found effective audit difficult to conduct, and thus problematised what they saw as deficiencies in record-keeping, oversight, and management documentation. In this case, potential obstacles to audit became legitimation for reforming care processes and structures, and for further audit itself.[118] It was a co-constructed pattern followed elsewhere.[119]

Auditing also had a close relationship with health services research that assessed the functioning of novel schemes for diabetes management. Though encompassing process measures, reviews of services also variously added intermediate outcome measures (such as HbA1c results) that may have formed part of local protocol standards.[120] Whilst such reviews were not always labelled 'auditing', participants expressly framed their investigations in relation to concerns about reformulated care responsibilities.[121] Reviews of novel programmes appeared within a few years of new arrangements being established, and were considered necessary 'to assess the efficacy' of schemes and even to provide 'baseline' information for ongoing evaluation.[122]

It was through this longitudinal assessment that investigative forms of review later became routine practice, providing a 'feedback loop' into clinical medicine.[123] Towards the end of the 1980s, assessments became more formally framed as audits, whilst incorporating measures pioneered in health services research and local protocol.[124] Although published, such work provided ongoing evaluation, as opposed to consisting of retrospective analyses that promoted or critiqued alternative forms of organisation. New guides to audit stressed the importance of this distinction, arguing that older forms of evaluation were helpful in 'focusing the subject', but were 'concerned with the success or failure of some aspects of diabetes care[,] rather than providing a continuing assessment of management of this chronic disease from which further improvements can be made'.[125] Using the tools developed within this research, this guide now promoted embedding review as part of new service organisation.

Conclusion: did structured care produce a new order?

The implementation of audit completed a major shift that had taken place in diabetes care after the 1960s. By the 1980s, discussions of 'good diabetes care' persistently invoked structured care. Systematic organisation, recording, and review provided signs of good practice, and practitioners believed them to be crucial to guaranteeing effective patient management. In part, hospital clinicians and GPs (supported by specialist nurses, Community Physicians, and other interested parties) had mobilised recall systems, specialist records, and care protocol to improve patient oversight. However, the combination of these instruments, especially with audit, inherently ordered medical labour. As criticism of professional competence spread across British society, designers of new systems intensified the regulatory aspects of the new instruments. When combined, these tools formed local organisational technologies constructed in the name of 'quality', just as clinical trials formed an organisational technology in pursuit of 'truth'.[126] Such technologies were reproduced throughout Britain, beginning in areas with motivated and experienced practitioners, before moving slowly into the 'periphery'.

The question that now needs to be answered, therefore, is: what effects – if any – did this new technology have on practice?

A traditional response might be framed in terms of 'success'. Did care improve? Practitioners assessing new approaches varied considerably on this point. Organisers of the Wolverhampton 'mini-clinic' scheme, for example, expressed consistently positive evaluations, in terms of both process and outcomes.[127] New tools apparently facilitated increased oversight, as well as successful co-operation between participants. Likewise, organisers of a community scheme in Norwich noted improvements in recording practices and follow-up, even though considerable omissions remained.[128] By contrast, reviewers of the nearby Ipswich scheme criticised GPs for continuously poor testing, follow-up, and record completion, despite agreed policies.[129] And in Sheffield, worse results followed.[130]

Yet posing this question – or at least answering it in terms of audit results – is an effect of the changes being discussed. Instead, a more pertinent route of enquiry might be to ask whether the new combinations of concepts, instruments, and actors produced a new, structured order in diabetes care.[131] Did the developments traced succeed in making new ways of working possible, and in introducing new forms of professional management on a local level?

Answers can be drawn only indirectly. For instance, discussions of deputation, routine, and repetition in medical texts indicate how some doctors reacted against the managerial effects of new technologies.

During the 1980s, for example, guides to establishing general practice diabetes care argued that 'nurses are generally better trained in the repetitive tasks of measuring height, blood pressure, etc, than doctors' and 'are more reliable at recording them'. Consequently, 'the doctor should do more complex clinical tests, assess the basic information collected by the nurse and decide on necessary changes in management', as well as organise referral.[132] The tasks deputed to nurses were those most heavily subject to new managerial pressures, whilst clinical assessment was less able to be reviewed critically. Such language mirrored that applied by consultants and specialists earlier in the century. As seen in Chapter 2, professionals responded to patient load by routinising care for certain patients, and clinicians tried to depute this work to either GPs or non-medical staff (such as dieticians).[133] By the later 1980s, the routinising pressures of protocol and records saw tasks deputed again, from GPs to nurses. GPs in certain schemes became mini-consultants, with specialist and practice nurses running their own clinics.[134] To be sure, deputation of work could indicate that practitioners had found a way to negotiate the management of their activities, both in hospital and in general practice. Deputation may also have been interpreted as a positive sign by doctors, freeing them for more complex parts of consultation, such as discussing wellbeing issues. Regardless, deputation provides a sign that managerial pressures had successfully altered care to the extent that negotiations were necessary.

Yet perhaps it is this view of care as constantly changing, but never quite fully changed, that is most productive. One study of audit cycles in a general practice provides insight here. Through the practice's first audit in 1983, the partners noted that there had been 'no structured diabetic care in the practice and the process of care was haphazard'. Accordingly, the practice subsequently developed a patient register and 'a protocol for the care of ... diabetic patients ... which included a routine format for history taking and regular examination, suggested biochemical aims of treatment, and gave aims for education and support'. In 1990, the partners undertook a second audit. They noted that 'the protocol developed after the 1983 audit changed and organised the process of care in the practice', but the new audit was designed to 'examin[e] whether the conclusions of the previous audit had been implemented and whether the defined standards for the process of care and outcome of care ... had all been achieved'.[135] To this, they concluded 'no'. Further work was required, and new discussions were held about 'changes in the protocol and its monitoring to improve future performance'.[136] In other words, the study revealed that diabetes care had not been completely reformulated. Standards were missed, and some processes remained unfulfilled. Yet standards and preformatted practices of care did now exist, and deviations were being captured, subject to review, and structures subsequently reformulated. Substantial change had been implemented, and the combination of new tools subjected local practice to management, but no endpoint had been reached.

That this audit was another of general practice raises the question of whether managerialised care was an imposition of specialists upon GPs. Contemporary sociological investigation of audit indicated that traditional hierarchies may have protected consultants from review in some institutions.[137] Furthermore, as hospital clinics had been considered the 'orthodox' site for diabetes care, it was general practice that had come under suspicion with reorganisation.

The role of professional elites in designing and promoting tools of national clinical governance will be discussed in the coming chapters. At the local level, assumptions that professional management was a hospital invention would overlook the complex dynamics at play. Regardless of their supposedly superior status, hospital practitioners were not the formal managers of GP labour. Consultants could not direct GPs – or punish them for deviations – in the same way as 'superiors' within a traditional bureaucratic chain. Integrated diabetes care depended upon voluntary arrangements, and less motivated GPs or hostile consultants tended to clash with agreed arrangements. One participant in the Sheffield scheme acknowledged the importance of such mutual investment, noting how consultants 'didn't think general practitioners could look after people with diabetes at all'.[138] As a result, something akin to 'turf wars' broke out before mobile specialist nurses eventually rescued the scheme.[139] By contrast, elsewhere GPs were part of committees for creating protocols and designing records, as well as undertaking audit. In fact, GPs were themselves pioneers in promoting such tools, and individual practitioners frequently reviewed and reorganised their own practice independently of any official community scheme.

Professional management in diabetes care at a local level, therefore, was generally constructed out of a shared sense of what 'good practice' meant, and relied upon charismatic pioneers and dedicated staff to work.[140] Debate existed about the importance of specific markers or how to measure potentially immeasurable elements, such as social and psychological wellbeing.[141] Nonetheless, over the decades following the 1960s many figures involved in diabetes care converged on an agreed set of quantifiable indicators, and placed great emphasis on the organisation and structure of care to secure quality. Designers of systematic schemes often adapted tools from existing instruments, reflecting – as did their drive to integrate care – their socialisation within a bureaucratic medical culture The reorganisation of the NHS in 1974 may even have supported such developments, bringing professionals with epidemiological and evaluative expertise closer to clinical institutions. Drawing on their abstractive, 'administrative way of knowing', such individuals were important facilitators and evaluators of new schemes.[142] When instruments for regulating time and co-ordinating activity were thus combined in coherent schemes with practices of review, the resulting technology subjected professional work to management, producing bureaucratising effects of codification, division, re-integration, and oversight. These effects were not totalising, but were nonetheless substantive, and diabetes provided a leading edge for their implementation.

In the chapters that follow, we will explore how support for managed care developed as a guarantor of quality. These chapters open up a broader vista on political and cultural context as well as international developments. This changing lens is necessary if we are to understand how local developments transformed into (and interacted with) national, and international, programmes of clinical governance. Before this latter history can be traced, however, it will be necessary to make a detour via diabetic retinopathy. Through studying the specific policy debates around retinopathy, we will see how the developments focused upon so far manifested in a single issue. We will also chart how diabetes returned to the policy agenda after the Ministry of Health issued its standards for diabetic clinics in 1953. This exploration will highlight the main players involved in shaping policy and how they interacted with one another, thereby providing a crucial map for historicising developments during the end of the twentieth century.

Notes

1 L. Winner, 'Do artifacts have politics?', *Daedalus*, 109:1 (1980), 121–36.
2 M. Foucault, *Discipline and Punish: The Birth of the Prison*, trans. A. Sheridan (London: Penguin, 1991 [1975]).

3 S. Timmermanns and M. Berg, *The Gold Standard: The Challenge of Evidence-Based Medicine and Standardization in Health Care* (Philadelphia: Temple University Press, 2003).
4 H. Marks, *The Progress of the Experiment: Science and Therapeutic Reform in the United States, 1900–1990* (Cambridge: Cambridge University Press, 1997). See also discussions of 'networks' and 'systems' in W. E. Bijker, T. P. Hughes, and T. Pinch (eds.), *The Social Construction of Technological Systems: New Directions in the Sociology and History of Technology*, Anniversary Edition (Cambridge, MA: MIT Press, 2012 [1987]), pp. 11–44, or of 'platforms' in P. Keating and A. Cambrosio, 'Cancer clinical trials: the emergence and development of a new style of practice', *Bulletin of the History of Medicine*, 81:1 (2007), 197–223, esp. pp. 198–9. Each term belongs to a specific theoretical school. My use of 'technology' derives from my interests as a social historian of medicine, and is to be differentiated from network and platform approaches.
5 M. Weber, *The Theory of Social and Economic Organisation*, trans. A. M. Henderson and T. Parsons, ed. T. Parsons (New York: Free Press, 1966 [1947]).
6 R. D. Hill, *Diabetes Health Care: A Guide to the Provision of Health Care Services* (London: Chapman and Hall, 1987), p. 21.
7 H. Valier and R. Bivins, 'Organization, ethnicity and the British National Health Service', in J. Stanton (ed.), *Innovations in Health and Medicine: Diffusion and Resistance in the Twentieth Century* (London: Routledge, 2002), pp. 37–64; C. Sinding, 'Flexible norms? From patients' values to physicians' standards', in W. Ernst (ed.), *Histories of the Normal and the Abnormal: Social and Cultural Histories of Norms and Normativity* (London: Routledge, 2006), pp. 225–44.
8 A. Mold, *Making the Patient-Consumer: Patient Organisations and Health Consumerism in Britain* (Manchester: Manchester University Press, 2015).
9 A. M. Brandt and M. Gardner, 'The golden age of medicine?', in R. Cooter and J. Pickstone (eds.), *Companion to Medicine in the Twentieth Century* (Abingdon: Routledge, 2003), pp. 29–34. See Chapter 5 below.
10 W. R. Arney and B. J. Bergen, *Medicine and the Management of Living: Taming the Last Great Beast* (Chicago: University of Chicago Press, 1985).
11 Sinding, 'Flexible norms?', p. 237; R. Tattersall, *Diabetes: The Biography* (Oxford: Oxford University Press, 2009), pp. 162–4.
12 Tattersall, *Diabetes*, p. 152.
13 J. T. Ireland, W. S. T. Thomson, and J. Williamson, *Diabetes Today: A Handbook for the Clinical Team* (Aylesbury: HM+M, 1980).
14 Hill, *Diabetes Health Care*, p. 21.
15 M. O. Aveline, D. K. McCulloch, and R. B. Tattersall, 'The practice of group psychotherapy with adult insulin-dependent diabetics', *Diabetic Medicine*, 2:3 (1985), 275–82.

16 Hill, *Diabetes Health Care*, p. 91.
17 Ibid., p. 37.
18 Ibid., p. 91.
19 R. D. Lawrence, *The Diabetic Life: Its Control by Diet and Insulin. A Concise Practical Manual for Practitioners and Patients*, 6th edition (London: J. & A. Churchill, 1931); J. Malins, *Clinical Diabetes Mellitus* (London: Eyre & Spottiswood, 1968).
20 H. P. Himsworth, 'Management of diabetes mellitus, part II', *BMJ*, 2:3942 (1936), 188.
21 'Organization of out-patient departments', *BMJ*, S.1:2665 (1956), 55.
22 G. Forsyth and R. Logan, *Gateway or Dividing Line? A Study of Hospital Outpatients in the 1960s* (Oxford: Oxford University Press for the Nuffield Provincial Hospitals Trust, 1968), p. 221; interview with J. Harkness conducted by the author. Harkness trained and worked as a manager in the NHS from the early 1970s to the 1990s.
23 D. Armstrong, 'Space and time in British general practice', *Social Science and Medicine*, 20:7 (1985), 659–66.
24 J. M. Wilks, 'Diabetes – a disease for general practice', *JRCGP*, 23:126 (1973), 46–54.
25 Ibid., p. 52.
26 On the importance of documentary technologies for maintaining visibility, and thus discipline: Foucault, *Discipline and Punish*, pp. 189–92.
27 G. Horobin and J. McIntosh, 'Time, risk and routine in general practice', *Sociology of Health and Illness*, 5:3 (1983), 312–31.
28 M. T. Wojciechowski, 'Systematic care of diabetic patients in a general practice', *JRCGP*, 32:242 (1982), 532.
29 J. D. Grene and J. M. Henderson, 'Automated recall in general practice', *JRCGP*, 21:107 (1971), 352–5.
30 R. L. Gibbins and J. Saunders, 'Develop diabetic care in general practice', *BMJ*, 297:6642 (1988), 187–9.
31 B. Hurwitz, C. Goodman, and J. Yudkin, 'Prompting the clinical care of non-insulin dependent (type-II) diabetic patients in an inner-city area: one model of community care', *BMJ*, 306:6878 (1993), 624–5.
32 Foucault, *Discipline and Punish*, p. 154.
33 Wilks, 'Diabetes', p. 46.
34 Interview with B. Potts conducted by the author.
35 E. Martin and S. Goodwin, 'Audit of diabetic care', *JRCGP*, 38:308 (1988), 124.
36 G. F. Morgan, D. A. Cadman, P. H. Edwards, T. C. O'Dowd, and R. Harvard Davis, 'Diabetes care: whose responsibility?', *BMJ*, 289:6454 (1984), 1310.
37 Gibbins and Saunders, 'Develop diabetic care in general practice', p. 189.

38 C. Pope, 'Trouble in store: some thoughts on the management of waiting lists', *Sociology of Health and Illness*, 13:2 (1991), 205–7.
39 T. Benson, 'Why general practitioners use computers and hospitals do not – part 1: incentives', *BMJ*, 325:7372 (2002), 1086–9; T. Benson, 'Why general practitioners use computers and hospitals do not – part 2: scalability', *BMJ*, 325:7372 (2002), 1090–3. The divergence in computerisation between general practice and hospitals has perhaps been the most striking inequality.
40 T. Pinch and W. E. Bijker, 'The social construction of facts and artifacts: or how the sociology of science and sociology of technology might benefit each other', in Bijker, Hughes, and Pinch (eds.), *The Social Construction of Technological Systems*, pp. 11–44.
41 B. Hurwitz and J. Yudkin, 'Diabetes care: whose responsibility?', *BMJ*, 289:6450 (1984), 1000–1.
42 Martin and Goodwin, 'Audit', p. 124.
43 See Chapters 1 and 2.
44 B. M. Doyle, *The Politics of Hospital Provision in Early Twentieth-Century Britain* (London: Pickering and Chatto, 2014).
45 R. Wall, 'Using bacteriology in elite hospital practice: London and Cambridge, 1880–1920', *Social History of Medicine*, 24:3 (2011), 776–95; A. Hull, 'Hector's house: Sir Hector Hetherington and the academization of Glasgow hospital medicine before the NHS', *Medical History*, 45:2 (2001), 232–6.
46 See Chapters 2 and 1 respectively.
47 B. L. Craig, 'The role of records and of record-keeping in the development of the modern hospital in London, England and Ontario, Canada', *Bulletin of the History of Medicine*, 65:3 (1991), 376–97; J. D. Howell, *Technology in the Hospital: Transforming Patient Care in the Early Twentieth Century* (Baltimore: Johns Hopkins University Press, 1995).
48 V. Hess and J. A. Mendelsohn, 'Case and series: medical knowledge and paper technology, 1600–1900', *History of Science*, 48:3 (2010), 304; B. L. Craig, 'Hospital records and record-keeping c.1850–c.1950, part 1: the development of records in hospitals', *Archivaria*, 29:1 (1989), 61–3. On casebooks: L. Kassell, 'Casebooks in early modern England: medicine, astrology and written records', *Bulletin of the History of Medicine*, 88:4 (2014), 595–625.
49 Craig, 'The role of records and of record-keeping', pp. 383–8; Howell, *Technology in the Hospital*, pp. 42–56.
50 Hess and Mendelsohn, 'Case and series', pp. 296–310; Craig, 'The role of records and of record-keeping', pp. 388–93; D. Cantor, 'Introduction: cancer control and prevention in the twentieth century', *Bulletin of the History of Medicine*, 81:3 (2007), 12–13.

51 G. Weisz, A. Cambrosio, P. Keating, L. Knaapen, T. Schlich, and V. J. Tournay, 'The emergence of clinical practice guidelines', *Milbank Quarterly*, 85:4 (2007), 691–727.
52 M. Edwards, *Control and the Therapeutic Trial: Rhetoric and Experimentation in Britain, 1918–48* (Amsterdam: Rodopi, 2007), pp. 93–119; M. Berg, 'Problems and promises of the protocol', *Social Science and Medicine*, 44:8 (1997), 1081–8.
53 D. Cantor, 'The MRC's support for experimental radiology during the inter-war years', in J. Austoker and L. Bryder (eds.), *Historical Perspectives on the Role of the MRC: Essays in the History of the Medical Research Council of the United Kingdom and its Predecessor, the Medical Research Committee, 1913–1953* (Oxford: Oxford University Press, 1989), pp. 199–200.
54 Standing Medical Advisory Committee of the CHSC, *The Standardization of Hospital Medical Records: Report of the Sub-Committee* (London: HMSO, 1965).
55 G. Rivett, *From Cradle to Grave: Fifty Years of the NHS* (London: King's Fund, 1998), pp. 96–7, 181–2; T. Osborne, 'Epidemiology as an investigative paradigm: the College of General Practitioners in the 1950s', *Social Science and Medicine*, 38:2 (1994), 317–26.
56 'Moving towards clinical integration', *BMJ*, 2:6402 (1976), 964.
57 Edwards, *Control and the Therapeutic Trial*; S. Sturdy and R. Cooter, 'Science, scientific management and the transformation of medicine in Britain, c.1870–1950', *History of Science*, 36:4 (1998), 429; C. Lawrence, *Rockefeller Money, The Laboratory and Medicine in Edinburgh, 1919–1930: New Science in an Old Country* (New York: University of Rochester Press, 2005), p. 269.
58 N. R. Eder, *National Health Insurance and the Medical Profession in Britain, 1913–39* (London: Garland, 1982), pp. 155–62.
59 S. Taylor, *Good General Practice: A Report on a Survey* (London: Oxford University Press, 1954), pp. 147–64, esp. pp. 148–9.
60 Ibid.; Standing Medical Advisory Committee of the CHSC, *The Standardization of Hospital Medical Records*.
61 Ibid.
62 TNA, MH 160/416, letter by Dr John Bingle to multiple recipients (including Dr Jarrett, Dr Pyke, and Dr Montgomery), untitled, 9 December 1968, p. 1.
63 TNA, MH 160/416, letter by Dr John Bingle to Dr Avery Jones (DHSS), untitled, 5 January 1969, p. 5.
64 TNA, MH 160/416, H/H.183/29, letter by Dr John Bingle to Mr Alderman (DHSS), 'Advisory committee on hospital medical records', 5 July 1969, p. 1.
65 See Chapter 1.

66 On the ways 'non-human' objects order action and knowledge: B. Latour, *Reassembling the Social: An Introduction to Actor-Network-Theory* (Oxford: Oxford University Press, 2005), pp. 70–85.
67 Albuminuria is the passing of protein into the urine, indicating kidney disease.
68 Howell, *Technology in the Hospital*, pp. 42–56.
69 A. P. Kratky, 'An audit of the care of diabetics in one general practice', *JRCGP*, 27:182 (1977), 536–43, esp. pp. 539–40.
70 Ibid., p. 540.
71 Ibid.
72 Ibid., p. 541.
73 Ibid., p. 540.
74 Ibid., p. 541.
75 M. Berg, 'Practices of reading and writing: the constitutive role of the patient record in medical work', *Sociology of Health and Illness*, 18:4 (1996), 499–524.
76 RCGP, *Diabetes Clinical Information Folder* (London: RCGP, 1988).
77 C. Waine, *Why Not Care for your Diabetic Patients?*, 2nd edition (London: RCGP, 1988), p. 2.
78 D. Irvine, *A Doctor's Tale: Professionalism and Public Trust* (Abingdon: Radcliffe Medical Press, 2003), pp. 11–21.
79 N. Bosanquet and C. Salisbury, 'The practice', in I. Loudon, J. Horder, and C. Webster (eds.), *General Practice under the National Health Service, 1948–1997* (Oxford: Oxford University Press, 1998), p. 53, appendix D.1.
80 J. T. Corbett, 'Keeping records in general practice', *JCGP*, 5:2 (1962), 270–1.
81 See Chapter 2.
82 C. E. Upton, 'Diabetic community care', *The Practitioner*, 215:1284 (1975), 83–6.
83 Ibid., p. 83.
84 R. D. Hill, 'Community care service for diabetics in the Poole area', *BMJ*, 1:6018 (1976), 1138.
85 P. Home and S. Walford, 'Diabetes care: whose responsibility?', *BMJ*, 289:6447 (1984), 713–14.
86 Hill, 'Community care service for diabetics', p. 1138.
87 Marking a comparative weakness in disciplinary relationships: Foucault, *Discipline and Punish*.
88 TNA, MH 150/953, report, 'The Community Care Service (CCS) for diabetics in the Poole area', 1983, pp. 10–12.
89 Hurwitz and Yudkin, 'Diabetes care'.
90 J. Day, H. Humphries, and H. Alban-Davies, 'Problems of comprehensive shared diabetes care', *BMJ*, 240:6587 (1987), 1591.
91 Waine, *Why Not Care for your Diabetic Patients?*, p. 28.

92 S. Ezedum and D. Kerr, 'Collaborative care of hypertensives, using a shared record', *BMJ*, 2:6099 (1977), 1402.
93 On NHS and research: H. Valier and C. Timmermann, 'Clinical trials and the reorganization of medical research in post-Second World War Britain', *Medical History*, 52:4 (2008), 493–510; Hull, 'Hector's house', pp. 236–40.
94 'Moving towards clinical integration', p. 964.
95 Hill, 'Community care service for diabetics', p. 1138.
96 Day et al., 'Problems of comprehensive shared diabetes care', pp. 1590–1.
97 Gibbins and Saunders, 'Develop diabetic care in general practice'.
98 'Diabetes: a protocol', in RCGP, *Diabetes Clinical Information Folder*, appendix 4.
99 J. C. Scott, *Seeing Like a State: How Certain Schemes to Improve the Human Condition Have Failed* (New Haven: Yale University Press, 1998).
100 R. Pinder, R. Petchey, S. Shaw, and Y. Carter, 'What's in a care pathway? Towards a cultural cartography of the new NHS', *Sociology of Health and Illness*, 27:6 (2005), 759–79.
101 'Diabetes: a protocol', in RCGP, *Diabetes Clinical Information Folder*, appendix 4, p. 8.
102 See Chapters 5 and 6 for the quantification and codification of good care after the mid-1980s.
103 See the box in Fig. 3.2 suggesting that patients 'Joi[n] the Diabetic Association'.
104 P. Day, R. Klein, and F. Miller, *A Comparative US–UK Study of Guidelines* (London: Nuffield Trust, 1998), pp. 13–14, 19.
105 C. O. Hawthorne, 'The freedom of medicine', *BMJ*, 2:3432 (1926), 705–8, esp. p. 706; C. Lawrence, 'Incommunicable knowledge: science, technology and the clinical art in Britain, 1850–1914', *Journal of Contemporary History*, 20:4 (1985), 503–20.
106 Foucault, *Discipline and Punish*. As was the case for patients: Sinding, 'Flexible norms?'
107 These were tools for cultivating the self-managing self: D. Willems, 'Managing one's body using self-management techniques: practicing autonomy', *Theoretical Medicine and Bioethics*, 21:1 (2000), 23–38.
108 Kratky, 'An audit of the care of diabetics in one general practice', pp. 536–7.
109 B. Essex, 'Records and audit', in RCGP, *Clinical Information Folder*, appendix 19, p. 1.
110 Foucault, *Discipline and Punish*.
111 'A medical audit', *The Lancet*, 280:7251 (1962), 339–40; I. McWhinney, 'Medical audit in North America', *BMJ*, 2:5808 (1972), 277–9; H. W. K. Acheson, 'Medical audit and general practice', *The Lancet*, 305:7905 (1975), 511–13. There were differences in aims and contexts, however: W. J. Jackson, A. S. Paterson, C. K. M. Pong, and S. Scarparo, 'Doctors under

the microscope: the birth of medical audit', *Accounting History Review*, 23:1 (2013), 23–47.
112 For instance, in the teaching profession: F. S. E. Hatfield, 'Monitoring general practitioners', *JRCGP*, 26:171 (1976), 764.
113 M. Power, *The Audit Society: Rituals of Verification* (Oxford: Oxford University Press, 1999); A. Digby, *The Evolution of British General Practice, 1850–1948* (Oxford: Oxford University Press, 1999).
114 Armstrong, 'Space and time in British general practice', p. 662; P. Sleight, J. A. Spencer, and E. W. Towler, 'Oxford and McKinsey: Cogwheel and beyond', *BMJ*, 1:5697 (1970), 682–4; B. L. E. Reedy, 'Morale and management in general practice', *JRCGP*, 16:1 (1968), 3–11.
115 T. Osborne, 'Power and persons: on ethical stylisation and person-centred medicine', *Sociology of Health and Illness*, 16:4 (1994), 529; J. N. Morris, *Uses of Epidemiology*, 2nd edition (London: E. & S. Livingstone, 1964); A. L. Cochrane, *Effectiveness and Efficiency: Random Reflections on the Health Services* (London: Nuffield Provincial Hospitals Trust, 1972).
116 B. J. Doney, 'An audit of the care of diabetics in a group practice', *JRCGP*, 26:171 (1976), 734–2, esp. p. 734.
117 Kratky, 'An audit of the care of diabetics in one general practice', p. 536.
118 Ibid., pp. 536–43.
119 Doney, 'An audit of the care of diabetics'.
120 D. R. R. Williams, C. Munroe, C. J. Hospesdales, and R. H. Greenwood, 'A three-year evaluation of the quality of diabetes care in the Norwich community care scheme', *Diabetic Medicine*, 7:1 (1990), 74–9.
121 T. M. Hayes and J. Harries, 'Randomised controlled trial of routine hospital clinic care versus routine general practice care for type-II diabetics', *BMJ*, 289:6447 (1984), 728.
122 J. S. Yudkin, B. J. Boucher, K. E. Schopflin, B. T. Harris, H. R. Claff, N. J. D. Whyte, B. Taylor, D. H. Mellins, A. B. Wootliff, J. G. Safir, and E. J. Jones, 'The quality of diabetic care in a London health district', *Journal of Epidemiology and Community Health*, 34:4 (1980), 277.
123 Valier and Bivins, 'Organization, ethnicity and the British National Health Service'.
124 P. J. Burrows, P. J. Gray, A.-L. Kinmonth, D. J. Payton, G. A. Walpole, R. J. Walton, D. Wilson, G. Woodbine, 'Who cares for the patient with diabetes? Presentation and follow-up in seven Southampton practices', *JRCGP*, 37:295 (1987), 65.
125 D. R. R. Williams, P. D. Home, and Members of a Working Group of the Research Unit of the RCP and BDA, 'A proposal for continuing audit of diabetes services', *Diabetic Medicine*, 9:8 (1992), 759–64, esp. p. 759.
126 Marks, *The Progress of the Experiment*.
127 P. A. Thorn and R. G. Russell, 'Diabetic clinics today and tomorrow: mini-clinics in general practice', *BMJ*, 2:5865 (1973), 534–6; B. Singh,

M. Holland, and P. Thorn, 'Metabolic control of diabetes in general practice clinics: comparison with a hospital clinic', *BMJ*, 289:6447 (1984), 726–8.
128 Williams et al., 'A three-year evaluation of the quality of diabetes care in the Norwich community care scheme'.
129 Day et al., 'Problems of comprehensive shared diabetes care'.
130 E. Wilkes and E. E. Lawton, 'The diabetic, the hospital and primary care', *JRCGP*, 30:213 (1980), 199–206.
131 Keating and Cambrosio, 'Cancer clinical trials'.
132 Gibbins and Saunders, 'Develop diabetic care in general practice', p. 189.
133 For the long history of distinguishing between testing and interpretation: S. J. Reiser, *Medicine and the Reign of Technology* (Cambridge: Cambridge University Press, 1978).
134 C. Bradshaw and J. Spencer, 'Nurse-run diabetic clinics in general practice', *Diabetic Medicine*, 7:7 (1990), 572–3.
135 T. J. Kemper and S. R. Hayter, 'Audit of diabetes in general practice', *BMJ*, 302:6774 (1991), 451–3, esp. p. 452.
136 Ibid., p. 453.
137 N. Black and E. Thompson, 'Obstacles to medical audit: British doctors speak', *Social Science and Medicine*, 36:7 (1993), 849–56.
138 Interview with M. MacKinnon conducted by the University of Oxford, 23 April 2007, available at: www.diabetes-stories.com/interview.asp?UID=62 (accessed April 2017).
139 M. MacKinnon, R. M. Wilson, C. A. Hardisty, and J. D. Ward, 'Novel role for specialist nurses in managing diabetes in the community', *BMJ*, 299:6698 (1989), 552–4.
140 On the role of key individuals working within a broader policy structure: M. Gorsky, '"To regulate and confirm inequality"? A regional history of geriatric hospitals under the English National Health Service, c.1948–1975', *Ageing & Society*, 33:4 (2013), 610–11.
141 K. Piwernetz, P. D. Home, O. Snorgaard, M. Antsiferov, K. Staehr-Johansen, and M. Krans for the DiabCare Monitoring Group of the St Vincent's Declaration Steering Committee, 'Monitoring the targets of the St Vincent Declaration and the implementation of the quality management in diabetes care: the DiabCare initiative', *Diabetic Medicine*, 10:4 (1993), 374.
142 Williams et al., 'A three-year evaluation of the quality of diabetes care in the Norwich community care scheme'. For the 'administrative way of knowing': Sturdy and Cooter, 'Science, scientific management and the transformation of medicine in Britain'.

4

Retinopathy screening and the new politics of prevention

With the emergence of structured diabetes management in general practice and the development of integrated care programmes, local medical practitioners had taken their first steps on the road to managed medical practice. A key driver for more expansive systems of care had been the growing emphasis on surveillance and prevention of diabetic complications in medical discourse. Over the 1970s and 1980s, hospital clinicians, GPs, ophthalmologists, and opticians all displayed particular concern with retinopathy (visual impairment and blindness following bleeds in the eye), and the BDA also strengthened its ongoing efforts to improve management of the issue.

Underpinning this interest was new evidence that the timely application of screening and photocoagulation (laser) therapy might prevent visual deterioration in patients with specific types of retinal lesions. Indeed, large-scale studies proved so convincing that diabetes specialists and ophthalmologists lobbied the DHSS during the late 1970s about establishing new centres for retinopathy prevention. Despite a change of government and a simultaneous shift in the trajectory of British politics, over the next decade retinopathy screening and treatment became the subject of much (albeit intermittent) policy discussion within the DHSS. By 1985 the DHSS had approved a trial programme for retinopathy screening and treatment under a Special Medical Development (SMD) grant, one intended to produce future regional standards.

Moving our focus from the clinic to Whitehall, this chapter reconstructs the shifting fortune of retinopathy screening trials within the DHSS, exploring the ways in which political change, financial constraints, and new understandings of prevention enhanced political interest in diabetes and reshaped policy around its management. Following the creation of regional standards for clinics in 1953, diabetes failed to generate substantial political interest in subsequent decades, certainly in comparison to other chronic diseases and risk factors with higher mortality rates or more influential lobbying interests.[1] Various aspects of diabetes care – from prescription charges to special foodstuffs – had been raised in Parliament during the 1960s and 1970s, and the DHSS and MRC had engaged with questions about drug safety.[2] However, there was little in the way of concerted government programmes or interventions. This changed considerably in the 1980s. The volume of parliamentary discussion increased greatly, as technological innovations and concerns about complications became subject to debate and the limitations of NHS resources.[3]

In part, this chapter argues, the reappearance of diabetes was predicated upon networks of exchange developed over the post-war period. For instance, between the 1960s and 1980s, a plethora of actors – including medical specialists, professional and non-governmental organisations, civil servants, Members of Parliament, and ministers – interacted to construct retinopathy as a political object. Action was provoked by new evidence about a hitherto marginal clinical technology, but the creation of novel programmes required persistent support and lobbying. Of equal importance to the political fortunes of diabetes, however, were the ways in which policy actors adapted to a changing political environment. The election of a Conservative government in 1979 intensified government dedication to reducing and reallocating state expenditure, posing problems for any potential initiative. In response, between 1977 and 1985, professional organisations and interested civil servants gradually developed bodies of evidence that reframed retinopathy screening and treatment in terms that were more convincing in the new political climate. Increasingly, policy participants stressed screening and photocoagulation therapy as a form of tertiary prevention, and suggested that intervention could reduce health and social welfare spending. As well as being a clinical and moral issue, management of retinopathy aligned with new political imperatives of retrenchment and national competition. It was this focus on preventive medicine and potential savings that attracted ministerial attention to organisational trials. Funding had been in doubt as late as 1983, but fresh political interest in the economic possibilities of prevention set retinopathy in a new light.

In examining these developments, this chapter does more than tell a story of policy networks.[4] Although the trials in question were not the most significant government intervention into diabetes management, tracing the tribulations of DHSS support enables us to explore how diabetes was politicised by the professional connections and changing conceptions of preventive health discussed in earlier chapters. Moreover, the work of influential organisations and dogged civil servants, like those discussed here, had longer-term impacts, with diabetes constructed as an object of prolonged interest to British governments. In the years after 1985, successive administrations engaged with diabetes management as a clinically and financially important concern. In the political arena, diabetes management itself was simultaneously transformed into a clinical and public health act, one which provided a promising laboratory for practices of clinical governance, service management, and NHS reform. Finally, in telling the story of central government interest in retinopathy, this chapter also begins to trace the importance of international conditions and British neoliberal politics to diabetes management, concerns that are taken up in Chapters 5 and 6. Before we can give this interest meaning, however, we must first understand how retinopathy emerged and developed as a medical concern.

Retinopathy and the clinic at the mid-century

Discussions of retinal changes in diabetes were commonplace in medical discourse by the 1950s.[5] Doctors practising in the late nineteenth century had first proposed the possible existence of a discrete 'diabetic retinitis' following the development of the ophthalmoscope.[6] However, the existence of similar lesions in other conditions – particularly the renal and arterial pathologies then common in older patients with diabetes – undermined consensus about whether specific ocular changes occurred in diabetes until the 1930s.[7] The development of insulin therapy provided the grounds for clinicians to resolve their disputes, as retinopathy was gradually noted in younger patients without associated pathologies, and specialist clinics concentrated patients for more refined research.[8] Doctors continued to disagree about the possible causes of retinopathy, a debate that became entangled with wider disputes about the relationship between long-term metabolic control and the onset of diabetic complications.[9] Nonetheless, medical agreement about the distinctiveness of diabetic retinopathy had been reached by the mid-century, and textbooks dedicated considerable space to describing characteristic pathological changes.

Retinopathy itself, mid-century doctors noted, involved different types of lesion in the eye. Microaneurysms (swelling of blood vessels), neovascularisation (growth of new blood vessels), and exudate (oozing fluid) of differing character were of special interest, and clinicians suggested that visual impairment followed from haemorrhages into the vitreous humour (the jelly substance between retina and lens). This bleed might clear after causing initial impairment. Nonetheless, clinicians read this development as a portent that further bleeds would ultimately result in permanent opacity and blindness, despite also admitting that the unpredictable course of retinal changes made prognosis and therapeutic assessment difficult.[10] In fact, although specialists remarked on the commonality of patients with retinopathy after the 1930s, by no means did the vast majority of patients go blind.[11] In the mid-1970s, for instance, one textbook estimated that 7 per cent of patients with diabetes for over thirty years would experience a loss of sight, and that 'in the majority of diabetics with retinopathy sight is unaffected'.[12]

Irrespective of such statistics, both patients and doctors feared finding retinopathy. For instance, one interviewee (diagnosed in 1973) remarked that she had remained on a strict dietary regimen for over thirty years because 'I am always terrified of going blind or losing my feet or something'.[13] Clinicians also admitted complex feelings towards retinal changes before the late 1970s. One doctor, for example, spoke of his 'dread' of the complication, whilst others admitted a sense of 'helplessness' in the presence of degenerative pathology.[14]

It was this 'helplessness in the face of progressive eye disease', one textbook suggested, 'rather than ... confidence in treatment', that led to recommendations of 'drastic procedures'.[15] A fatalism surrounded retinopathy during early post-war decades. 'In practice', wrote one authority, 'few would have the courage to neglect strict control as a part of the treatment of retinopathy although it clearly has no striking effect if any on the course of the disease.'[16] Yet the alternatives to strict control were often risky and of uncertain value.[17] On the one hand, doctors during the 1950s and 1960s experimented with dietary and pharmacological attempts to lower blood lipids, believing that retinopathy was connected with arteriosclerosis. Such efforts were often found to have inconsistent effects, and visual improvements were not demonstrated.[18] On the other hand, doctors and patients could turn to more radical interventions, most prominently pituitary ablation (hypophysectomy) or adrenalectomy. Although the effects in some young patients could be stark, these treatments held the inherent risks of dramatic surgery. One symposium on hypophysectomy held in 1962 indicated an 11.2 per cent postoperative death rate (15 of 134 cases), with a further 29 per cent of patients dying after six years (39 of 134 cases).[19] Beyond mortality, surgery also had significant side effects, such as worsening hypoglycaemia, impotence, and the reliance on replacement therapy. Aware of the dangers and uncertainties, senior British doctors were seemingly reluctant to use these more drastic interventions. Whilst some avoided them completely, others considered for surgery only those 'rare' patients whose retinopathy had met the possible criteria for intervention: 'young people in which new vessels rapidly sprout up all over the retina and, untreated, lead to blindness within a year'.[20] In other words, before the late 1970s, doctors considered 'prevention ... difficult and treatment unsatisfactory'.[21]

Politicising treatment: retinopathy, photocoagulation, and the BDA

One treatment for retinopathy that had been experimented with, and often dismissed, during these early post-war decades was photocoagulation. The first tests with light-focused therapy had taken place in Germany during the 1950s. The practice cauterised new vessels, with the aim of preventing the haemorrhages that produced visual impairment.[22] By the early 1970s, thousands of photocoagulation procedures had occurred internationally, but in Britain (as elsewhere) as late as 1972 ophthalmologists still suggested that 'the place of light coagulation in treating retinopathy remained doubtful'.[23] It was the emergence of new studies in the 1970s that altered this perception, and in Britain the BDA used the results to politicise screening and treatment as a moral imperative.

As noted in earlier chapters, large-scale trials and epidemiological studies came to play an increasingly important role in medical epistemology over the initial post-war decades.[24] Clinical experience and judgement remained integral parts of medical knowledge, and GPs stressed the importance of knowing patients as individuals.[25] Moreover, trial results did not translate easily into practice given the artificiality of study protocol, and the data (and interpretations) of different studies could conflict.[26] Nonetheless, academic doctors in particular placed a strong emphasis on universalisable, statistically validated evidence (alongside other forms of basic scientific research) in debates about medical truth, treatment, and disease causation.[27]

Thus, when a large-scale American trial of photocoagulation therapy for diabetic retinopathy published its findings during the mid-1970s,

British doctors were quickly convinced of the technology's efficacy, despite earlier reservations. Within a changing epistemological landscape, the trial's methodological innovations proved crucial to its acceptance. Firstly, the study was predicated upon a standard definition of retinopathy, produced by respected participants. The reputation of the architects secured external credibility, whilst standardisation enabled large-scale co-ordination between practitioners, and comparison between and subjects.[28] Secondly, with increasing importance being attached to case-controlled studies in scientific debates, the trial's employment of single-eye treatments – which constituted a subject's second eye as a control – proved convincing.[29] The study was thus able to alleviate previous uncertainties over whether individually variable natural remissions affected outcome more than treatment. Undertaken in cases with severe 'background' retinopathy and proliferative changes, the trial indicated that photocoagulation would 'approximately halve the risk of catastrophic visual loss' when it reported towards the end of the 1970s, and the findings found support from influential figures and publications in British medicine.[30]

Results from contemporaneous trials in the UK supported the American findings, and the new evidence raised pressing ethical and political questions.[31] As one prominent clinician and member of the BDA, Arnold Bloom (Whittington Hospital, London), put it in the *Lancet*: 'it has now been demonstrated that photocoagulation is effective in delaying visual deterioration in some types of diabetic retinopathy. This being so, we have a plain duty to make available this treatment to all diabetics who can benefit from it.'[32] But, as the reference to 'some types' of retinopathy made clear, these trials indicated that treatment would benefit only patients with particular retinal changes.[33] Given the speed and unpredictability of these changes, both the medical press and senior figures like Bloom pointed out that new screening and surveillance arrangements would be necessary.[34] Finding and monitoring the 'higher risk' population would offer the best possibility of detecting problems at their earliest stage, as well as fulfilling another ethical aim: avoiding harm to patients who could not be helped by removing them from consideration.[35]

These moral imperatives had political implications within a collectivised system. During the late 1970s and the 1980s, the resources and expertise to conduct screening and treatment were in short supply.[36] Interlocutors on the issue had already conceded that the new evidence demanded a redistribution of tools, personnel, and activity, a process that could often be intensely fraught.[37] Nonetheless, questions remained about the most effective form of organisation, and it soon became clear that extra resources might be required to establish an efficacious and equitable system within the NHS. Political authorities would need to be engaged.

One party interested in recent therapeutic developments was the BDA, which, along with British ophthalmologists, had co-ordinated the UK photocoagulation studies.[38] The BDA had long been interested in the problems of blindness, and had established its own Committee on Blindness to consider issues of prevalence, incidence, clinical management, and social services between 1967 and 1969.[39] Once again international connections were important. The BDA established the Committee following resolutions on blindness passed at the 1967 congress of the International Diabetes Federation, a body composed of representatives of national diabetes associations from across the world.[40]

In terms of later political work, however, the Committee's report is notable for two reasons. Firstly, the report heavily revised existing estimates of blindness due to diabetes. Feeling that official methods of assessment (based on registrations for welfare services) underplayed the prevalence of diabetes-related blindness, the Committee conducted a sample survey of diabetic clinics. The results nearly doubled estimates of prevalence (to around 5,700 individuals), amplifying the size of the problem and introducing demographic disaggregation by identifying retinopathy as the leading cause of blindness in women during their seventh decade.[41] Later research would refine demographic arguments to produce considerably more noticeable claims, but the medical press reported the increased estimates of retinopathy-related blindness.[42]

The second notable part of the Committee's report was the national network of institutions from which it emerged. The Committee received evidence from the DHSS, the Central Office of Information, and the Government Social Survey, and had close connections with the Royal National Institute for the Blind.[43] In addition, we have already noted how BDA involvement in trials had forged connections with leading ophthalmologists. The co-operation from such bodies speaks to a broader point about the BDA's authority on diabetes management in Britain. The organisation had a considerable professional membership, and its mix of annual events and support for research enabled doctors and epidemiologists to forge important connections.[44] Beyond the profession, the Committee's work reveals how the Association's influence also spread to central government departments. The DHSS and other state-funded bodies were aware that policy decisions about diabetes would ideally have Association input. This is not to say that relations between such agencies were always cordial. For instance, during a long and tortuous attempt to establish a trial on the safety and efficacy of oral hypoglycaemic drugs, the MRC had predicted 'trouble' with the BDA from the start, whilst senior figures in the Association spoke in frustration of delays and the continued 'digest[ion]' of proposals 'by the bureaucrats'.[45] Nonetheless, perhaps more telling of the BDA's position was the admission by the MRC and DHSS that that they 'would need full BDA cooperation if the trial is to be successful'.[46] It was a sentiment that neatly indicated the extent of the connections based on the Association's moral and scientific authority.

Establishing retinopathy as a political problem: diabetic eye centres and the DHSS, 1976–1977

Following the American and British trial results, the BDA and senior British ophthalmologists worked to establish retinopathy screening and photocoagulation as concerns for the DHSS. Diabetic retinopathy had appeared indirectly in parliamentary discussion in June 1976, when a question about government research on causes of blindness revealed MRC and DHSS funding for investigations on specific forms of retinopathy.[47] The BDA, however, made more substantive moves on screening and photocoagulation during 1977. Its Medical and Scientific Section held a symposium on the subject in March, attended by the most influential figures in diabetology from across the country. Here, a unanimous decision was taken to initiate further collaboration with ophthalmologists and the DHSS in a bid to establish 'Regional Diabetic Eye Centres' (DECs) across Britain.[48] In preparation, two senior figures in the fields of diabetology and ophthalmology, Dr Arnold Bloom and Mr Rolf Blach (Moorfields Eye Hospital, London), sent letters to all the RHAs and the most significant ophthalmologists and diabetic departments. They enquired about the possibility of establishing such centres, where they might be located, and what resources would be needed.[49] In general, the RHAs forwarded the letters to their medical advisory committees, and senior medical figures responded favourably to the proposals for centres. All, however, commented on the need for extra finance and staffing for plans to be put into practice.[50] Some correspondents indicated that photocoagulation had been discussed already within various fora, including doctors making contact with the DHSS.

The extent to which this action was independent of the BDA, though (given its professional membership), is uncertain.[51]

The final step in these early moves around photocoagulation treatment involved the Faculty of Ophthalmologists (at this time, one of two professional organisations for ophthalmologists in Britain) contacting the DHSS to 'assess the provision of facilities following the publication of [a] leading article in the *Lancet*' (mentioned above).[52] In response, the DHSS called a meeting of leading specialists in diabetes and ophthalmology in November 1977, and the issue of retinopathy treatment also appeared (albeit in a non-committed manner) in the White Paper *Prevention and Health*, published at the end of December 1977.[53] By late 1977, therefore, key specialist bodies, a lay-professional organisation, and influential practitioners had formed connections with interested civil servants, and the issue was of demonstrable practical concern within health authorities and their medical advisory committees. DECs now became of political interest.[54]

The basis of the first DHSS meeting on retinopathy and photocoagulation was a position paper produced by the chair, Dr G. Pincherle, a Senior Medical Officer in the DHSS and a person with diabetes.[55] Although not explicitly framed in ethical terms, the paper presumed that new evidence about the preventive and ameliorative powers of photocoagulation had created a new 'need', and that the DHSS should assist in some way.[56] On this basis, Pincherle set about estimating the possible extent of the problem, and the potential labour requirements for meeting any increase in workload. His paper succeeded in highlighting a significant lack of information on the issue. The paper cited no epidemiological or clinical surveys, and instead used registrations of blindness and estimates of diabetes' prevalence in England and Wales to assess resource requirements. With the labour divided between thirty to forty centres, Pincherle estimated that the work would require one to two whole time equivalent (WTE) staff per centre, with most staff being new appointments trained in the requisite techniques.[57] Pincherle made clear, however, that the meeting and paper would not signify a government commitment, and no new resources would be found centrally. Instead – declaring that the work would probably cover areas established under the 1976 planning and priorities system – Pincherle indicated that health authorities could reasonably be expected to bear the burden.[58] The purpose of the meeting would be to assess the estimates made and talk further about resource requirements, as well as to discuss possible changes in organisation, training, and staffing (such as the use of general ophthalmic service opticians, rather than consultants).

The meeting followed the pattern Pincherle laid out. New BDA figures about the incidence of diabetic retinopathy were introduced, and the Association's estimates of need (screening all 1 million people with diabetes, twice a year) and required personnel (100 WTE staff initially, 36 after backlog) were considerably larger than those in the DHSS paper. Following this, discussion then turned to who should conduct screening, with participants disagreeing about the abilities of ophthalmologists, physicians, and opticians. Both sides of the debate agreed, nonetheless, that the contrast between the monotony of the work and the need to maintain vigilance meant that the workload should be shared to prevent mistakes. Moreover, all participants concurred with the BDA's position that specialist DECs were necessary, and should receive referrals from clinics, GPs, and ophthalmologists without requisite equipment. In other words, the meeting demonstrated considerable interest in questions of organisation, management, division of labour, and hierarchy, which, as previous chapters have shown, were being worked out elsewhere in diabetes care and British medicine.

The main outcome of the meeting was that DHSS staff committed themselves to 'look favourably on applications for research grants to assist the establishment of 2–3 pilot centres as a means to assessing the most suitable means of organising ... a service'.[59] The findings would influence debates about training, and it was noted that 'if the pilot schemes showed that a change in [position] was desirable' then the Special Advisory Committee 'would no doubt give serious consideration' to incorporating screening skills into the 'basic training for consultants'.[60] It was on the basis of funding two or three demonstration centres that an administrative civil servant in the meeting forwarded on plans for SMD funds within the DHSS. In light of straitened finances, the plans stressed careful site selection, proposing to establish test centres 'within hospitals which already specialised in the treatment of diabetic eye conditions'. In this way, an 'extremely worthwhile candidate for SMD funds' would require only a 'very modest bid'.[61]

The support for SMD funding of pilot DECs at this juncture should not be a surprise. Firstly, the parlous state of government finances during the late 1970s made retinopathy prevention enticing, but ruled out more extensive options. The government's need to ease anxious capital markets and maintain a stable currency undermined room for policy manoeuvre, with drastic expenditure cuts compounded by conditions attached to an International Monetary Fund loan in 1976.[62] In such conditions, preventive medical activity became of interest 'both on humanitarian and economic grounds', though only limited resources were available for innovation.[63]

Secondly, the BDA was well represented in the meeting. Amongst the attendees were five ophthalmologists (including Mr Blach) and two diabetologists (Professor J. Malins, along with Dr Bloom), with at least five of the eight medical and surgical invitees connected to the BDA.[64] Crucially, as we have seen, these individuals had also been a part of high-level discussion within the Association, and promoted regional organisation in the medical press. They had therefore helped construct the BDA's position on DECs, which was upheld in the meeting and which remained steady over the following five years.

Finally, Labour Party policy on the NHS also meant that DHSS staff were attracted by DECs. The perceived predominance of retinopathy amongst the elderly dovetailed with the new priorities and planning system. Furthermore, the potential position of 'the region' in screening and treatment proved important. Although heavily questioned within NHS reform debates, regional machinery had emerged relatively unscathed from the 1974 NHS changes, and RHAs were central to priority-setting and planning.[65] The idea of regionally organised centres aligned neatly with the politics of the health service at this time, and with the old tradition of technocratic planning within the DHSS.[66] The DEC plan thus gained traction with interested officials, who felt 'one of the attractions at our meeting the other day was the prospect of getting this going in the Regions'.[67] Such favourability did not mean that interested DHSS officials were willing to back any potential applicant. The DHSS received several proposals for DEC funding towards the end of the 1970s that officials deemed inappropriate for support.[68] Nonetheless, this civil service investment proved crucial to the survival of SMD applications during a change of government, even as party policies moved the goalposts for officials.

DECs, neoliberalism, and SMD funding, 1979–1984

Despite support within and without the DHSS, initial discussions over DECs did not lead to earmarked funds for the following year.[69] Almost as soon as momentum for DECs was building, the political and policy context within which advocates for DECs had to function changed considerably.

The general election of 1979 returned the Conservative Party to government, and installed Margaret Thatcher as Prime Minister. Early academic analyses cast the policies and rhetoric of Thatcher's subsequent administrations (1979–90) as an 'end of consensus'. This work suggested that, after 1979, retrenchment and a policy dedication to individualism and free market economics replaced a cross-party, cross-Whitehall policy paradigm which had been forged after the Second World War, built around state intervention in industry and a Keynesian commitment to full employment, as well as generous support for a social wage and the welfare state.[70] Such assessments were consciously put forward by Margaret Thatcher herself, and were in part derived from the critique espoused by leading Conservative figures from 1974 onwards.[71] After the mid-1970s, Thatcher, along with Sir Keith Joseph, vigorously attacked 'the state', its socialist architects, and an undemocratic corporatism with unions as the causes of Britain's ills.[72] State responsibility, they proposed, sapped Britons of their self-discipline and entrepreneurial initiative; robbed individuals and families of choice over schools and parenting; created corrosive 'dependency' amongst social security recipients; failed to confront criminality and delinquency; 'crowded out' businesses from wealth-creating activities; and provided the conditions in which markets – crucial moral and economic technologies – could no longer function.[73]

Although acknowledging that considerable shifts in policy and political discourse took place, scholarship since the 1990s has queried earlier assumptions of consensus or political revolution. These accounts have highlighted significant policy disagreement, change, and opportunism (rather than conviction) before and after 1979.[74] Such work has doubted the extent to which Keynesianism, planning, or economic corporatism had ever been consistently or effectively applied, as well as tracing policies and rhetoric around economic freedom across the post-war period.[75] Likewise, just as the three decades after 1945 were not truly marked by consensus, the two decades after 1979 were not quite as radical as some scholarship would suggest.[76] Conservative administrations certainly incorporated neoliberal analyses into policy-making: critiques of state and economy within which competition and enterprise are considered the most efficacious forms of allocating resources and guaranteeing individual freedom.[77] Yet, rather than supporting efforts to 'roll back the state' *per se*, neoliberal rationalities prompted the creation of an interventionist architecture of monitoring and regulation in the name of competition.[78] Efforts to denationalise industries or introduce market-like mechanisms into welfare services rarely translated into complete freedom from government intervention, and the distance between planning and management practices was perhaps not as great as might have been expected.

This is not to say that the political situation in Britain was unchanged after 1979. Under the Conservatives many areas of policy – from industry and union regulation to social security, finance, and local government – experienced considerable transformation.[79] Nonetheless, some policy modifications had a longer trajectory than a change of government, and many interventions were adjusted considerably in implementation.[80] Equally, the profound social and economic transformations of post-war Britain – as well as the development of government policies – had as much to do with broader international climate, long-term social and cultural trends, party-political strategy, non-governmental organisations, ministerial personalities, and other influences as they did with the Conservative government's particular ideological predilections.[81] Considerable political shifts occurred, but change was rarely as systematic or as ground-breaking as an earlier literature has suggested.[82]

In terms of DECs, along with professional, BDA, and civil service support, the fate of SMD funding was tied closely to shifts in health policy, especially political orientations to welfare service oversight and government spending. The period between 1979 and 1982 witnessed little discussion of SMD funding, even though exchange over trial centres continued. For instance, DHSS officials were in constant contact with the BDA, specialists, and authorities who might potentially house trial DECs.[83] They even brought the problem of retinopathy to the attention of new ministers where possible.[84] Responses to a number of enquiries at this time, however, indicated that attitudes to funding and provision were influenced by a broader government policy of decentralisation in the health services.[85] Partially mirroring the approach taken under the previous administration, DHSS civil servants could offer encouragement to bodies looking to establish specialist screening and treatment services, but no more. Funding decisions were for local authorities, as was made clear in government correspondence and parliamentary replies on issues of retinopathy and diabetes management.[86]

This policy disposition slowly changed after 1982, alongside government interest in NHS managerial reform, but parties interested in SMD funding still faced problems of state finance.[87] On the one hand, there was the issue of spending constraints. Despite intended budget cuts, government expenditure rose in real terms almost every year during Thatcher's premiership.[88] However, spending decreased as a proportion of GDP, and real-terms figures probably reflected shifting demographics and uneven expenditure. Increases in unemployment and retirement, for instance, meant that rising social security payments offset deep cuts elsewhere, and much of the safeguarded NHS expenditure for the early 1980s funded wage increases rather than services.[89] In other words, successive administrations sought to reduce spending on activities that they deemed ineffective or iatrogenic. Although not a high-spending area, DHSS-funded research felt the pinch: as Dr Pincherle explained to colleagues in 1982, initial efforts at pilot studies for retinopathy screening and treatment were 'victims of cuts in research budget[s]'.[90]

On the other hand, as well as imposing financial restraints, the Conservative governments of the 1980s also sought to reform how money was allocated. For a host of individual social security benefits, Conservative administrations expanded extant administrative procedures (such as means testing), introduced taxation and new eligibility criteria, and altered cost-indexing to reverse, freeze, or slow increases.[91] These changes in allocative practices were also applied systemically, encouraged by shifts in political discourse and institutions outside the Conservative Party leadership. The Thatcher administrations allied cash-limited budgeting (introduced to departments under previous Labour governments) with more intense programme review analyses; at the same time, parliamentary reforms of select committees encouraged more rigorous monitoring of the effects of government spending.[92] Policy drives to reallocate government intervention, and increase competition and labour mobility, therefore, were supported by old Treasury concerns about government expenditure and broader emphases on value for money.

It was in this context that DEC planning received a boost in the summer of 1982. In August, Wallace Foulds, Professor of Ophthalmology at the University of Glasgow, sent Pincherle, and contacts at the Scottish Home and Health Department (SHHD), a pre-publication paper on retinopathy prevalence and incidence, with particular focus on the potential costs of a screening and treatment programme for the west of Scotland.[93] Demonstrating the ways in which personnel and research moved across Britain as a whole, Foulds had participated in the initial DHSS panel to discuss DECs in 1977.[94] The networks of interested parties supporting DECs before 1979 had thus held fast, ensuring broad support for the idea across the intervening period.

Moreover, the interconnected structure of British medicine and administrative machinery ensured that, whilst the Scottish health services were in many respects distinct from those of England and Wales, the boundaries separating the NHS's constituent elements could easily be crossed in the right circumstances.[95]

Between the consultation meeting in 1977 and Foulds's paper in 1982, DHSS officials had become aware of numerous publications and projects on retinopathy and its detection and treatment.[96] Foulds's paper, however, was the first substantive piece of work seen by officials that drew together large-scale investigation of prevalence and incidence with costed comparisons of tests, screening staff, and equipment.[97] One medical civil servant who received the paper even suggested that it was 'one of the most exciting [papers] in practical terms I have seen in some time' and exactly 'the sort of health services research we need more of'.[98]

To some extent, the paper confirmed findings from smaller-scale projects and the previous 'best guesses' made by DHSS staff.[99] From a sample of around 1,200 patients, the study estimated the prevalence of different types of retinopathy at 30 per cent, with 10 per cent of people with diabetes estimated to have retinopathy serious enough to go blind. (This was similar to the proportion estimated in 1977, though for different reasons.) Foulds's team found a fresh incidence of retinopathy to be around 5.5–8 per cent, estimating that around 1.2 per cent of patients would have serious cases.[100] At the same time, marking a more overt recognition of economic arguments in motivating change, they noted that 'diabetic retinopathy was the leading cause of blindness in the age groups 20–44 and 45–64[,] underlying the important economic fact that diabetic blindness is the commonest cause of blindness amongst those of working age'.[101] Extrapolating these figures to the west of Scotland region (2.5 million population), the paper then estimated the likely workload for a new system that screened 25,000 people diagnosed with diabetes (1 per cent prevalence) annually. In the first two years, the programme would encounter a backlog of 8,300 patients with retinopathy, of which 2,500 would have serious cases and 1,250 would be treatable. Once these were cleared, the authors then expected to find 300 patients with serious retinopathy per year, of which 150 would need laser therapy.[102]

The respective methods applied to calculating staffing requirements in the Foulds and Pincherle papers make their estimates incomparable. More important for the DHSS staff, however, were Foulds's estimated comparative costs of the scheme if different workers were to undertake

Table 4.1 Estimated costs of different screening modalities

Staff screening	Cost per person screened	Cost per patient identified	Cost per patient treated	Cost-benefit (£)
Physicians	£2.30	£193	£387	1:3.3
Hospital opticians	£1.20	£99.40	£199	1:6.5
General ophthalmic service opticians	£6.84	£570	£1,141	1:1.1

Source: TNA, final report, 'An investigation of the prevalence of diabetic retinopathy'.

screening and treatment.[103] The paper even estimated the total savings in social security arising from preventing blindness through screening and treatment, and provided cost-benefit ratios for each possible alternative. For physicians as screeners, for instance, £3.30 would be saved from social security for every £1 spent (see Table 4.1). Added to these were psychological and social losses to blindness that 'cannot be assessed in economic terms', and the potential earnings (and thus tax revenue) of now employable non-blind persons.[104]

Taken on its own merits, the new paper possessed several logical and practical limitations, given its extrapolation from one small sample to a much larger presumed population. However, within the context of the Conservatives' fiscal management, the considerable excitement amongst DHSS officials is understandable. Almost immediately upon receipt, DHSS staff re-engaged with the SMD grant proposals that they had begun to draw up in 1977. Pincherle forwarded the evidence to colleagues, who recommended preparing a paper for ministers.[105] Pincherle also arranged a meeting of DHSS officials in December 1982 and prepared a fresh paper to present. Reflecting the intensified emphasis on economy within central government, this paper was written with advice from the Economic Advisers' Office.[106] Although health economics did not always prove influential in service reform, the input of economists – and languages of costs and savings – were important here.[107] The new paper broadly used Foulds's figures for incidence and prevalence, but extrapolated for the whole of the UK, and estimated a higher rate of treatability on the basis that regular screening would catch problems earlier.[108] The meeting, which included input from the DHSS Ophthalmological Consultant Adviser, made no considerable alterations to Pincherle's paper, and participants mostly discussed issues of personnel (ratio of staff to patient population, suitable work to be undertaken).[109] With a broad consensus reached, the meeting endorsed Pincherle's suggestion to contact the Finance Division to discuss funding.

The financial prospects did not initially appear favourable. In October 1982, staff received a memo on Centrally Reserved Funds (including those for SMD), which spoke of the assessor's 'generally unfriendly attitude to centrally financed services in the current climate'.[110] After receiving notification that a bid might be made in July 1983, a DHSS advisor 'counsel[led] caution in going very far at this stage in working up detailed bids'. The author cited 'the Chancellor's statement on public expenditure reductions', and remarked that 'when Ministers come to consider bids for central funding there is likely to be very little room to manoeuvre'. In so doing, the correspondent did not seek to close the door on opportunities 'if [a bid] can be demonstrated to be a potentially cost-effective use of central funds'. Rather, 'what it does mean', they concluded, 'is that it would probably not be sensible, or at least it would run the risk of generating false expectations and wasting effort, if work was done at this stage ... [preparing] schemes which are critically dependent on central support'.[111]

Whilst Pincherle did not significantly alter the proposal paper in response, pressure from financial advisors had been anticipated in early drafts of associated documents. A cover note on 'diabetic retinopathy', for instance, repeated Foulds's claims about the epidemiology of blindness, stressing that 'diabetic retinopathy is the most common cause of registered blindness in the 16–64 age group'.[112] A revised paper took references to labour market loss even further. It added that diabetic retinopathy accounted for 'some 2,100 people in the economically active age group becoming blind each year', but that prevention would save on social security 'payments and special facilities for the blind which will [now] not be required'.[113] Moreover, speaking specifically to health service concerns, it suggested that even the NHS might save money. Pincherle was careful not to commit the DHSS to any larger programme, noting how 'any adoption by health authorities of the results of this study, if successful, must of course be a further call upon their resources'.[114] However, by operating more efficiently in the process of screening, he suggested that immediate savings would accrue, and a good service would also gradually free up beds otherwise taken by blind persons.

The discursive frameworks for the study, in other words, were subtly different in tone from those of the late 1970s. Whereas talk had previously been of need, with some reference to economic benefits of prevention, now there was substantial discussion of cost-effectiveness and social security savings. The previous Labour administration had become increasingly interested in such matters when confronting economic turbulence. However, the Conservative government's ideological principles saw it pursue expenditure reductions much more vigorously, and it demonstrated considerable interest in social security reductions, especially during 1982–83.[115] As one medical civil servant declared after receiving the Foulds paper: 'The humanitarian aspect [of improving facilities] is important and continuing' as it had been in earlier years. But the Foulds paper motivated new action because, the official noted, 'for a change and a bonus establishing a programme could actually save money'.[116] Moreover, this focus consolidated views of diabetes management as preventive health practice, ideas which had been discussed in the 1977 White Paper but which did not link to firm action.[117] Neither the control of diabetes nor even avoiding its associated pathologies was of issue here. Retinopathy of some form already had to be present to trigger intervention. Discussions thus centred upon the tertiary prevention of disability. Equally, in linking prevention in diabetes management to costs and savings in the health and social services, the new framework around retinopathy screening programmes also connected health services management with chronic disease control and public health medicine (see Chapter 6).

This is not to deny the influence of other political concerns. The cover note made it clear that inaction might produce very visible and unwelcome inequalities, resulting in 'uneven service development across the country'. Furthermore, 'in this particular case – preventable blindness', the paper warned that 'failure to take an initiative would be particularly embarrassing to both Ministers and this Department'.[118] Though these were seemingly strong words, the tone had been tempered from an earlier draft which suggested that 'where people become blind in circumstances where it need not have happened, they remain a reproach to those responsible, possibly for many years', in contrast to situations where shortages resulted in death. For moral and public relations purposes, the draft thus concluded, 'there does not appear to be the option of doing nothing'.[119] Whilst softening this rhetoric in the final draft, officials nonetheless played heavily on images of an uncaring government that probaby had considerable currency amid rising unemployment and economic dislocation.[120]

This reframing of the issue by civil servants and their professional interlocutors appeared to succeed. The proposal eventually gained the backing of the Office of the Chief Scientist, which administered SMD funding and would provide support for project evaluation. At a meeting in August 1983, the Chief Scientist gathered staff from their Office, the Economic Advisers' Office, and DHSS administrative and medical divisions.[121] Participants noted the foreboding financial advice, but felt that DEC trials would be needed before the DHSS could issue advice on service organisation to RHAs.[122] The meeting devised study parameters, which would form the basis of an SMD application supported by the Office of the Chief Scientist. The project itself would involve three centres (as suggested in 1977) comparing the organisation, costs, and benefits of four type of screeners: ophthalmologists, diabetologists, hospital-based ophthalmic opticians, and general ophthalmic service opticians.[123] With this support gained, Pincherle revised the DHSS paper, and a senior administrative official completed the application. This submission passed up the chain and received ministerial backing in April 1984.[124] Securing additional support from the BDA, the programme was established in 1985, and began reporting its results in 1990–91.[125]

Conclusion: DEC trials, 'New Right' politics, and diabetes

After all the build-up to the DEC trials, the results of the SMD study did not deliver definitive answers. Study centres were established in Sheffield, Oxford, and Exeter, and assessed the sensitivity of different potential screeners (hospital physician, GP, ophthalmic optician) and screening methods in five different patient groups. Ultimately, it was suggested that 'on the evidence' of the studies 'the routine use of any of these screening methods will fail to detect a large proportion of cases with sight threatening diabetic retinopathy'.[126] Equally, the costs for the initial cases found were considerably higher than previous estimates, and the researchers suggested that 'before any policy decisions can be made about a screening programme ... alternative screening strategies need to be evaluated'.[127] By 1995, there was still no national system for diabetic retinopathy in place, and debate continued about who should provide screening.[128]

Regardless, debates about SMD funding formed part of diabetes' return to policy discussion during the 1980s. The creation of a durable policy network around the issue was crucial in this regard. Spurred on by international interest in blindness during the 1960s, and Anglo-American evidence for the effectiveness of retinopathy treatment in the 1970s, medical specialists, professional organisations, and an influential lay-professional non-governmental organisation helped promote the issue to contacts within the DHSS. Behind the scenes, officials retained contact with these agencies, and promoted the cause within the Department prior to ministerial consideration. Figures outside the DHSS were also able to bring forth new evidence bases and promote the issue to the profession and health services. It was a network that spanned Britain, with evidence from Scotland and elsewhere providing momentum to efforts to secure SMD funding for DECs.

Despite the intensity of clinical concern about retinopathy, DHSS support for centres was not easily secured. In a period of financial retrenchment, and shifts in how and where government money was spent, the construction of retinopathy screening within government was crucial. Although economic concerns and disease prevention had been part of discussions before the 1980s, officials responded to growing central concerns about health and welfare expenditure by positioning such issues as the major themes of any debate on retinopathy screening and treatment. By the middle of the 1980s, the second Thatcher administration had also begun to think more seriously about preventive medicine, though the major reforms on this front would wait until the third Thatcher government.[129] As noted in Chapters 2 and 3, this orientation to prevention followed growing international emphasis on health promotion and primary care, as well as being motivated by potential cost reduction in acute care. Such thinking may have influenced ministerial decisions on SMD funding. The personal staff of the Minister for Health, for instance, questioned officials in 1984 about whether the DEC trial might be included in a press release on preventive medicine innovations within the Department.[130] On this occasion, DHSS personnel felt it would be too early to make announcements: funding had been secured, but the programme had yet to choose trial sites and recruit professional staff, with effective decisions here crucial to producing meaningful service standards.[131] Nonetheless, the fact that a pronouncement was considered speaks to how the politics around prevention had made DEC trials attractive.

It is this fusion of cost-reduction, preventive medicine, clinical care, and health service management that gives this episode in diabetes care significance. By the 1980s, doctors had framed surveillance and treatment of diabetes and its sequelae as preventive, as well as clinical, medicine. On a local level, success in secondary and tertiary preventive efforts had been gradually linked to questions of organisation, integration, and management of care. In terms of retinopathy, we can see how such equations were making their way into central government. SMD funding was predicated upon the idea that, once new evidence was produced, new guidance could be offered to health authorities on the most effective means for dividing professional labour. Research would create guidance to manage healthcare activity, resulting in improved health and cost savings.

The way in which DECs were discussed, and SMD funding granted, was informed by previous changes in the relationship between diabetes, clinical medicine, and prevention between the 1960s and early 1980s. It was also indicative of the way in which organisations like the BDA and Royal Colleges were thinking about diabetes more broadly. As we will see in the following chapters, during the 1980s and 1990s this reframing of relations provided the basis for a new role in healthcare governance for these bodies, and their views were transmitted into government via the networks discussed above.

In terms of diabetes, interested politicians like Dr Roger Thomas (Labour, Carmarthen) raised questions about its management and surveillance in Parliament, to some extent forcing government attention onto the issue.[132] Yet diabetes' position at the intersection of cost-reduction, preventive medicine, clinical care, chronic disease, and health service management saw state bodies become interested in the condition as an early testing ground for developing new approaches to managing medicine.

Although not determinative of government direction, neoliberal critiques of welfare were particularly influential here. As noted above, reforms of the health service in the 1980s and 1990s were not implemented according to any blueprint. Nor were they purely 'neoliberal' according to any abstract criteria. However, characteristic of 'New Right' reforms in Britain, these policies did emerge from neoliberal-inspired analyses, and involved considerable transformation of NHS machinery. As a disease already heavily subject to monitoring and management within the health services, diabetes became an interesting testing ground for the new way of governing healthcare. In collaboration with leading professional bodies and other interested parties, the state would produce national standards of process, outcome, and audit, which would inform new contracting arrangements. Likewise, national audits would support local measures to ensure functionality and inform ongoing changes. The specific dynamics of these developments will be explored in the next two chapters. The position of diabetes within new government and professional ideas for health service management and public health, however, began with projects like those funded in retinopathy discussed here.

Notes

1 V. Berridge, *Marketing Health: Smoking and the Discourse of Public Health in Britain, 1945–2000* (Oxford: Oxford University Press, 2007); M. Bufton and V. Berridge, 'Post-war nutrition science and policy making in Britain c.1945–1994: the case of diet and heart disease', in D. Smith and J. Phillips (eds.), *Food, Science, Policy and Regulation in the Twentieth Century: International and Comparative Perspectives* (London: Routledge, 2000), pp. 207–22; A. Mold, '"Everybody likes a drink. Nobody likes a drunk": alcohol, health education, and the public in 1970s Britain', *Social History of Medicine*, 30:3 (2017), 612–36.
2 TNA, FD 23/1442, 20, memo for Dr Owen, 'Meeting on oral hypoglycaemic agents', 5 October 1972.
3 A keyword search for 'diabetes' in Hansard revealed a notable step change in interest, returning 172 results in the 1960s, 187 hits in the 1970s, and 634 hits in the 1980s: http://hansard.millbanksystems.com/search/diabetes (accessed May 2017). Issues of technology and complications were considerable talking points.
4 For post-war health policy networks: V. Berridge (ed.), *Making Health Policy: Networks in Research and Policy after 1945* (Amsterdam: Rodopi, 2005).
5 The retina is a thin layer of light sensitive tissue behind the cornea, iris, and lens of the eye.
6 C. O. Hawthorne, 'On peripheral neuritis and retinal changes in diabetes mellitus', *The Lancet*, 154:3970 (1899), 876–7.
7 S. West, 'Notes on diabetic retinits', *The Lancet*, 183:4728 (1914), 1034–5; R. B. Tattersall, *Diabetes: The Biography* (Oxford: Oxford University Press, 2009), p. 26.
8 Tattersall, *Diabetes*, pp. 82–3.
9 'Retinal changes in diabetes', *The Lancet*, 246:6361 (1945), 114; T. Dornan and S. Vernon, 'Diabetes and the eye', in R. B. Tattersall and E. A. M. Gale (eds.), *Diabetes Clinical Management* (Edinburgh: Churchill Livingstone,

1990), pp. 263–6. See the discussion of control and complications in Chapter 2.
10 J. Malins, *Clinical Diabetes Mellitus* (London: Eyre & Spottiswoode, 1968), pp. 191–8.
11 Ibid., p. 202; 'High carbohydrate diets in diabetes', *The Lancet*, 222:5740 (1933), 538.
12 W. G. Oakley, D. A. Pyke, and K. W. Taylor, *Diabetes and its Management*, 2nd edition (Oxford: Blackwell Scientific Publications, 1975), pp. 119, 127.
13 Interview with Shirley conducted by the University of Oxford, 22 March 2004, available at: www.diabetes-stories.com/interview.asp?UID=4 (accessed April 2017); C. Feudtner, *Bittersweet: Diabetes, Insulin and the Transformation of Illness* (Chapel Hill: University of North Carolina Press, 2003).
14 Respectively: G. Graham, 'The diet in diabetes', *BMJ*, 2:4307 (1943), 116; Oakley et al., *Diabetes and its Management*, 2nd edition, p. 126.
15 Oakley et al., *Diabetes and its Management*, 2nd edition.
16 Malins, *Clinical Diabetes Mellitus*, p. 198.
17 Tattersall, *Diabetes*, pp. 98–100.
18 Malins, *Clinical Diabetes Mellitus*, pp. 198–9.
19 Ibid., pp. 199–202, esp. p. 199.
20 Oakley et al., *Diabetes and its Management*, 2nd edition, p. 126; Malins, *Clinical Diabetes Mellitus*, p. 201.
21 Malins, *Clinical Diabetes Mellitus*, p. 125.
22 Tattersall, *Diabetes*, pp. 101–2.
23 'Retinopathy', *The Lancet*, 299:7758 (1972), 1004.
24 J. Daly, *Evidence-Based Medicine and the Search for a Science of Clinical Care* (Berkeley: University of California Press, 2005).
25 I. Löwy, 'The experimental body', in R. Cooter and J. Pickstone (eds.), *Companion to Medicine in the Twentieth Century* (Abingdon: Routledge, 2003), pp. 443–4. See Chapter 2 above.
26 H. Valier and C. Timmermann, 'Clinical trials and the reorganization of medical research in post-Second World War Britain', *Medical History*, 52:4 (2008), 493–510; J. A. Greene, *Prescribing by Numbers: Drugs and the Definition of Disease* (Baltimore: Johns Hopkins University Press, 2007), pp. 115–47.
27 J. N. Morris, *Uses of Epidemiology*, 2nd edition (Edinburgh: E. & S. Livingstone, 1964); A. L. Cochrane, *Effectiveness and Efficiency: Random Reflections on the Health Services* (London: Nuffield Provincial Hospitals Trust, 1972). On quantification in medicine: G. Weisz, 'From clinical counting to Evidence-Based Medicine', in G. Forland, A. Opinel, and G. Weisz (eds.), *Body Counts: Medical Quantification in Historical and Sociological Perspectives* (Montreal: McGill University Press, 2005), pp. 377–93.

28 Both co-ordination and comparison were essential in securing multiple participating centres, and thus in increasing the power of the study through higher rates of subject enrolment. As Tattersall makes clear, the absence of a standard definition for what was being treated had made drawing conclusions from a mixture of earlier reports impossible: Tattersall, *Diabetes*, pp. 102–3.
29 'Photocoagulation for diabetic retinopathy', *The Lancet*, 308:7976 (1976), 77–8, esp. p. 77.
30 Ibid.
31 Ibid.; Tattersall, *Diabetes*, p. 102.
32 A. Bloom, 'Photocoagulation for diabetic retinopathy', *The Lancet*, 308:7978 (1976), 206.
33 E. M. Kohner and P. J. Barry, 'Prevention of blindness in diabetic retinopathy', *Diabetologia*, 26:3 (1984), 173–9.
34 Bloom, 'Photocoagulation for diabetic retinopathy'; 'Photocoagulation for diabetic retinopathy', p. 78.
35 Though anxiety might arise in some patients as they 'observ[e] the increased interest and activity centred on [their] eyes': ibid. 'Photocoagulation for diabetic retinopathy', p. 78.
36 C. J. Burns-Cox, 'Early detection of diabetic retinopathy', *The Lancet*, 324:8404 (1984), 693–4.
37 H. Valier and R. Bivins, 'Organization, ethnicity and the British National Health Service', in J. Stanton (ed.), *Innovations in Health and Medicine: Diffusion and Resistance in the Twentieth Century* (London: Routledge, 2002), pp. 37–64.
38 'Diabetic retinopathy', *The Lancet*, 296:7682 (1970), 1073–4.
39 Wellcome Library Archive, London (WLA, PP/ASH/A/3, BDA Committee on Blindness 1967–1969, *A Report on Diabetic Blindness in the United Kingdom* (London: BDA, c.1970).
40 WLA, *A Report on Diabetic Blindness*, p. 9.
41 Ibid., pp. 10–13.
42 'Diabetic retinopathy', p. 1073.
43 WLA, *A Report on Diabetic Blindness*, pp. 10–13.
44 J. G. L. Jackson, 'The formation of the Medical and Scientific Section of the British Diabetic Association', *Diabetic Medicine*, 14:10 (1997), 886–91.
45 Respectively: TNA, FD 23/1442, 5294/17 [29], memo by D.M.G.M. to Dr Godfrey, 'Oral hypoglycaemic agents in the treatment of diabetes', 16 January 1973, p. 2; TNA, FD 23/1442, 39, Medical and Scientific Section, BDA, 'Secretary's report for the year ended the 31st December 1972', undated, p. 1. The trial had been sparked by British uncertainty over a major US trial, which indicated that oral hypoglycaemic agents might increase mortality: Greene, *Prescribing by Numbers*, pp. 115–47; Tattersall, *Diabetes*, pp. 131–5.

46 TNA, memo for Dr Owen, 'Meeting on oral hypoglycaemic agents'.
47 Hansard, HC, vol. 912, cols. 1186–9, 8 June 1976.
48 TNA, MH 150/953, letter by Dr Arnold Bloom and Mr Rolf Blach, untitled, 1977, 1. On the Medical and Scientific Section: Jackson, 'The formation of the Medical and Scientific Section', pp. 886–91.
49 TNA, MH 150/953, letter by Dr Arnold Bloom and Mr Rolf Blach. As a consultant surgeon, Mr Blach forwent the title 'doctor'.
50 See responses in file TNA, MH 150/953, 'Hospital Eye Service: facilities for the detection and treatment of diabetic retinopathy; proposed pilot project', 1977–84.
51 TNA, MH 150/953, RJH/JMH, letter by R. J. Hutchinson (Specialist in Community Medicine, Yorkshire RHA) to Dr A. Bloom and Mr. R. Blach, untitled, 13 July 1977; TNA, MH 150/953, EMK/FMH, letter by E. Kohner (Senior Lecturer in Medicine, Royal Postgraduate Medical School, Hammersmith Hospital) to Dr A. Bloom, untitled, 9 June 1977.
52 TNA, MH 150/953, 8B, meeting note, 'Facilities for the detection and treatment of diabetic retinopathy', 1977, p. 1.
53 Ibid.; DHSS, Department of Education and Science, Scottish Office, and Welsh Office, *Prevention and Health*, Cmnd 7047 (London: HMSO, 1977), p. 71.
54 On the importance of post-war lobbying and health policy networks: Berridge, *Marketing Health*.
55 TNA, MH 150/953, 4B, Dr G. Pincherle, draft discussion paper, 'Facilities for the detection and treatment of diabetic retinopathy', 17 November 1977. My thanks to Professor Roberta Bivins for sharing this biographical information.
56 TNA, Pincherle, draft discussion paper, 'Facilities for the detection and treatment of diabetic retinopathy', pp. 1–4, esp. p. 3.
57 WTE was a unit indicating the workload of a full-time member of staff. As members of the clinical team would not be employed solely for this work, predictions used WTE to estimate costs rather than new members of staff *per se*.
58 Services for the elderly, children, and people with mental health and cognitive challenges were the initial priority areas: G. Rivett, *From Cradle to Grave: Fifty Years of the NHS* (London: King's Fund, 1998), pp. 272–5.
59 TNA, meeting note, 'Facilities for the detection and treatment of diabetic retinopathy', p. 1.
60 Ibid., p. 2.
61 TNA, MH 150/953, 5A, memo by N. L. J. Montagu to Mr Mayoh, 'Special Medical Developments: diabetic eye centres', 2 December 1977.
62 P. Addison, *No Turning Back: The Peacetime Revolutions of Post-War Britain* (Oxford: Oxford University Press, 2010), pp. 270–1.

63 DHSS et al., *Prevention and Health*, p. 71.
64 Another prominent diabetes specialist, J. Nabarro, was invited but could not attend.
65 C. Webster, *The Health Services since the War*, vol. 2: *Government and Health Care, the British National Health Service, 1958–1979* (London: HMSO, 1996), pp. 453–579, esp. pp. 507–8, 606–13.
66 R. Klein, *The New Politics of the NHS: From Creation to Reinvention*, 5th edition (Oxford: Radcliffe, 2006), pp. 1–21, 46–75.
67 TNA, MH 150/953, 9A, memo by N. L. J. Montagu to Dr Pincherle, 'Proposed diabetic eye centre: St George's Tooting', 10 January 1978.
68 For instance: TNA, MH 150/953, 10A, memo by L. B. Hunt to Dr Pincherle, 'Proposal for the establishment of a diabetic regional eye centre at St George's Hospital', 11 January 1978.
69 TNA, MH 150/953, file note by R. Weighton for Dr Pincherle, untitled, 5, 3 March 1978.
70 P. Addison, *The Road to 1945: British Politics and the Second World War* (London: Pimlico, 1994 [1975]); D. Kavanagh and P. Morris, *Consensus Politics from Attlee to Major*, 2nd edition (Oxford: Blackwell, 1995).
71 P. Kerr, *Post-War British Politics: From Conflict to Consensus* (London: Routledge, 2001).
72 R. Saunders, '"Crisis? What crisis?" Thatcherism and the seventies', in B. Jackson and R. Saunders (eds.), *Making Thatcher's Britain* (Cambridge: Cambridge University Press, 2012), pp. 25–42, esp. p. 34.
73 M. Thatcher, 'It's your freedom they hate', *Sunday Express*, 23 November 1975, *Margaret Thatcher Foundation*, available at: www.margaretthatcher.org/document/102808 (accessed April 2017); M. Thatcher, 'My kind of Tory Party?', *Daily Telegraph*, 30 January 1975, *Margaret Thatcher Foundation*, available at: www.margaretthatcher.org/document/102600 (accessed April 2017); Sir K. Joseph, speech given at Edgbaston, 19 October 1974, *Margaret Thatcher Foundation*, available at: www.margaretthatcher.org/document/101830 (accessed April 2017); M. Thatcher, speech given in Derby, 2 May 1975, *Margaret Thatcher Foundation*, available at: www.margaretthatcher.org/document/102458 (accessed April 2017). See also S. Hall, 'The great moving right show', in S. Hall and M. Jacques (eds.), *The Politics of Thatcherism* (London: Lawrence and Wishart in Association with Marxism Today, 1983), pp. 19–39; N. Timmins, *The Five Giants: A Biography of the Welfare State* (London: Fontana Press, 1996), pp. 356–60.
74 Kerr, *Post-War British Politics*. For economic policy: R. Lowe, *The Welfare State in Britain since 1945*, 3rd edition (Basingstoke: Palgrave Macmillan, 2005), pp. 125–6.
75 J. Tomlinson, 'Why was there never a "Keynesian revolution" in economic policy?', *Economy and Society*, 10:1 (1981), 72–87; N. Rollings,

'Poor Mr Butskell: a short life, wrecked by schizophrenia?', *Twentieth Century British History*, 5:2 (1994), 183–205; G. O'Hara, *From Dreams to Disillusionment: Economic and Social Planning in the 1960s* (Basingstoke: Palgrave Macmillan, 2007); N. Rollings, 'Cracks in the post-war Keynesian settlement? The role of organised business in Britain in the rise of neoliberalism before Margaret Thatcher', *Twentieth Century British History*, 24:4 (2013), 637–59.
76 On 'Thatcherism' and its literature: C. Hay, 'Whatever happened to Thatcherism?', *Political Studies Review*, 5:2 (2007), 183–201.
77 D. Stedman Jones, *Masters of the Universe: Hayek, Friedman, and the Birth of Neoliberal Politics* (Princeton: Princeton University Press, 2014); M. Foucault, *The Birth of Biopolitics: Lectures at the Collège de France, 1978–79*, trans. G. Burchell, ed. M. Senellart (Basingstoke: Palgrave Macmillan, 2008).
78 Cf. D. Harvey, *A Brief History of Neoliberalism* (Oxford University Press, 2005).
79 Addison, *No Turning Back*, pp. 259–314; Timmins, *The Five Giants*, pp. 369–494.
80 D. Marsh and R. A. W. Rhodes (eds.), *Implementing Thatcherite Policies: Audit of an Era* (Buckingham: Open University Press, 1992).
81 A. Gamble, *The Free Economy and the Strong State: The Politics of Thatcherism*, 2nd edition (Basingstoke: Macmillan, 1994); Timmins, *The Five Giants*, 369–494; Klein, *The New Politics of the NHS*, pp. 140–86.
82 B. Jackson and R. Saunders (eds.), *Making Thatcher's Britain* (Cambridge: Cambridge University Press, 2012).
83 TNA, MH 150/953, 23A, memo by Dr Pincherle to Mr Saville and Dr Buxton (DHSS), untitled, 2 December 1980; TNA, MH 150/953, 33A, minutes of a meeting on 8 June 1982, 'Economic appraisal of screening and early treatment of diabetic retinal blood vessel disorders', 9 July 1982.
84 TNA, MH 150/953, 21B, note by A. G. Saville to Dr Pincherle (and response), untitled, 26 June 1979; TNA, MH 150/953, 22A, note by Dr Pincherle to Mr Godfrey, untitled, 9 July 1979.
85 Klein, *The New Politics of the NHS*, pp. 96–101.
86 TNA, MH 150/953, 19A, letter by G. Pincherle to Dr M. Hartog (Honorary Consultant Physician, Southmead Hospital, Bristol), untitled, 23 March 1979; Hansard, HC, vol. 32, col. 495W, 24 November 1982.
87 Klein, *The New Politics of the NHS*, pp. 114–23.
88 R. Chote, R. Crawford, C. Emmerson, and G. Tetlow, *IFS Briefing Note 5: Public Spending Under Labour* (London: Institute for Fiscal Studies: 2010), pp. 3–4, available at: https://www.ifs.org.uk/bns/bn92.pdf (accessed May 2017).
89 J. Bradshaw, 'Social security', in Marsh and Rhodes (eds.), *Implementing Thatcherite Policies*, pp. 85–6; Timmins, *The Five Giants*, p. 385. Spending

as a proportion of GDP decreased from 48.1 per cent in 1982–83 to 39.2 per cent in 1989–90.
90 TNA, MH 150/953, 15, note at front of file by Dr Pincherle for Mr Saville, untitled, 7 April 1982.
91 P. Pierson, *Dismantling the Welfare State? Thatcher, Reagan and the Politics of Retrenchment* (Cambridge: Cambridge University Press, 1994).
92 Timmins, *The Five Giants*, p. 381; P. Hennessey, *Whitehall* (London: Fontana Press, 1990), pp. 330–7.
93 TNA, MH 150/953, 35C, final report, 'An investigation of the prevalence of diabetic retinopathy among patients attending a diabetic clinic and the cost effectiveness of its identification and treatment', undated (c.August 1982).
94 TNA, MH 150/953, 35B, letter by Professor W. S. Foulds (University of Glasgow) to Dr G. Pincherle, untitled, 20 August 1982.
95 J. Stewart, 'The National Health Service in Scotland, 1947–74: Scottish or British', *Historical Research*, 76:193 (2003), 389–410.
96 For instance, see papers listed at 18A and 20A in file TNA, MH 150/953.
97 TNA, MH 150/953, minutes of a meeting on 8 June 1982; TNA, MH 150/953, 57A, memo by Dr Pincherle to Mr Mancini (Economic Advisers' Office), 28 September 1983. Prior discussion with the BDA about comparative screening costs in Stoke Mandeville had proved disappointing.
98 TNA, MH 150/953, 35B, memo by Dr Sweeney to Dr Pincherle, 'Treatment of diabetic retinopathy', 20 September 1982.
99 TNA, final report, 'An investigation of the prevalence of diabetic retinopathy'.
100 Ibid., pp. 3–4 for raw figures, p. 1 for summaries.
101 Ibid., p. 10.
102 Ibid., pp. 9–10.
103 Ibid., pp. 11–13.
104 Ibid., pp. 13–14.
105 TNA, MH 150/953, 35A, memo by Dr Pincherle to Mr Saville, Dr Sweeney, Dr Ford, and Mr Ratcliffe, 'Treatment of diabetic retinopathy', 13 September 1982; TNA, memo by Dr Sweeney, 'Treatment of diabetic retinopathy'.
106 TNA, MH 150/953, 40A, memo by A. Burchell (Economic Advisers' Office, DHSS) to Dr Pincherle, 'Diabetic retinopathy', 6 December 1982. See also the attached paper, pp. 1–2.
107 S. Sheard, 'Space, place and (waiting) time: reflections on health policy and politics', *Health Economics, Policy and Law*, 13:3–4 (2018), 226–50. My thanks to Professor Sheard for allowing me advance access. Cf. J. Stanton, 'The cost of living: kidney dialysis, rationing and health

economics in Britain, 1965–1996', *Social Science & Medicine*, 49:9 (1999), 1169–82.
108 TNA, MH 150/953, 43C, meeting paper by Dr Pincherle, 'Diabetic retinopathy – screening and treatment', c. December 1982, p. 2.
109 TNA, MH 150/953, 43B, meeting note, 'Diabetic retinopathy', c.December 1982, pp. 1–2.
110 TNA, MH 150/953, 37C, memo by Mr Jewesbury, 'Centrally Reserved Funds', 20 October 1982.
111 TNA, MH 150/953, 47A, memo by T. J. Mathews to Dr Pincherle, 'Screening of diabetic retinopathy', 19 July 1983.
112 TNA, MH 150/953, 44A, cover note, 'Diabetic retinopathy', c.December 1982, p. 1.
113 TNA, MH 150/953, 66B, memo by T. E. Nodder to Mr Alcock on central funding bids, untitled, 21 March 1984, p. 3.
114 Ibid.
115 I. Kirkpatrick, S. Ackroyd, and R. Walker, *The New Managerialism and Public Service Professions: Change in Health, Social Services and Housing* (Basingstoke: Palgrave Macmillan, 2005), p. 52.
116 TNA, memo by Dr Sweeney to Dr Pincherle, 'Treatment of diabetic retinopathy'.
117 DHSS et al., *Prevention and Health*, pp. 71, 82.
118 TNA, memo by T. E. Nodder to Mr Alcock, p. 4.
119 TNA, cover note, 'Diabetic retinopathy', p. 2.
120 Addison, *No Turning Back*, pp. 279–84.
121 TNA, MH 150/953, 54D, minutes, 'Note of a meeting held on 22 August 1983', pp. 1–3.
122 Ibid., p. 1.
123 Ibid., pp. 1–3.
124 TNA, memo by T. E. Nodder to Mr Alcock; TNA, MH 150/953, 6/18, memo by Mr Alcock to Mr Nodder, 'Prevention of inherited disease; diabetic retinopathy screening', 10 April 1984.
125 M. J. Buxton, M. J. Sculpher, B. A. Ferguson, J. E. Humphreys, J. F. B. Altman, D. J. Spiegelhalter, A. J. Kirby, J. S. Jacob, H. Bacon, S. B. Dudbridge, J. W. Stead, T. G. Feest, H. Cheng, S. L. Franklin, P. Courtney, J. F. Talbot, R. Ahmed, and T. R. Dabbs, 'Screening for treatable diabetic retinopathy: a comparison of different methods', *Diabetic Medicine*, 8:4 (1991), 371–7.
126 Ibid., pp. 371–7, quotation at p. 376.
127 M. J. Buxton, M. J. Sculpher, B. A. Ferguson, J. E. Humphreys, J. F. B. Altman, D. J. Spiegelhalter, A. J. Kirby, J. S. Jacob, H. Bacon, S. B. Dudbridge, J. W. Stead, T. G. Feest, H. Cheng, S. L. Franklin, P. Courtney, J. F. Talbot, R. Ahmed, and T. R. Dabbs, 'A relative cost-effectiveness

analysis of different methods of screening for diabetic retinopathy', *Diabetic Medicine*, 8:7 (1991), 644–50, quotation at p. 650.
128 P. M. Hart, D. B. Archer, and A. B. Atkinson, 'Diabetic patients should continue to be assessed by direct ophthalmoscopy', *BMJ*, 312:7047 (1996), 1670.
129 Klein, *The New Politics of the NHS*, pp. 133–5.
130 TNA, MH 150/953, memo by J. P. Cashman to Dr Halliday, 'Diabetic retinopathy screening', 68A, 14 May 1984.
131 TNA, MH 150/953, 70B, memo by N. P. Halliday to Mr Cashman, 'Screening for diabetic retinopathy', 15 May 1984; TNA, MH 150/953, 70C, memo by Dr Pincherle to Dr Halliday, 'Screening for diabetic retinopathy', 14 May 1984.
132 Hansard, HC, vol. 988, cols. 146–7W, 8 July 1980.

5

Constructing standards at a time of crisis

Projects like the SMD-funded retinopathy screening trials reflected the British state's growing engagement with diabetes during the 1980s. In that specific instance, the DHSS's hopes for generating organisational guidance for the NHS were disappointed. Central state interest in diabetes management, however, remained undimmed, and much more extensive standards for diabetes care would be produced by the new millennium.

The work of elite practitioners and specialists proved integral to maintaining state interest in both diabetes and service guidance. Reflecting their historic concerns with service organisation, and engaging with mounting critiques of medicine made from within and without the profession, various professional bodies, international organisations, and the BDA became increasingly concerned about standards of diabetes care over the last quarter of the twentieth century. The Royal Colleges and BDA, for instance, collaborated in drawing up guidance on service organisation in 1977, and audited the staffing and facilities available for NHS diabetes management in 1984. Into the early 1990s, these bodies devised more formal clinical guidelines: specialised documents providing specific advice on acceptable standards of disease management, encompassing not just organisation, but also process and outcomes.[1] As discussed in Chapter 3, since the 1970s some innovative practitioners had come to see structured care – built around locally codified protocol and audit – as the embodiment of good diabetes management. During the late 1980s and early 1990s, however, the production of guidelines increased to a rate hitherto unknown, both within diabetes care and in British medicine in general.[2] Guidelines and their standards, in other words, entered the very fabric of medical practice.

Examining a mixture of published and unpublished guidelines, this chapter traces the development of standards documents in British diabetes care from the late 1970s to the early 1990s. It argues, firstly, that the nature of guidance shifted dramatically over these decades, developing in ways that opened care to external management and challenged traditional views about clinical decision-making.[3] Initially covering ideal facilities and staffing, the parameters of guidance expanded to encompass standards for care process and targets for therapeutic outcomes as concerns over clinical standards and professional accountability grew. Moreover, indicative of novel visions of professionalism that emphasised self-reflection and peer critique, the new documents covered not just disease management, but also the process of review; they aimed to structure care and audit, and to provide benchmarks against which performance (and by extension, professionals themselves) could be managed.

Secondly, this chapter underlines the centrality of elite medical professionals to the production of national guidance on best practice during the 1980s and 1990s, beginning a process that would fundamentally alter the regulation of British medicine in the following decades. Operating within nationally focused organisations like the BDA and Royal Colleges, as well as international agencies like the WHO, groups of specialists and prominent British doctors created early guidelines to structure the work of fellow physicians. They did so, moreover, in the name of 'quality'. During the mid-twentieth century, most doctors saw the quality of medicine as dependent upon the employment of sufficient numbers of trained and experienced professionals, often working together, with access to the latest diagnostic and therapeutic technologies. However, amid growing popular, political, and medical criticisms of clinical practice, academic doctors in particular began to reframe concepts of quality during the last decades of the twentieth century. Drawing on concepts and technologies developed in medical research and education, elite practitioners cast quality as measurable, assessed in relation to defined outcome measures, and best secured by following agreed protocol standards and undertaking regular review. Pre-war clinical medicine had been subject to external constraints and peer discussion, but in issuing guidance post-war specialists and their organisations began to add layers to existing, informal regimes of clinical government. During the late 1980s and the 1990s, that is, elite medical professionals produced national standards to directly inform local protocols (previously devised through experience and negotiation) and provide the basis for effective audit. In fact, moves to establish national strategies to guide and monitor the performance of health authorities could be seen in the changing form of guidelines, which shifted from published reports to consensus statements and technical documents. Thus, though not connected to a formal structure or hierarchy at this point, leading specialists (along with the range of bodies to which they were attached) were part of a project to restratify the government of British medicine. Whilst not entirely successful, by the mid-1990s their efforts created the political space for more the fulsome regulatory architecture of clinical governance that emerged at the turn of the millennium.

In taking a deeper look at guidelines within diabetes management, this chapter explores their expanding remit and the ways in which they made certain forms of work and organisation possible.[4] It also traces the roots of a more fundamental reorganisation of medicine in Britain at the end of the twentieth century, one structured by political, cultural, and social trends, but nonetheless driven in part by medical practitioners themselves. Finally, although providing an important window onto broader changes, this chapter also highlights how diabetes management – along with chronic disease management more broadly – was deeply embedded within the guideline movement. In so doing, it provides the groundwork for assessing how specialists and their various institutions opened space for, and intersected with, government efforts at professional regulation, which are explored in Chapter 6.

British medicine under fire: regulating quality in medicine

By the 1970s, questions about the quality of care provided by British doctors had begun to be raised from numerous quarters. Not all concerns were related to clinical decision-making. Some focused on the demeanour of staff, whilst others related to access to services and distribution of resources. Nonetheless, this 'crisis of quality' intersected with several other debates – most notably those concerning the costs of care and the need for greater accountability in public life – to undermine faith in long-established mechanisms of training and licensing.[5] It was this conflation of debates over quality, cost, and accountability that produced calls for more formal systems of regulation for British medicine, and that set the stage for the construction of clinical guidelines.

Sustained public concerns over standards in British medicine first emerged during the late 1960s, propelled by an increasingly critical British media. Popular media interest in healthcare had increased over the post-war period. Whilst some doctors, particularly those involved in public health campaigns, could turn public curiosity to their advantage, increased attention also brought heightened scrutiny of medical practice.[6] Towards the end of the 1960s, journalists investigated reports of appalling conditions within long-stay and psychiatric hospitals, and the resulting exposés sparked political reactions.[7] The DHSS launched its own reviews and attempted to subject hospitals to inspection and independent advice. It also reformed complaints mechanisms, notably creating an ombudsman.[8] Intended reforms were attenuated in practice. For instance, the ombudsman could not examine complaints concerning clinical decision-making. Nonetheless, continual media attention ensured that 'scandals' became a regular feature of reportage into the 1980s, and doctors became subject to public criticism.[9] Campaigns for change emerged out of such scrutiny, and throughout the 1980s parliamentary figures pressured the General Medical Council to clarify minimum standards for ethics and professional conduct and to bring incompetence into the disciplinary arena.[10]

The weakness of complaints mechanisms available to professionals and the public sat at the heart of many scandals, and the issue greatly concerned bodies claiming to speak for patient-consumers. The emergence of these organisations during the 1960s coincided with the broader professionalisation of collective consumer voices in post-war Britain and their institutionalisation within state bodies.[11] Moreover, groups like the Patients' Association built upon contemporaneous public demands for autonomy and political accountability. Recent research on the 1970s and 1980s, for instance, has traced the migration of accountability practices from financial institutions to public and commercial life and examined the reformulation of auditing practices within government.[12] Such work has also examined the ways in which 'ordinary' people came to express desire for greater control over their lives, and to reinterpret collective identities in terms of individual rights.[13] The creation of the NHS had recast health as a basic social right within the public imagination, and demands for professional accountability and patient rights can be seen in the work of patient organisations.[14] These agencies helped to move complaints beyond long-stay hospitals, assisting patients with individual grievances and building campaigns to reform procedures.[15] Along with Community Health

Councils (created in 1974 to represent consumer voices in the NHS), these organisations also surveyed patient opinions on health services, identified areas for improvement, and worked with health service bodies to implement changes.[16] Whilst not always critical of medical performance, this work added to concerns about service quality.

Anxieties about quality were not only expressed by public and political bodies. By the 1970s, certain sections of the medical profession had also questioned the capacity of certification, informal regulation, and discipline to effectively ensure quality care. During the mid-century, for instance, dissatisfied GPs, registrars, and consultants expressed numerous frustrations with the NHS, ranging from underinvestment and poor resource distribution to colleagues' attitudes to patients and – particularly in general practice – the detrimental impact of professional isolation on care.[17] Quality practice was seen to depend on more than just trained professionals with good character, also requiring effective distribution and combination of staff as well as access to up-to-date facilities and treatments. For the most part, however, these criticisms left the existing framework of regulation alone. Despite dissatisfaction with elements of medical education, critics trusted the system to produce practitioners whose clinical judgements could be relied upon.[18]

Later criticisms, by contrast, focused upon questions of knowledge and performance at the heart of this traditional model. From the late 1950s onwards, a small number of doctors and academics began to make uncomfortable criticisms about the efficacy of medical practices and the inconsistency of doctors' decision-making. Such assessments developed out of older conflicts between cultures of individual expertise and universal knowledge in medicine.[19] By the 1960s and 1970s, British epidemiologists and clinical researchers began to use trials and, to a lesser degree, observational studies as a basis for criticising much medical practice.[20] Perhaps most famously, Archie Cochrane suggested that many services and treatments – including those in diabetes – had not been proved effective via 'scientific' experimentation grounded in statistical theory.[21] As a result, he argued that considerable sums of public monies were either being wasted on potentially inefficacious treatment (based on fallible experience and tradition) or were being deployed inefficiently (because the best means of deploying effective tests or therapies had not been established).

Similar critiques were voiced by practitioners of newly institutionalised disciplines, such as health economics and health service research, that took the delivery of care as their object of study.[22] Academic units in York and London, as well as think-tanks like the Office for Health Economics, became sites for raising questions about large variations in healthcare, in part building upon epidemiological studies of variation in diagnostic testing and interpretation.[23] Contributing to longer-term trends in the standardisation of categories and techniques of investigation, these disciplines problematised clinical decision-making and sought to find practices offering the most efficient outcomes for routine care.[24] In so doing, they further undermined the idea that high standards could emerge solely from the effective distribution of well-trained practitioners and high-technology medicine. Cochrane himself even recommended a loose system of monitoring, guideline production, and protocol dissemination using the existing architecture of Hospital Activity Analysis data systems, scientific papers, and 'Cogwheel' clinical management committees.[25] He also considered the loss of clinical and administrative freedoms resulting from setting and reviewing parameters to be worthwhile if outcomes were improved.[26]

Finally, these discussions about standards of care and regulation of medical professionals were closely connected to other concerns about health service costs and broader debates about accountability. As discussed in Chapter 1, the unexpected costs of the NHS during the late 1940s and early 1950s provoked widespread political concerns about the service's viability. We have already noted how state agencies responded in the 1960s and 1970s, seeking to incorporate professionals into hospital administrative structures and hoping that increased information about clinical decisions and resource use would encourage better self-management and reduce costs.[27] As we will see in Chapter 6, in the decades following the 1970s, governments took even more strident moves in this direction, with neoliberal analyses of professional self-interest and market efficiency underpinning the use of new accountability techniques.

Again, however, elite medical professionals and academic researchers had linked discussions of quality with concerns about public expenditure and accountability ahead of political developments. As well as generating parliamentary attention, the problems facing the new service drew interest from researchers and practitioners, and especially from academics politically dedicated to the pursuit of social equality. Alongside emergent health economists and service researchers, this small group of professionals connected questions over service finance with critiques of clinical practice, and from the late 1950s fostered new academic disciplines from the search for service stability and improvement.[28]

In 1957, for instance, the pioneer GP and primary care researcher John Fry reflected upon the way in which GPs received remuneration amid financial disputes with the then Conservative government.[29] In a letter to the *Lancet*, he mused upon a 'lack of supervision' in current arrangements. Whilst 'freedom of the individual to practise medicine according to his own views and principles must be jealously guarded', Fry wrote, 'we are being paid out of public monies to care for our patients'. It thus 'seems only right that some steps be taken to ensure that the public is receiving a sufficient standard of medical care', none of which were presently in place.[30] Admitting that 'no-one likes "controls"', he went on to suggest that 'there exist innumerable safeguards in hospital practice to see that suitable standards are being maintained and these are accepted as inevitable and reasonable interferences'. In the case of general practice, he recommended a mix of reforms. These included some pay-for-performance activities – 'whereby the practitioner who is providing a high standard of care would have a scale of increased remuneration based on some agreed standards' (for instance, related to the organisation of practices) – as well as the limiting of certain drugs for 'use in specific diseases'. Along with reforms to hospital prescribing and administration, the latter might provide some remedy for 'the ever rising cost' of 'the whole service'.[31]

Jerry Morris, a qualified clinician and renowned epidemiologist, echoed Fry's views.[32] As one summary of a lecture, also given in 1957, put it: 'Every system, in Dr Morris's view, needs itself to be regularly scrutinised, and routine systems need built-in controls of quality.' Connecting these views to broader medical and business culture, Dr Morris went on to suggest that 'this is widely accepted in industry, in biochemistry, and in bacteriology; and there is great scope for its application in clinical medicine and the health services'. The cost of the NHS was not far from his thoughts. 'At present remarkably little attempt is being made to ascertain how our £500 million health service is working, what are the needs to be met, and how well they are being met.' Comparing variations in 'the average prescription rate' in different cities and areas of the country, he asked, 'what do these figures mean? Would not a coöperative [sic] inquiry by the local medical committees of these towns ... be of more local value – not only in showing answers but in showing how to tackle such questions[?]'[33]

The challenge of such views to predominant thinking about professional practice should not be downplayed. The invocation of controls or investigations had been strongly feared by doctors who were sceptical – or even simply hesitant – about employment in state-funded services during the 1940s and early 1950s. These concerns had been particularly strong amongst GPs, many of whom had joined the NHS only on the proviso that they would operate as 'independent unit[s]', 'not subject in ... purely professional judgements to any lay authority or ... superior medical officer'.[34] Such freedom was necessary, firstly, because clinical medicine was considered irreducible to rigid formula. Revitalising a powerful turn of-the-century rhetoric, opponents of universal state service spoke of how 'the practice of medicine' was 'more of an art than a science' and 'an art, moreover, applied in an intimate personal relationship between doctor and patient'.[35] The variability of clinical disease, in other words, meant that experience provided the soundest basis for decision-making, and only a doctor who knew the individual peculiarities of their patient could determine the appropriate course of action in any given case. References to 'intimate' relationships, moreover, recalled the ethical obligation of the doctor to the patient that lay at the heart of the professional encounter. Medical practitioners were duty-bound to do what they felt was in the best interests of the patient, and if clinical autonomy were curtailed they could neither be fully accountable for their care nor effectively fulfil their professional commitments.

Secondly, the inviolability of clinical autonomy touched the very heart of professional self-image. GPs dissatisfied with restrictions in the early NHS, for instance, referred to 'charge[s] of excessive prescribing' as 'degrading and insulting' and as indicative of a lack of 'trust [in] the clinical acumen of the doctor'. Already frustrated about their exclusion from the hospital, they wondered where 'the intrusion on our liberty' would 'cease', and feared becoming 'an outcast of the profession'.[36] Similarly, despite hospitals having well-established clinical hierarchies to oversee the practice of junior clinicians, anxieties about controls also existed within hospital practice.[37] For example, when the Ministry of Health recommended that NHS bodies appoint 'consultant[s] in administrative charge' to improve co-ordination of hospital work during the early 1950s, civil servants also felt compelled to clarify that the appointment of such figures was not intended to 'confer any authority over the clinical freedom of other consultants in the[ir] department'.[38] Across the profession, therefore, freedom of action was a mark of status as well as being central to views of good and ethical medicine.

In light of such views, it is unsurprising that the majority of doctors were initially lukewarm to critiques of medical care.[39] However, facing mounting political and academic critique in the decades after the 1950s, some British practitioners – often GPs involved in innovative training programmes, or clinicians with experience of trial work and international practice – began to respond proactively to concerns about standards and the need for review.[40] As noted in Chapter 3, hospital clinicians and GPs engaged with 'medical audit' after the 1960s, drawing on developments in market-oriented and insurance-based systems.[41] Similarly, as the pressures of resource constraints built during the 1970s and 1980s, debates about clinical autonomy became more intense.[42] Leading journals and academic practitioners developed earlier arguments, suggesting that the financial insufficiencies in the NHS made setting limits to clinical activity in individual cases an ethical responsibility to protect the collective.[43] More strident voices even echoed Cochrane's assault on individual judgement, suggesting that clinical decisions should now follow only where trials had proved measures effective.[44] Criticisms of the profession and the drive for audit were also reinforced by philosophers, sociologists, and political scientists publishing in popular books and journals, exposing doctors to outside perspectives on accountability and 'quality.'[45]

This was the context within which guidelines emerged. Critiques had been made about the nature, cost, and quality of medical practice from within medicine and without. A small minority of doctors and academics tried to address their concerns through novel methods for some time, but external pressure from patients and political bodies accelerated the process and informed responses. Guidelines had been mooted as a sensible way to steer practitioners in certain situations, and local protocol had already been devised in some locations to manage care. A drive for better monitoring of care as an educational aid also encouraged the development of standards. In the case of diabetes, tentative guidelines (and allied auditing systems) began with service facilities and staffing before moving on to process and outcomes. This shift itself marked a significant transformation in the nature of medical regulation and autonomy. However, attention also needs to be paid to the agencies involved in guideline production. The lead taken by professional bodies, international organisations, and the BDA not only highlighted the prominence of professionals themselves in the reformulation of managed medicine. It also marked a shift in the organisation of British medicine, with elite agencies laiming to more formally regulate the activity of local practitioners.

The emergence of guidelines in diabetes care: facilities, staffing, and nomenclature

As Chapter 1 outlined, the first official guidance on diabetes care emerged from professional advisory mechanisms that were embedded in the early NHS. Coming in the form of a Ministry of Health circular, it was not extensive. Over its eight points and three sub-points, the two-page document offered health authorities advice on organisation, bed requirements, and staffing of regional services. Although offering one quantified norm on the provision of beds (one bed per every fifty patients with diabetes), the circular's vague advice was respectful of decentralised decision-making and mindful of the way specialist services were structured around regional hierarchies of hospital provision.[46] As such, the guidance focused upon how authorities might scale up provision at different levels of the service. For instance, the circular advised that local clinics should have 'facilities for urine testing and blood sugar estimations, and in addition to medical staff should have a sister trained in dietetics and insulin administration as well as one or more other nurses'. For larger centres, dealing with greater numbers of complex patients, a 'full range of ancillary facilities, notably pathological and radiological' should be complemented by 'necessary nursing staff and dietitians and probably a part-time almoner and also chiropodist'.[47] Finally, the circular advised that the largest centres – at the apex of the system, and probably based 'in Teaching Hospitals' – should each be run by a diabetes specialist, or at least 'a general physician with a special interest in the condition'.[48] The circular then concluded by proposing that in 'each hospital region there should be a scheme, drawn up by the Regional Hospital Board in consultation with Boards of Governors, for the provision of special facilities'.[49]

The circular itself did not carry the word 'guideline'. Indeed, the term did not appear to be commonly deployed in British medical discourse until around the 1970s, and even then it initially operated with a number of interconnected meanings.[50] During the 1960s and early 1970s, for instance, 'guideline' could refer to physical signs indicative of future diagnostic or therapeutic action; general rules of thumb guiding clinical practice; or principles, papers, or pieces of evidence that could aid

Constructing standards at a time of crisis 189

clinical decision-making.[51] It was not until the mid-1970s that the term 'guideline' was used for a specific type of document and official regulation, predominantly concerning service organisation.[52]

Nonetheless, despite the 1953 circular neither being called a guideline nor resembling later algorithmic forms, it reflected a new type of documentary advice to hospital doctors and administrators designing services.[53] It was produced specifically to offer external advice on the organisation of care, even if the Ministry itself ultimately lacked the mechanisms and political interest to ensure take-up.[54] Moreover, though further state-funded guidance on diabetes care would not be issued until the mid-1980s, the circular also marked the beginning of a process in which numerous agencies set standards for diabetes care.

In general, the guidance produced for the next three decades sat within the same framework as the 1953 guidance. Most took the form of reports and focused on facilities, staffing, and organisation, setting aside issues of clinical decision-making. There were some variations. For instance, in light of rising prevalence estimates in colonial and international surveys, in 1965 the WHO brought together an expert committee on diabetes which included British representation.[55] Although it covered a host of topics, the WHO was interested in the accumulation of accurate and comparable data between locations, seeing it as central to 'motivat[ing] action to resolve' the 'public health problems of diabetes'.[56] As a result, along with very detailed guidance on establishing screening services, the committee produced clear provisional nomenclature standards for different stages of diabetes, and recommended quantified thresholds for definitively ruling out and providing diagnoses.[57] The hope in fixing such criteria would be to standardise units for statistical comparison (providing a powerful conceptual and practical precedent for managing medical practice).[58]

Ultimately, the WHO standards appeared to make little immediate impact upon clinical care. Textbooks continued to use discordant terminology and diagnostic criteria, and the report itself was inconsistently cited.[59] Instead, the report's standards laid the foundations for important research programmes, and for more influential diagnostic criteria produced in 1980 and revised in 1985.[60] Though the 1965 report exercised little influence, it – and its successors – marked an attempt to set standards that possessed clinical implications. The production and reception of all three WHO reports also signified the increased movement of British diabetologists into expanding transnational networks, and the way in which international organisations like the WHO would exercise influence on British diabetes policy (as discussed further in Chapter 6).[61]

Perhaps more typical of guidelines in this period, however, was the 1977 report from a working party of the Standing Committee on Endocrinology and Diabetes Mellitus of the Royal College of Physicians of London (RCP), in which the focus remained upon facilities and staffing.[62] The Standing Committee itself emerged from elite diabetologists and endocrinologists across the UK, who lobbied the RCP to establish a committee following the closure of a counterpart in the MRC.[63] The Standing Committee intended to offer leadership in the field, advising the College on all matters concerning endocrinology (particularly training programmes and resources), co-ordinating research efforts, and maintaining the existing high standard of practice in clinical endocrinology.[64] No doubt connected with this last point was a specific reference to 'keep under constant review[,] and advise on[,] the facilities required by Clinical Endocrinologists and General Physicians with a special interest and experience in endocrinology working in different types of hospitals in this country'.[65]

The Committee's working group on diabetes contained two prominent diabetologists, Dr John Nabarro and Professor J. M. Malins, who, as we have already seen, were at the leading edge of innovative clinical practice and service organisation, and were also involved in policy discussions with the DHSS.[66] Their report was much firmer than earlier documents on questions of personnel and facilities required for quality care. The group's most direct suggestion was that a general physician with an interest in diabetes (and, where possible, endocrinology) 'should be appointed in each NHS District' (the most local level of administration introduced during the 1974 reorganisation). Alongside 'taking a full part in the general medical work of the District', this physician would also 'be responsible for promoting a service to diabetic patients in the community and in the hospital'.[67] Clinical work would not be undertaken alone. In the clinic, the authors recommended that the physician in charge 'will need at least two experienced doctors' to cope with the '3,600' follow-up appointments generated by a 'District of 250,000' population.[68] These doctors, moreover, would lead a 'Diabetic Team', including 'nurses, a dietician and a chiropodist', as well as a medical secretary.[69] Similarly, the physician would support the development of services outside the clinic, and would in turn be supported by GPs, district nurses, and health visitors.[70]

Constructing standards at a time of crisis 191

The report also offered greater clarity on equipment and the distribution of expertise than earlier guidance. Reflecting the importance of surveillance to patient management, district clinics would require specific 'accommodation and equipment', including 'a separate room in the clinic' for each doctor; 'two examination rooms'; a 'dark room for ophthalmoscopy'; 'appropriate facilities' for analysing urine for 'glucose, ketones, and protein'; and access to the 'Biochemistry Department' and either an 'hospital autoanalyser service' or a 'rapid glucose oxidase machine' for timely 'blood sugar examinations'.[71] Alongside these more routine instruments and spaces, new evidence concerning 'diabetic retinitis' meant that 'regular supervision', particularly of 'the younger diabetic', was 'of great importance'. To this end, the report suggested that 'the Physician in Charge of the Diabetic Clinic must establish close liaison with his ophthalmological colleague[s]' and arrange access to laser equipment, which, along with the expertise to use it, would 'only be available in a limited number of centres'.[72] In cases of retinopathy, patients might, therefore, be passed on to one of the centres existing in 'most regions' where 'difficult problems may be referred'. These centres were 'usually ... in the Teaching Hospital of the Region' and had 'physicians with very wide range experience of the problems of diabetics'.[73]

In many respects, the RCP report updated arrangements first considered in 1953, responding to renewed policy interest in planning as well as to changes in clinical technologies and the care team over the intervening period. It was therefore dominated by issues of staffing, facilities, and service organisation, but now reflective of different institutional arrangements, and with more prescriptive recommendations. The 1977 report also gave greater consideration to divisions of labour than the Ministry's guidance. For instance, the physician was to depute 'the slow and patient education of the diabetic to look after his or her condition' to nurses, and instead take a role in promoting community services and educating staff.[74] Likewise, though some patients would be seen by their GP 'whenever possible', the report also noted that physician follow-up would be required regularly, between every three and every twelve months.[75] Notably, like the 1953 guidance, this report did not seek to infringe upon the content of clinical care, or set standards for expected outcomes. Instead, the target audience consisted of those clinicians, Community Physicians, and others involved in the planning of NHS services. In this sense, it mirrored simultaneous efforts by the

DHSS to provide guidance on staffing and priorities, and to introduce better technocratic management to the health service.[76]

Nonetheless, this report was significant in one respect: it saw the tentative entrance of elite diabetologists and professional bodies into the realm of standard-setting and guidance production, following specialists in other fields.[77] As noted above, specialists had been central to the production of earlier guidance on diabetes care, but the resulting documents derived legitimacy from the statutory powers of the CHSC and the Ministry of Health. Similarly, whilst the Royal Colleges had played historic roles in maintaining professional standards, they had hitherto pursued their aims through certification, education, and their influence over policy committees and NHS bodies.[78] The 1977 guidance, therefore, represented diabetes specialists' adoption of more formal technologies for managing care, and the beginning of a move by elite professional bodies to govern ongoing medical practice more directly.

Although the RCP report focused only on the structural elements of care, it nonetheless set a precedent. Through the creation of clinical guidelines and audit programmes over the next two decades, the College and other elite bodies would extend their managerial interests into the process and outcomes of care, features of medical practice once considered the sovereign domain of the individual professional. Such national efforts at regulating care in the name of quality were designed to influence local practices and establish some form of national system for tracking care provision. They would also provide space for further government efforts into the 1990s.

This is not to say that state-sponsored guidance completely disappeared in the 1970s and 1980s. Reflecting the more co-operative relationships between central government, health authorities, and healthcare professionals in Scotland, the National Medical Consultative Committee of the SHHD commissioned a working group in 1984 to 'prepare guidelines for improved care of patients with diabetes' with consideration to integrated care, technology, and resource costs.[79] Senior figures in general practice, diabetology, paediatrics, health economics, nursing, and community medicine made up the membership of the working group, with a Senior Medical Officer of the SHHD on the secretariat. Creating the guideline involved approximately a year of evidence-gathering from key figures and organisations, and the Committee drew on several reports produced across Britain and the WHO.[80] Once again, the guideline primarily focused on staffing, education, facilities, and relationships between various sectors of the healthcare system. However, reflecting a growing managerialisation of British medicine, it also recommended the production of performance indicators for outcomes and process to facilitate national audit. A minority of its final recommendations caused friction in the SHHD because of concerns over costs, but the guideline was revised and published in 1986 with the SHHD's approval.[81] During the 1990s, this form of guideline commissioning and evidence-gathering would become more popular across Britain, though taking place within new state agencies independent from government. However, this future work would also target the content of clinical care with greater vigour, and the involvement of leading specialists and professional bodies gave such work legitimacy.

Guidelines and audit in the 1980s: process, outputs, and outcomes

The SHHD report's call for performance indicators signified the changing nature of the guidance being produced in the 1980s and early 1990s. In short, elite guideline-creating bodies increasingly produced prescriptions for the content of clinical practice, and in so doing challenged the concepts and structures of clinical autonomy at the core of traditional views of medical professionalism.

One of the earliest movements in this direction came from the BDA. In view of its strong links with elite specialists and its dedication to improving care for patients with diabetes, it was perhaps unsurprising that the Association would be at the forefront of guidance production. In 1982, the BDA published a 'policy statement' on dietary recommendations for the decade that became widely cited.[82] Produced by an expert committee that considered a large body of published research, this work built on the state-backed guidelines for diet of the 1970s and 1980s, and brought recommendations for individuals with diabetes roughly into line with advice for the rest of the population.[83] To provide the clearest possible advice, the guidance contained specific, quantified recommendations for constructing patient diets: 50 per cent of daily energy intake was to be derived from carbohydrate, 30 per cent from fat, and 20 per cent from protein. In some respects, this guidance thus marked a novel and more confident take on dietary proposals. However, the Association had given recommendations on diet before, and it was not necessarily an area which doctors assumed responsibility for or valued as part of their clinical autonomy.[84]

Perhaps a more significant intervention in this regard was the 'protocol' (later renamed 'guideline') for diabetes care produced by the RCGP in 1986 as part of its Quality Initiative (and related Clinical Information Folders).[85] By comparison with the looser norms and organisational focus of earlier guidance, the College guideline adopted a more prescriptive form, containing step-by-step, algorithmic guidance on how to manage diabetes within general practice. Beginning with 'identification', it advised GPs to create a register of patients already diagnosed with diabetes. Then, using WHO criteria, it detailed the diagnostic process, and outlined the possible interpretations to make within four specified situations: fasting blood glucose results of 'over 8 mmol/l' or random results 'over 11 mmol/l' were declared to be 'almost always indicative of diabetes', whilst diabetes was considered 'unlikely if the fasting blood glucose is below 6 mmol/l or the random blood glucose below 8 mmol/l'. Only in cases of uncertainty – where symptoms were absent and results fell between thresholds – were oral glucose tolerance tests 'justified'.[86]

Mirroring an abstract idealisation of the developing clinical encounter, the text then moved from diagnosis to disease management, setting out a precise programme for establishing appropriate treatment:

> if the patient is overweight (i.e. 20% above ideal body weight) try diet alone for three months. At the end of this period, review diet, weight loss and assess compliance. If control has not been achieved and the fasting blood glucose is above 8 mmol/l consider adding Metformin starting with 500 mg b.d. (always check blood urea and serum creatinine first and remember that metformin should not be used in patients with renal or hepatic impairment nor in those with an alcohol problem).

'If hyperglycaemia persists after a month' on the highest possible dose of metformin, it concluded, the criteria had been met for specialist referral.

Although demurring from directive language in favour of suggestive phrases (such as 'consider adding'), the guideline's formulaic 'if/then' structure was indicative of the way in which standards documents were becoming more explicit about the 'correct' clinical actions to be taken in given situations. As suggested above, such codification of disease management clearly contested visions of clinical practice as inherently variable and unavoidably individual, and provided the foundations on which the autonomy at the heart of professionalism could be structured and subject to review.

Perhaps the apogee of the guideline's ambition and prescriptivism, however, was located in the advice given for the process of patient review. Alongside detailed discussions about the conditions under which certain laboratory tests were needed, the RCGP documents disaggregated and codified the actions to be undertaken at each consultation in considerable detail:

At each consultation there should be consideration of:

(a) well-being, number of hypo attacks, days off work/school, presence or absence of nocturnal frequency, visual problems etc.
(b) review of blood glucose or urine tests
(c) review of diet and/or medication
(d) review of patient's smoking habits
(e) check of weight
(f) inspection of feet and review of the need for chiropody
(g) test urine for protein
(h) review of injection sites
(i) review of urine
(j) review of urine testing or blood testing technique
(k) check on the need for pre-conception counselling
(l) check of patient's understanding of their diabetes
(m) if appropriate, set further goals for treatment
(n) discuss specific problems and arrange follow-up.[87]

Whilst later revisions were updated in line with recent research and thinking – for instance, adding patient-focused elements, such as 'the patient's perceived problems' and 'educational needs' – the new texts retained the layout and tone of the original.[88]

Without any commentary by the College on its use, the guideline may have embodied the worst fears of mid-century practitioners. As will be noted below, the proliferation of guidelines into other areas of practice certainly drew complaints about curtailed autonomy and laments that the 'inflexibility' of guidelines made them 'clumsy' in the face of patients' uniqueness.[89] The College recognised some limits to its vision and reach, however. To avoid offending the sensibilities of more individualist practitioners, the guideline's introductory segments included disclaimers to dispel fears that it would be determinative of practice. The College suggested that 'no protocol can cover every situation', and whilst diabetes was 'a marvellous example of a condition which lends itself to team care', the documents declared that 'no attempt is made to define the responsibilities for individual members'. It was 'better', the authors felt, 'that they [the team members] agree these amongst themselves'.[90] A joint RCP, BDA, and RCGP guideline published in 1993, which assumed similarly prescriptive form, came to the same conclusion.[91]

Crucially, neither the RCGP guideline nor the joint guideline was designed to directly influence practice in the sense of replacing local frameworks and tools. Rather, these documents were intended to inform the protocols structuring local systems. Though modified to suit local situations, these guidelines were to provide a uniform standard around which doctors and agencies could organise their work. In this sense, the creators of national standards sought to subject local care to greater regulation, but believed that local ownership of clinical protocol might make adoption and adaptation of guidelines more likely.

The RCGP and joint RCP–BDA–RCGP guidelines were created at a time when 'how-to' guides for establishing quality diabetes services began to appear with great regularity. The College's publications probably carried greatest authority, being grounded in multi-disciplinary experience and accumulation of various sorts of evidence. However, the involvement of the BDA in guideline production was also notable, marking a move into a new role. Over the 1980s and into the 1990s, the Association self-consciously reframed its work, discursively positioning itself as 'active in improving standards of care provided for people with diabetes in the National Health Service'.[92] In part, this involved continuing its traditional role of gathering information on services and providing advice and support to the public and its patient membership.

In later decades, though, the BDA believed that improving the quality of care required the codification of process standards, and not just for professionals. In line with its role as a patient advisory body, it developed guidance for patients themselves, informing them, as individuals, on 'what diabetic care to expect'.[93] These leaflets outlined in clear and prescriptive bullet-points the types of supervisory processes professionals should perform. For instance, they declared that 'when you have just been diagnosed you should have':

1. A full medical examination.
2. An explanation of what diabetes is and what treatment you are likely to need: diet alone, diet and tablets, or diet and insulin.
3. A talk with a dietitian, who will want to know what you are used to eating and will give you basic advice on what to eat in the future. A follow-up meeting should be arranged for more detailed advice ...

Constructing standards at a time of crisis

This section went on to cover a further six points, taking in treatment modality, self-monitoring, social and financial implications of diagnosis, and ongoing education. The next segment, entitled 'Once your diabetes is reasonably controlled', included a further four points about annual supervisory check-ups, ongoing education, accessibility of specialist staff, and a formal annual review. Finally, this last topic was then broken down into nine sub-points detailing how:

At this review:

- Your weight should be recorded.
- Your urine should be tested for ketones and protein.
- Your blood should be tested to measure long term control.
- You should discuss control, including your home monitoring results

...

The list ran on to describe other tests and how a consultation should include 'the opportunity to discuss how you are coping at home and at work'.[94] Notably, the guide closed with the lines 'the control of diabetes is important, and so is the detection and treatment of any complications. Make sure you are getting the medical care and education you need to ensure you stay healthy.'[95]

Clearly, these leaflets emerged from the Association's fear that patchy service from doctors and health authorities might result in missed supervision and support. The codification and supply of knowledge were therefore important because not all healthcare providers could be relied upon. Yet, in trying to persuade patients to insist upon their rights, the Association was also cultivating a particular type of patient, one who was not just an informed part of a team but also demanded submission to review.[96] Although seemingly contradictory on the surface – at once empowered and subjectified – this patient emerged from deeply held convictions about the importance of oversight in diabetes care. Moreover, in the context of both neoliberal health service reform and a growing political and grassroots emphasis on patient consumerism, the Association's vigilant and vocal patient was also to offer a solution to concerns about medical practice. Informed and active patients were to add another layer of regulation to care: they would call certain forms of action into question, and encourage practitioners to behave in approved manners. Guidelines from above and protocol designed with peers would be enforced by patients below. If everyone was aware of expectations, then surveillance could come from all directions.

Through this emphasis on monitoring, the BDA and elite professional bodies sought to make the final move into the realm of healthcare government. As noted in Chapter 3, to some extent the drive for local audit provided a motivation to create practice protocols: sets of standards against which measurement could take place. However, during the 1980s and early 1990s, elite professional and specialist organisations began to audit whole systems. Some looked nationally, others on a smaller scale; some surveyed facilities and staffing, whilst others worked with performance benchmarks for process and outcomes. Regardless, the institution of regular review added new layers to healthcare regulation.

Once again, the BDA played a central role. Its UK-wide review of staffing and facilities in hospital services, undertaken with the RCP and published in 1984, marked an important take-off point for placing national diabetes management under scrutiny.[97] The survey emerged, in part, from the RCP's efforts to improve standards in clinical endocrinology, which, as we have seen, involved monitoring and promoting the employment of specialists across the health service. Similarly, specialists associated with both the RCP and BDA were concerned about how UK hospitals had responded to recent developments in clinical diabetology, fearing considerable regional variations and inequalities.[98] The review thus surveyed medical professionals across the NHS to generate baseline data, and simultaneously updated and transformed the recommendations of the RCP's 1977 report, turning them into benchmarks for minimum requirements. The report noted, for example, how 'in 30 health districts in the United Kingdom there are no physicians specialising in diabetes', and highlighted the fact that 'of 428 respondents ... 48% do NOT have [a] dark room for retinal examination.'[99]

The staffing element of this research was followed up several years later, with only minimal progress made towards greater equality.[100] As noted above, though, professionals involved in bodies like the National Medical Consultative Committee of the SHHD working group had sought to expand audit's remit in the intervening period, taking process and outcome into account. Rooting itself within interlocking contexts of Scottish, British, and international medicine, the SHHD report noted that some indicators had already been recommended elsewhere in the world. English access measures, it had recalled, were devised to facilitate comparison between health districts, but 'Scottish health boards were too diverse for comparison between areas'. Thus the authors suggested that longitudinal measures for 'all Scotland' would be preferable, and 'access measures for the process of care' could allow for intra-area comparison. As for the metrics to be chosen, the report drew on American suggestions, with the United States National Diabetes Advisory Board proposing 'five major indicators of the quality of care': visual impairment, perinatal morbidity and mortality, amputations, end-stage renal failure and diabetic ketoacidosis (an acute metabolic crisis potentially resulting in coma).[101]

In the event, admission to hospital for diabetic ketoacidosis did become a 'clinical outcome indicator' in Scotland during the early 1990s.[102] The Clinical Outcomes Working Group of the SHHD's Clinical Resources and Audit Group annually published a series of indicator metrics. These measures in themselves were not taken to be a guarantee of quality: 'we must emphasise', the authors suggested, 'that no conclusions can or should be drawn from the comparisons in this report about the quality or efficacy of the treatment provided for the populations of different Health Boards'. Rather, it was hoped that the 'disparities' in this series of indicators might lead boards and clinicians to review their performance, and subsequently to 'correc[t]' those 'deficiencies in service provision or therapeutic regimes' that were uncovered.[103] For four years, admissions for diabetic ketoacidosis provided one such measure, being easily quantified and providing a possible sign of problematic care prior to hospitalisation. Although this metric was dropped in 1996 after an overhaul of the measures used, its early use nonetheless reflected how widespread the desire to audit diabetes services had become.[104]

Once again, the role of central government agencies in facilitating performance indication was reflective of Scotland's earlier move into state-backed guideline and audit production. However, as will be discussed in Chapter 6, similar processes were underway in England and Wales. The RCP and BDA were keen to develop a national dataset and protocol for diabetes auditing, with the Department of Health providing funding for this work.

Furthermore, the eagerness to audit itself came from clinicians. As noted above, doctors increasingly deployed audit at local levels during the 1980s, slowly institutionalising the practice within hospitals, general practice, and integrated care programmes as a path to better self-management. Into the 1990s, reviews expanded to include outcome measures, both intermediate (like average HbA1c readings) and 'end-point' (mortality from complications). In this regard, audits of diabetes care benefited from the highly quantified culture of diabetes management, a heritage of its previous grounding in physiological concepts and practices.

Moves towards audit were supported in 1989 by the St Vincent Declaration, a document emerging from a joint International Diabetes Federation–WHO (Europe) initiative that aimed to reduce morbidity and mortality from diabetes through target-setting. Blindness, renal failure, and neuropathy all received quantified reduction targets, and the Declaration included a promise to embark on auditing programmes.[105] The Declaration was signed not only by representatives of national diabetes associations, but also by government delegates. As we shall see in Chapter 6, a host of initiatives originated from the St Vincent Declaration in Britain, even though its targets were later criticised. An important element of its influence, however, was the creation of a standardised dataset for audit purposes.[106] The development of audit programmes, then, emerged from bodies at a local, national, and international level, linking professional organisations, non-governmental bodies, and groups of specialists who promoted audit as a basis for quality care. In short, as well as constructing guidelines to inform local protocol, the profession itself was pushing for audit of process and outcomes as the means by which to ensure quality care from trained professionals.

Conclusion: guidelines, audit, and regulating medicine

What, then, did this shift of regulatory architecture mean? What are we to make of the role of elite professional and specialist bodies in constructing it? And how could new tools to structure and review care be squared with traditional views of professionals as trained experts, trusted to serve their patients and distinguished by their autonomy?

To some extent, the late-century pursuit of guideline construction by bodies like the Royal Colleges forms part of a longer history. Colleges and their specialists had produced service guidance during the mid-twentieth century as part of their efforts to maintain high standards in their respective fields. Indeed, some of these guidelines even recommended pursuing forms of peer conference and integrated care solutions a decade before similar suggestions in diabetes care.[107] Yet the move to include the process and outcomes of clinical care within these guidelines, and to set benchmarks for future review, indicated a significant change in remit. Traditional views of professionalism – both within and without medicine – stressed that the esoteric knowledge of certain occupations justified collective regulation, as only members of these professions could set and judge reasonable standards. Throughout the first half of the twentieth century, these understandings of professionalism also suggested that the variability of the problems faced necessitated freedom for individuals to exercise autonomous judgement. Finally, professionals were deemed, by dint of their education and character, to be trustworthy.[108] External practices of prescribing roles would thus be counterproductive, and techniques of accounting unnecessary. Making these claims may have been ideological acts, attempts to turn supposedly esoteric knowledge into control over market functions and work processes.[109] Nonetheless, they played an important symbolic role in identity construction and had material impact in medicine.[110] The construction of guidelines and auditing frameworks, therefore, seemingly contested these myths and experiences of medical professional life, formalising trust into a process of accounting and providing codified norms of practice against which actual performance could be measured.

Debates about the role of guidelines in British medicine at the beginning of the 1990s captured the possible extent of this challenge. As hitherto the least managed medical practitioners, GPs and consultants in these years criticised the 'increasing flood of guidelines and protocols issued by royal colleges and other organisations' and expressed concerns about how such tools might limit cherished professional freedoms and weaken medical authority.[111] Some doctors, for instance, were concerned about the potential accountability issues that guidance documents raised beyond self-audit and peer review. At one meeting between senior medical representatives and the Chief Medical Officer in 1993, interlocutors voiced worries 'about the medicolegal aspect if [guidelines] were not followed to the letter'.[112] The fear of legal action was probably heightened amid ongoing medical scandals, but such a worry also spoke to broader apprehensions about external limits on the hallmark of clinical freedom. Such constraints were at the heart of contemporary sociological theories concerning 'deprofessionalisation', and found echoes in the complaints of a surgeon at another meeting of senior consultants.[113] Linking the development of guidelines with the recent introduction of general management and internal markets (see Chapter 6), this practitioner warned of the coming of '"cookbook medicine", with doctors being given clinical protocols on the most economical way to treat patients'.[114] As work on the emergence of Evidence-Based Medicine has demonstrated, the concept of 'cookbook medicine' provided a common filter for concerns about the creation of bureaucratised, unthinking provision, and one editorial of the early 1990s summed up such anxieties with the question 'if doctors are not required to exercise judgement what are they there for?'[115] Even practitioners sympathetic to guidelines approvingly commended advocates for reassuring doctors that 'guidelines are not intended to replace clinical judgement ... and that practising medicine in the 1990s remains an art'.[116]

And yet many of the complaints about guidelines, at least in the medical press, did not concern the principles of codifying statements of good care, or of professionals reviewing their practice. As one of the critics quoted above suggested, 'no one objected to broad recommendations on what was acceptable', and we have seen that there were powerful voices supporting new trends.[117] Instead, criticisms of guidelines often concerned the sheer number being produced, the frequency of disagreement, the poor evidence on which they could be based, the remoteness of their production, their potential inflexibility and limitation of innovation, and the lack of consideration given to implementation.[118] By the early 1990s, debates about the potential problems and mechanics of guidelines were still in their infancy, but a consensus was forming around the idea that they could, theoretically at least, help to secure high standards of care.

In part, the support for guidelines and audit could be interpreted as part of a change in the precise meaning attached to the concept of 'high standards' over the twentieth century. The notion of 'quality care' emerged within a context of managerial reform and broader professional, public, and political concerns about professional performance. Elite professional bodies pioneered efforts to remake practice, responding to this crisis of collective regulation by constructing new tools for formal professional management. Appeals to quality here served to reframe traditional concepts of professionalism, and to transmute old features.[119] A service ethic had been a key feature of older discourses of professionalism. Now, however, this selflessness could be used to justify the codification of previously individualised clinical decision-making and the use of new quality-assurance tools. Discussing its ideal GP, the RCGP suggested that 'he [sic] subjects his work to critical self-scrutiny and peer review, and accepts a commitment to improve his skills and widen his range of services in response to newly disclosed needs'.[120] The author of the College's diabetes materials translated this ideal when discussing calls for protocol and audit in the NHS reforms of the early 1990s: 'intrinsic in many of the government's proposals ... is the theme of accountability. This theme does not frighten me: does it frighten you?' 'Surely', he went on, 'the way forward must be for the nurses, the dieticians, the chiropodists, the patients to unite with the doctors in the production of suitable guidelines.' He then closed with an appeal to that most traditional figure, Hippocrates: 'of the recent achievements of science, the emancipation of the human mind from a servile adherence to the opinions of antiquity is one of the most important'.[121]

Of course, given the local use of protocol and audit since the late 1970s, the potential challenge to individual clinical autonomy from new guidelines was not novel. Though having reservations about the extent to which autonomy would become structured and performance reviewed, many rank-and-file practitioners shared the broad outlines of new visions for professionalism. Rather, the involvement of specialist bodies like the BDA and Royal Colleges in the production of formal regulatory tools was significant for how it opened the way for a transformation in the government of British medicine.

Crucially, as we will see in the next chapter, the involvement of elite professional and specialist bodies in setting and reviewing standards in diabetes care legitimated these tools as means for managing and regulating medicine. On the one hand, it provided a seal of approval for local efforts. On the other, these elite practitioners' attempts to produce tools that informed local systems marked the emergence of what would later be called clinical governance architecture: namely, institutions whose role was to ensure that local systems had standards and accountability measures in place, and to assess whether these local structures functioned effectively. Doctors may have firmly resisted the encroachment of 'lay' or 'state' management of their work. Many did not, however, actively oppose medically led local systems for managing medical labour; nor did they disagree with the construction of frameworks that sought to inform and reinforce these local professional structures.[122] Of course, the ways in which discourses of medical professionalism had been reframed over the second half of the twentieth century opened the opportunity for greater lay, external management. Moreover, audit provided the basis on which political actors could co-operate with elite practitioners to reframe clinical governance, linking it with broader structures for cost-control and welfare management. Although not sacrificing individual clinical autonomy or formalising stratifications within the profession to the extent suggested in contemporary sociological work, these developments did consolidate major changes in how British medicine was managed and regulated.[123]

Notes

1 The terms 'protocol' and 'guidelines' have historically been interchangeable. This chapter, however, uses 'guideline' to refer to texts produced nationally or internationally for the sole purpose of assisting clinical decision-making and the organisation of care in specific conditions (exclusive of other aids, such as textbooks or journal articles). 'Protocol', by contrast, refers to local documents, usually more precise than guidelines, indicating specific responsibilities for staff and providing detailed steps to be taken in precise circumstances during the clinical management of disease. Guidelines, then, tend to inform protocol, although – as will be seen in this and the next chapter – protocols have also been used by doctors and other interested parties to create guidelines.
2 Clinical Standards Advisory Group (CSAG), *Standards of Clinical Care for People with Diabetes* (London: HMSO, 1994), pp. 18, 30–1. This report reviewed over nineteen documents created between 1987 and 1992 alone. P. Day, R. Klein, and F. Miller, *A Comparative US–UK Study of Guidelines* (London: Nuffield Trust, 1998), pp. 15–16.
3 D. Armstrong, 'Clinical sense and clinical science', *Social Science and Medicine*, 11:11–13 (1977), 599–601.
4 S. Timmermanns and M. Berg, *The Gold Standard: The Challenge of Evidence-Based Medicine and Standardization in Health Care* (Philadelphia: Temple University Press, 2003), pp. 55–81; P. Keating and A. Cambrosio, 'Cancer clinical trials: the emergence and development of a new style of practice', *Bulletin of the History of Medicine*, 81:1 (2007), 197–223.
5 Broadly, these were the arrangements established under the 1858 Medical Act, with subsequent amendments. See discussion in the Introduction and in M. Stacey, *Regulating British Medicine: The General Medical Council* (Chichester: John Wiley & Sons, 1992), pp. 17–23.
6 V. Berridge and K. Loughlin (eds.), *Medicine, the Market and the Mass Media: Producing Health in the Twentieth Century* (London: Routledge, 2005); L. Diack and D. F. Smith, 'Professional strategies of Medical Officers of Health in the post-war period – 1: "innovative traditionalism": the case of Dr Ian MacQueen, MOH for Aberdeen, 1952–1974, a "bull-dog" with the "hide of a rhinoceros"', *Journal of Public Health Medicine*, 24:2 (2002), 123–9; G. Millward, *Vaccinating Britain: Mass Vaccination and the Public since the Second World War* (Manchester: Manchester University Press, 2019).
7 A. Mold, *Making the Patient-Consumer: Patient Organisations and Health Consumerism in Britain* (Manchester: Manchester University Press, 2015), pp. 72–3; S. Sheard, *The Passionate Economist: How Brian Abel-Smith Shaped Global Health Policy and Social Welfare* (Bristol: Policy Press, 2013), pp. 233–9.

8 C. Webster, *The Health Services since the War*, vol. 2: *Government and Health Care: The British National Health Service, 1958–1979* (London: HMSO, 1996), pp. 227–41, 399–414, 635–60.
9 Stacey, *Regulating British Medicine*, pp. 181–90; D. Irvine, *A Doctor's Tale: Professionalism and Public Trust* (Abingdon: Radcliffe Medical Press, 2003), pp. 121–35.
10 Irvine, *A Doctor's Tale*, pp. 75–80. Previously, the General Medical Council had restricted disciplinary cases to advertising, sexual encounters with patients, collusion with irregular practitioners, drug and alcohol abuse, prescribing dangerous drugs without cause, and gross misconduct (such as non-attendance to patients): Stacey, *Regulating British Medicine*, pp. 139–78, 182–6.
11 M. Hilton, *Consumerism in Twentieth-Century Britain* (Cambridge: Cambridge University Press, 2003).
12 M. Power, *The Audit Society: Rituals of Verification* (Oxford: Oxford University Press, 1999); D. Dewar and W. Funnell, *A History of British National Audit: The Pursuit of Accountability* (Oxford: Oxford University Press, 2017), pp. 196–230.
13 E. Robinson, C. Schofield, F. Sutcliffe-Brown, and N. Thomlinson, 'Telling stories about post-war Britain: popular individualism and the "crisis" of the 1970s', *Twentieth Century British History*, 28:2 (2017), 286–304.
14 T. H. Marshall, *Citizenship and Social Class and Other Essays* (Cambridge: Cambridge University Press, 1950).
15 Mold, *Making the Patient-Consumer*, pp. 69–93.
16 Ibid., pp. 117–26; G. O'Hara, 'The complexities of "consumerism": choice, collectivism and participation within Britain's National Health Service, c.1961–c.1979', *Social History of Medicine*, 26:2 (2013), 288–304.
17 I. C. Gilliland, 'Registrars', *The Lancet*, 256:6640 (1950), 710; 'Better general practice', *The Lancet*, 263:6813 (1954), 659–60; S. Taylor, *Good General Practice: A Report on a Survey* (London: Oxford University Press, 1954); Senior Registrar, 'Consultant and specialist', *The Lancet*, 270:6990 (1957), 338; 'The teaching hospitals', *The Lancet*, 270:6989 (1957), 277–8; E. Geiringer, 'Murder at the cross-roads or the decapitation of general practice', *The Lancet*, 273:7081 (1959), 1039–45. See the responses by M. B. Clyne, J. Fry, E. J. Raffle, and W. Tait: 'Murder at the cross-roads', *The Lancet*, 273:7083 (1959), 1146–9; J. S. Collings, 'Group practice: existing patterns and future policies', *The Lancet*, 262:6775 (1953), 31–3.
18 See discussion of the pre-registration year in Stacey, *Regulating British Medicine*, pp. 112–23.
19 C. Lawrence, *Rockefeller Money, The Laboratory and Medicine in Edinburgh, 1919–1930: New Science in an Old Country* (New York: University of Rochester Press, 2005).

20 This was part of an international phenomenon: J. Daly, *Evidence-Based Medicine and the Search for a Science of Clinical Care* (Berkeley: University of California Press, 2005). pp. 129–43.
21 A. L. Cochrane, *Effectiveness and Efficiency: Random Reflections on the Health Services* (London: Nuffield Provincial Hospitals Trust, 1972); for references to diabetes, pp. 54–7. On the power and historical elasticity of the term 'science' in medicine: J. H. Warner, 'The history of science and the sciences of medicine', *Osiris*, 10 (1995), 164–93.
22 On the development of these disciplines: Sheard, *The Passionate Economist*. For the influence on Cochrane: Cochrane, *Effectiveness and Efficiency*, pp. 70–7.
23 J. Welshman, 'Inequalities, regions and hospitals: the Resource Allocation Working Party', in M. Gorsky and S. Sheard (eds.), *Financing Medicine: The British Experience since 1750* (Oxford: Routledge, 2006), pp. 221–41; C. Cook, 'Oral history – Walter Holland', *Journal of Public Health*, 26:2 (2004), 121–9.
24 J. N. Morris, *Uses of Epidemiology*, 3rd edition (Edinburgh: Churchill Livingstone, 1975), pp. 71–98; G. Weisz, A. Cambrosio, P. Keating, L. Knaapen, T. Schlich, and V. J. Tournay, 'The emergence of clinical practice guidelines', *Milbank Quarterly*, 85:4 (2007), 691–727.
25 Cochrane, *Effectiveness and Efficiency*, p. 80.
26 Ibid., pp. 81–2.
27 See Chapter 2.
28 Daly, *Evidence-Based Medicine*.
29 On the disputes: C. Webster, *The Health Services since the War*, vol. 1: *Problems of Health Care: The National Health Service before 1957* (London: HMSO, 1988), pp. 227–33.
30 J. Fry, 'Government and profession', *The Lancet*, 269:6970 (1957), 690.
31 Ibid.
32 Morris would become famed for his work on chronic disease epidemiology, especially on heart disease and exercise. He was, moreover, a strong advocate of social equality: A. Oakley, 'Appreciation: Jerry [Jeremiah Noah] Morris, 1910–2009', *International Journal of Epidemiology*, 39:1 (2010), 274–6.
33 'Improvement of the N.H.S.', *The Lancet*, 269:6958 (1957), 41.
34 The quotation is from a statement by a branch of GPs in Lancashire issued in response to the first post-war White Paper. It neatly summarises the emphasis that GPs placed on their 'independence' in acceding to join the NHS, however. 'Panel conference: motions', *BMJ*, 2:4372, S.85 (1944), 91. See Chapter 1 for further discussion.
35 O. C. Carter, 'The 100% issue', *BMJ*, 2:4354, S.103 (1944), 101; C. Lawrence, 'Incommunicable knowledge: science, technology and the clinical art in Britain, 1850–1914', *Journal of Contemporary History*, 20:4 (1985), 503–20.

36 D. L. Brick, J. Brick, and J. W. Richardson, 'Fining the doctor', *BMJ*, 2:4902, S.233 (1954), 241.
37 Though perhaps one explanation for the divergence between practice and responses lay in the connections between voluntary institutions and autonomy in the professional imagination: S. Hastings, 'Scientific freedom and social medicine', *BMJ*, 1:4290 (1943), 392–3.
38 'Administration of special departments', *BMJ*, 2:4784, S.2486 (1952), 126.
39 Evidence for the reception amongst doctors is difficult to ascertain. Cochrane, his biographers, and others promoting guidelines and audit suggest that clinicians often resisted these ideas: Daly, *Evidence-Based Medicine*, pp. 130–41; Irvine, *A Doctor's Tale*, pp. 51–82. Also, medical professionals and epidemiologists were hesitant about political demands for enhanced NHS monitoring (though not service surveillance *per se*): R. Doll, 'Monitoring the National Health Service', *Proceedings of the Royal Society of Medicine*, 66:8 (1973), 729–40. On the other hand, Morris, Fry, and Cochrane received considerable financial support from several quarters and were very well connected. *Effectiveness and Efficiency* received favourable reviews in *The Lancet* and the *BMJ*: C. T. Dollery, 'Constructive attack', *BMJ*, 2:5804 (1972), 56; '*Effectiveness and Efficiency*', *The Lancet*, 299:7752 (1972), 668–9.
40 H. Dudley, 'Necessity for surgical audit', *BMJ*, 1: 5902 (1974), 275–7; R. Hoffenberg, *Clinical Freedom* (London: Nuffield Provincial Hospitals Trust, 1987). On GPs and new practices: Irvine, *A Doctor's Tale*, pp. 51–82.
41 I. McWhinney, 'Medical audit in North America', *BMJ*, 2:5808 (1972), 277–9; H. W. K. Acheson, 'Medical audit and general practice', *The Lancet*, 305:7905 (1975), 511–13. But not all US doctors were satisfied with their systems: P. N. Karnauchow, 'Medical audit', *The Lancet*, 305:7914 (1975), 1029–30.
42 Hoffenberg, *Clinical Freedom*.
43 They also proposed that curtailing autonomy collectively would prevent external limitations by lay managers: 'When wild ideas make sense', *BMJ*, 2:6204 (1979), 1532; J. R. Hampton, 'The end of clinical freedom', *BMJ*, 287:6401 (1983), 1237–8.
44 Hampton, 'The end of clinical freedom'.
45 For instance: I. Illich, *Limits to Medicine: Medical Nemesis – the Expropriation of Health* (Harmondsworth: Penguin, 1977); R. Klein, 'Auditing the NHS', *BMJ*, 285:6343 (1982), 672–3. These figures, and others, were cited in discussions about audit and quality: 'Towards medical audit', *BMJ*, 1:5903 (1974), 256; R. Johnson, 'Medical audit', *The Lancet*, 305:7908 (1975), 679; Irvine, *A Doctor's Tale*, pp. 20–1.
46 See Chapter 2. Regionalisation of specialist services was based on the rarity of need, with provision calculated according to population size needed to sustain efficient practice. On the origin of regional hierarchies:

D. Fox, *Health Policies, Health Politics: The British and American Experience, 1911–1965* (Princeton: Princeton University Press, 1986).
47 TNA, BD 18/793, R.H.B. (53) 66, Ministry of Health circular, 'National Health Service: regional planning of diabetic services', 1953, pp. 1–2.
48 Ibid.
49 Ibid.
50 A keyword search for 'guideline' and 'guide-line' in *The Lancet* and *BMJ* found no recorded usages before 1960, 16 uses in 1960–69, 80 in 1970–79, and 203 uses in 1980–89. Because of database functionality there were numerous repetitions, but the low rate of use before the 1970s is still telling.
51 E. Friedman, E. Grable, and J. Fine, 'Central venous pressure and direct serial measurements as guides in blood volume replacement', *The Lancet*, 288:7464 (1966), 611; P. N. Dixon, 'Work of a nurse in a health centre treatment room', *BMJ*, 4:5678 (1969), 293; 'Death of Proplist', *The Lancet*, 296:7679 (1970), 918; D. Corless, 'Diet in the elderly', *BMJ*, 4:5885 (1973), 160; 'Do anticoagulant drugs prevent complications?', *BMJ*, 4:5888 (1973), 352; V. Kempi, W. Van der Linden, and C. Von Schéele, 'Diagnosis of deep vein thrombosis with ^{99m}Tc-streptokinase: a clinical comparison with phlebography', *BMJ*, 4:5947 (1974), 749; H. Brown, 'Hand injuries', *BMJ*, 3:5927 (1974), 403.
52 C. J. H. Williams and T. A. Rathwell, 'Could the consultative document have its priorities wrong?', *BMJ*, 2:6041 (1976), 956–7; 'NHS reorganisation, planning, and priorities', *BMJ*, 281:6250 (1980), 1300.
53 Algorithmic guidelines work on an 'if/if not, then' system, wherein specific courses of action are recommended in the presence or absence of certain circumstances.
54 See Chapter 1.
55 WHO, *Diabetes Mellitus: Report of a WHO Expert Committee*, Technical Report Series, 310 (Geneva, WHO: 1965); for attendees, p. 2. The committee contained both Professor W. J. H. Butterfield – a well-known researcher involved in the Bedford study noted in Chapters 1 and 2 – and Professor J. A. Tulloch, a researcher and clinician in Uganda, who trained in Scotland and possessed colonial experience in Jamaica.
56 Ibid., p. 6.
57 Ibid., pp. 6–15, 25–31, esp. p. 28.
58 Weisz et al., 'The emergence of clinical practice guidelines'.
59 J. Malins, *Clinical Diabetes Mellitus* (London: Eyre & Spottiswoode, 1968), pp. 64–80; W. G. Oakley, D. A. Pyke, and K. W. Taylor, *Diabetes and its Management*, 2nd edition (London: Blackwell Scientific Publications, 1975), pp. 39–50.
60 WHO, *WHO Expert Committee on Diabetes Mellitus: Second Report*, Technical Report Series, 646 (Geneva: WHO, 1980), pp. 8–14, esp. table 1, p.

10; WHO, *Diabetes Mellitus: Report of a WHO Study Group*, Technical Report Series, 727 (Geneva: WHO, 1985), pp. 9–20, esp. figure 1 and table 1, p. 11. The 1985 report updated technical specifications. For citations in British medicine: 'Acute myocardial infarction and pre-existing diabetes', *The Lancet*, 322:8347 (1983), 451; SHHD, Scottish Health Service Planning Council, *Report of the Working Group on the Management of Diabetes* (Edinburgh: HMSO, 1987), p. 20; C. Waine, *Diabetes in General Practice*, 3rd edition (London: RCGP, 1992), pp. 6–7, 44. The research and take-up are discussed in Chapter 2 above.
61 Professors Harry Keen and K. G. M. M. Alberti were both involved in the 1980 and 1985 reports. They were highly influential clinicians and researchers, in Britain and internationally. British doctors had moved in international organisations for decades, and trained and practised in different countries and colonial locales for centuries: A. Hardy, 'Beriberi, vitamin B1 and world food policy, 1925–1970', *Medical History*, 39:1 (1995), 61–77. They had even commented on 'tropical diabetes' in the 1920s: D. Arnold, 'Diabetes in the tropics: race, place, and class in India, 1880–1965', *Social History of Medicine*, 22:2 (2009), 245–61. It was only in the 1950s and beyond, however, that diabetes specialists moved within dedicated colonial research structures, and within international health bodies after broad-scale decolonisation.
62 TNA, FD 7/2606, 5, report, J. D. N. Nabarro, J. M. Malins, and J. R. Hearnshaw, 'Medical care of patients with diabetes mellitus', 1977.
63 TNA, FD 7/206, minutes, 'A meeting of the College Standing Committee on Endocrinology and Diabetes Mellitus 23 February 1976', 1976, pp. 1–3; TNA, FD 7/2606, 6, 'Comments on draft RCP report on care of patients with diabetes', 1976, p. 1.
64 TNA, FD 7/2606, 1, letter, J. D. N. Nabarro to Sir C. Clarke (President, RCP), untitled, 27 August 1974, pp. 1–2; TNA, FD 7/2606, 2, letter, J. D. N. Nabarro to Sir S. Howarth (MRC), untitled, 14 February 1975, p. 1.
65 TNA, Nabarro to Clarke, p. 1.
66 See Chapter 2 and Chapter 4.
67 TNA, Nabarro et al., 'Medical care of patients with diabetes mellitus', p. 1.
68 Ibid., p. 2.
69 Ibid., pp. 2–3.
70 Ibid., p. 5.
71 Ibid., p. 3.
72 Ibid., p. 4.
73 Ibid., p. 5.
74 Ibid., pp. 2, 5.
75 Ibid.

76 Webster, *The Health Services since the War*, vol. 2, pp. 606–13. See Chapter 2 above.
77 WLA, SA/CMO/C/60 – Box 27, Royal College of Obstetricians and Gynaecologists, 'Recommendations on the principles and organisation of general practitioner maternity units and their relation to specialist maternity units', 1962.
78 G. Clarke, 'History of the Royal College of Physicians of London', *BMJ*, 1:5427 (1965), 79–82. The RCP also increasingly cultivated a public-facing role in health education: V. Berridge, 'Medicine and the public: the 1962 report of the Royal College of Physicians and the new public health', *Bulletin of the History of Medicine*, 81:1 (2007), 286–311.
79 SHHD et al., *Report of the Working Group on the Management of Diabetes*, p. 11. On Scotland and guideline production: Day et al., *A Comparative US–UK Study of Guidelines*, pp. 32–5.
80 See papers in National Records of Scotland, Edinburgh (NRS), HH98/242, National Medical Consultative Committee, 1985. For the rest of the guideline production: NRS, HH98/631, National Medical Consultative Committee, 1985–86; NRS, HH98/632, National Medical Consultative Committee, 1986; NRS, HH98/453, National Medical Consultative Committee, 1986–87; NRS, HH98/454, National Medical Consultative Committee, 1986–87.
81 NRS, HH98/454, 49, letter by C. F. Fleming (Medical Secretary) to Working Group, 'The management of diabetes', 23 December 1986, p. 1.
82 WLA, P9997, Nutritional Subcommittee of the BDA, 'Dietary recommendations for the 1980s – a policy statement by the British Diabetic Association', 1982. For citations: SHHD et al., *Report of the Working Group on the Management of Diabetes*, pp. 34–5; M. E. J. Lean and W. P. T. James, 'Prescription of diabetic diets in the 1980s', *BMJ*, 292:6524 (1986), 723–5.
83 Lean and James, 'Prescription of diabetic diets in the 1980s', p. 723. On dietary policy-making and its difficulties: M. Bufton and V. Berridge, 'Post-war nutrition science and policy making in Britain c.1945–1994: the case of diet and heart disease', in D. Smith and J. Phillips (eds.), *Food, Science, Policy and Regulation in the Twentieth Century: International and Comparative Perspectives* (London: Routledge, 2000), pp. 207–22.
84 WLA, EPH546, R. D. Lawrence, 'The Line-Ration Scheme', c.1951, pp. 1–4; WLA, EPH546, BDA, 'Basic exchange list for diabetics', c.1967, pp. 1–2. Doctors regularly deputed dietary composition, finding it 'tedious' work: J. Walker, 'Sociological implications of diabetes', *BMJ*, 2:4934 (1955), 318.
85 See Chapters 2 and 3. The 1986 folder was cited in SHHD et al., *Report of the Working Group on the Management of Diabetes*, p. 50. The protocol was later revised: 'Diabetes: a protocol', in RCGP, *Diabetes Clinical*

Information Folder (London: RCGP, 1988), appendix 4. It was then incorporated as a guideline within a chapter of an associated book: Waine, *Diabetes in General Practice*, 3rd edition, pp. v, 43–9. The protocol and guideline differed so little that 'guideline' will be used to discuss all three revisions to minimise confusion.

86 A tolerance test is a procedure in which a patient is fasted, 'stressed' with a glucose load, and assessed for metabolic capacities.
87 RCGP, 'Diabetes: a protocol', appendix 4, p. 8. Emphasis in original.
88 Waine, *Diabetes in General Practice*, p. 47.
89 P. Kinnersley, P. Owen, C. Wilkinson, and J. Richards, 'Set menus and clinical freedom', *BMJ*, 303:6806 (1991), 857–8.
90 RCGP, 'Diabetes: a protocol', appendix 4, p. 1.
91 WLA, BDA, RCP, and RCGP, 'Guidelines: good practice in the diagnosis and treatment of non-insulin dependent diabetes mellitus' (London: RCP, 1993).
92 J. Nabarro, 'BDA present and future', *Diabetic Medicine*, 7:6 (1990), 476.
93 S. Redmond, 'What diabetic care to expect', *Diabetic Medicine*, 7:6 (1990), 554.
94 Ibid.
95 Ibid.
96 In Foucauldian terms, the Association formed part of broader programmes to conduct patient conduct: M. Dean, *Governmentality: Power and Rule in Modern Society* (London: SAGE, 2010). The extent to which this practice of governmentality aligned with neoliberal political rationalities – cultivating agents to act free of government 'interference' – is debatable, however. These patients were to assume new levels of self-responsibility for ensuring effective care, but their demands for oversight would inevitably mean greater state support (and possibly expenditure) for the provision of health services.
97 RCP and BDA, *The Provision of Medical Care for Adult Diabetic Patients in the United Kingdom* (London: BDA, 1984).
98 The surveyors expressed common concerns about resource allocation and health inequalities in this regard: Welshman, 'Inequalities, regions and hospitals'; see also contributions to *Contemporary British History*, 16:3 (2002).
99 RCP and BDA, *The Provision of Medical Care for Adult Diabetic Patients*, pp. 9, 5 respectively.
100 P. D. Home and W. M. G. Tunbridge, 'Appointments and turnover of consultants and senior registrars in diabetes and endocrinology in the UK, 1984 and 1985', *Diabetic Medicine*, 4:1 (1987), 79–82.
101 SHHD et al., *Report of the Working Group on the Management of Diabetes*, p. 71.

102 NRS, HH48/112/5, Scottish Office, 'Clinical outcome indicators', December 1995, pp. 13–14.
103 Ibid., p. 2.
104 NRS, HH48/112/5, Scottish Office, 'Clinical outcome indicators', July 1996.
105 G. E. Reiber and H. King, *Guidelines for the Development of a National Programme for Diabetes Mellitus* (Geneva: WHO, 1991), annex 5, pp. 61–2.
106 Ibid.
107 WLA, Royal College of Obstetricians and Gynaecologists, 'Recommendations on the principles and organisation of general practitioner maternity units', p. 11.
108 For a review of the 'traits' literature: T. J. Johnson, *Professions and Power* (London: Macmillan, 1972).
109 M. S. Larson, *The Rise of Professionalism: A Sociological Analysis* (Berkeley: University of California Press, 1977).
110 E. Freidson, *Profession of Medicine: A Study of the Sociology of Applied Knowledge* (Chicago: University of Chicago Press, 1988 [1970]).
111 'Functions review is vital', *BMJ*, 307:6895 (1993), 69.
112 Ibid.
113 D. Light and S. Levine, 'The changing character of the medical profession: a theoretical overview', *Milbank Quarterly*, 66:2 (1988), 10–32.
114 'Clinicians must be involved in purchasing', *BMJ*, 306:6882 (1993), 935.
115 T. Delamothe, 'Wanted: guidelines that doctors will follow', *BMJ*, 307:6898 (1993), 218; G. Weisz, 'From clinical counting to Evidence-Based Medicine', in G. Forland, A. Opinel, and G. Weisz (eds.), *Body Counts: Medical Quantification in Historical and Sociological Perspectives* (Montreal: McGill University Press, 2005), pp. 377–93.
116 S. Wallace and R. Gullan, 'Mild head injury: guidelines should be flexible', *BMJ*, 307:6901 (1993), 447–8, quotation at p. 448.
117 'Functions review is vital'.
118 Delamothe, 'Wanted'.
119 F. Moffatt, P. Martin, and S. Timmons, 'Constructing notions of health care productivity: the call for a new professionalism?', *Sociology of Health and Illness*, 36:5 (2014), 686–702.
120 RCGP, *What Sort of Doctor? Assessing Quality of Care in General Practice* (London: RCGP, 1985), p. 2.
121 C. Waine, 'Diabetes and the NHS Bill', *Diabetic Medicine*, 8:3 (1991), 285.
122 This is not to say that doctors did not need persuading. One member of a local medical audit committee in the early 1990s recalls that some were initially suspicious but were later convinced by the practice once it was trialled: interview with B. Potts conducted by the author.
123 E. Freidson, 'The reorganization of the medical profession', *Medical Care Research and Review*, 42:1 (1985), 11–35, esp. pp. 27–8.

6

Making managerial policy in the neoliberal moment

By the 1990s, a consensus was emerging in British medicine about the need for new instruments of professional management and clinical regulation. In the four decades after the 1950s, professional, political, and public anxieties about standards of medical practice had grown inexorably. Critiques of variations and evidence in medical care had joined with concerns about cost and professional accountability to produce a 'crisis' over quality. Locally, some practitioners responded by intensifying projects for structured care, creating more precise protocols and undertaking institutional audits. Nationally, elite professional bodies and leading specialists produced guidelines to inform local developments, and sought to establish national datasets and audit systems. Through these changes, previously informal measures regulating clinical activity became explicit, and the rhythms and content of care became subject to new forms of structure and review.

The Conservative governments of the 1980s and 1990s had also become interested in guidelines and medical audit. Motivated by historic drives to control costs and increase efficiency in the health service – as well as by neoliberal critiques of state and economy – the Thatcher and Major administrations substantially remade the dynamics of the NHS. Inspired by the novel concept of internal markets in public services, extensive reforms converted health authorities from planning and management bodies into state-funded healthcare purchasers, and transformed hospitals and community care agencies into trusts that secured finance through procuring contracts from purchasing bodies.[1] In primary care, larger general practices were encouraged to operate as purchasers of certain hospital services (such as outpatient care), and new GP contracts introduced enhanced pay-for-performance elements.[2] Guidelines and medical audit were to play important roles in the new system. Although remaining under the control of professional bodies, these instruments would enhance professional accountability and provide standards against which care could be measured before payments were made. The earliest moves in this direction were made in relation to chronic disease, with diabetes a prominent target. Long-term conditions were costly problems, and better management promised to improve prevention of expensive sequelae. Furthermore, as diseases that crossed institutional lines, intervention enabled governments to tackle the thorny GP–hospital divide. Measures to confront these problems were included in the 1990 GP contract (and subsequent revisions), as well as forming the basis of reviews into clinical standards in the mid-1990s. By the late 1990s, diabetes had become one of the first conditions to be subject to a National Service Framework (NSF).

Given the contrast between professional and government political projects, this chapter explores how management of professional labour became government policy during the 1980s and 1990s. Despite disparities in aims, specialists and elite professional bodies found common ground with government and state agencies over the production of guidelines and audit structures. All parties saw benefits in co-operation and actively sought collaboration. Reliant upon medical professionals to construct new tools, government often acted through financial support for local programmes, supplemented by assistance for projects undertaken in national bodies. These efforts, moreover, were cultivated by key specialists and professional organisations, who sought resources and authority to develop new instruments. The creation of managerial policy, in other words, was co-constructed. Furthermore, this chapter stresses that elite bodies and leading specialists were crucial to initiating and connecting local, national, and international efforts to manage diabetes and its doctors. Personnel overlaps ensured strong consensus over the nature of reform across different scales of policy creation and service delivery. It was through mobile and influential figures, then, that government and professional projects were aligned enough for management of professional labour to become policy. Of course, the actual and intended effects of policy could be subverted by either government or profession, and the efforts of both sides could be mediated in practice. Nonetheless, their co-operation secured the basis for managerial policy and set the stage for more extensive future reform.

Finally, this chapter suggests that the policy networks surrounding diabetes noted in Chapter 4 were essential in establishing the condition at the forefront of new managerial policies. As a costly, cross-sectoral problem, diabetes – and chronic disease more broadly – provided an important entry point for promoting managerial technologies in the health service. In part, such intervention was facilitated by the institutional and technological groundwork laid in earlier decades. However, governments were also concerned about the possible financial and political costs of intervening in certain areas, meaning that state–professional relations were not always smooth. It was here that the strength of the diabetes policy community became important. Through a vocal lay-professional organisation, interested civil servants, persuasive specialist advocates, and international pressure (especially from the WHO), diabetes was established as an important subject for novel managerial technologies. Diabetes thus provides a lens through which to view managerial policy, not only because of how it was conceived as a possible model for change, but also because of the ways in which it became an object of political interest.

Managing British medicine before 1979

The 1980s and early 1990s were a period of radical innovation in British health policy.[3] During these years, Conservative administrations significantly altered the institutional configuration and dynamics of British healthcare, transforming the role of health authorities and central government in delivering health services. Neoliberal analyses of professionals, bureaucracy, state, and economy provided a broad underpinning for much reform. However, the Thatcher and Major governments were also motivated by a long-held desire of the British state to control NHS costs, and later initiatives built upon developments that took place before the 1980s.

Parliament and the Treasury had placed constant pressure on NHS budgets since 1948. Initial hopes that expenditure would decline as national health improved were dashed very quickly. Governments tried numerous strategies over the post-war period to control costs, ranging from the introduction of charges (most notably for prescriptions in the 1950s) to the application of innovative budgetary rules, such as the Labour government's cash-limited budgeting of the mid-1970s.[4] Maintaining satisfactory levels of provision, however, required considerable resources, and efficiency savings could stretch only so far.

Civil servants, politicians, think-tanks, and professional advisory bodies had noted the problematic connection between resource use and clinical decision-making soon after the creation of the NHS. However, the Ministry (and later Department) of Health felt unable to directly intervene in clinical judgement, given the poor quality of information available and the strength of anxiety that interference would generate backlash from both the public and the profession alike.[5] Instead, until the 1980s, state bodies and central professional advisory agencies sought to confront the issue of costs through improved service monitoring systems, and by encouraging clinicians to use institutional and comparative data to reform their own practices. These efforts began in the early 1950s. During these years, the CHSC sponsored the King's Fund and Nuffield Provincial Hospitals Trust to research alternative accounting systems within hospitals. New schemes linked costs with activity, enabling administrators to compare expenditure longitudinally and between institutions and to highlight possible areas for efficiency. Although they were trialled in various hospitals, implementation costs and administrative concerns about clinician interest resulted in less effective compromises being adopted.[6] Likewise, efforts to control prescribing costs in the 1950s were predicated upon exhortations about 'excessive prescribing' from the Chief Medical Officer in the Ministry of Health and on statistical analyses sent to GPs of their prescribing costs relative to other practitioners.[7] It was hoped that GPs would reflect on this information and alter their practices if their supposed deviations from common practice resulted in greater expenditure. The increasing costs of the drug bill indicate that such efforts did not achieve their ultimate objectives.[8]

Similar, if more complex, techniques were applied to the problem of clinically driven costs in the 1960s and 1970s. The Ministry of Health's Hospital Plan, launched in 1962, loosely practised budget planning, linking finance to specified outcomes and producing national bed norms per population.[9] The Plan itself emerged during a decade within which programme planning, budgeting, and review became more common within Whitehall.[10] Similarly, during the mid- to late 1960s the Ministry developed a new hospital information system, in which hospitals attached data sheets to each inpatient case file and sent 'returns' to RHBs for statistical analysis. Although it experienced problems of timeliness and accuracy, through this Hospital Activity Analysis 'for the first time it was possible, in theory, for consultants to relate the use of resources to the characteristics of their patients, their diagnoses, and their treatments'.[11] This new data system was entangled with attempts to incorporate clinicians into management structures, such as Cogwheel divisions or the consensus management groups upon which the 1974 NHS reforms were built. Improved monitoring was also needed for Labour's turn to priority-setting and planning in the 1970s.[12] Information provision and professional self-management sat at the heart of all such activities, with the hope that self-regulation could bring expenditure under greater control.

Neoliberalism, welfare reform, and the management of British medicine

Political concerns about the relationship between clinical decision-making and resource use continued after the election of Margaret Thatcher in 1979. Comments from parliamentary select committees during this period indicate that traditional fiscal conservatives and social democrats were united in a desire to, at the very least, map the effects of NHS expenditure – in short, to better understand what the benefits of state expenditure actually were.[13] However, the connection between professional autonomy and NHS expenditure disturbed successive Conservative administrations for reasons beyond traditional anxieties about public finances. Rather, the Party, and leading ministers, were increasingly influenced by neoliberal critiques of self-interested welfare professionals and state over-extension during the 1980s and 1990s. Such thinking shaped government policy, with reform packages inflected by debates about the efficiency of markets and the political importance of enterprise. In terms of the NHS, Conservative administrations developed attempts to promote professional self-management, but connected health policy with a broader remaking of the state. Before examining how these critiques informed health policy after 1979, it is worth returning to the often vexed question of 'neoliberalism', which we began to explore in Chapter 4.[14]

Although not gaining political currency in Britain for decades, neoliberal critiques first emerged in the 1930s and 1940s.[15] At this time, a small number of economists and political philosophers reacted against what they saw as a crisis of liberalism, in which liberal governments created mechanisms for securing individual freedom (from disease or old age) by collectivising social risks.[16] Faced with post-war planning and destructive totalitarian regimes, neoliberal theorists sought to rethink liberalism, and recast state interventions in social and economic realms as a risk to the individualised self-determination supposedly at the heart of Western civilisation.[17] Markets in such analyses represented not only the most efficient means for allocating resources, but also a political bulwark. Economic freedom and competition provided the basis for all liberty, and state encroachment here would inevitably result in political authoritarianism.[18] Moreover, in simple economic terms, thinkers such as Friedrich Hayek suggested that central planning and bureaucracy stunted creativity and spontaneous order, and crucially lacked the means to create and process all the information required for efficient production and consumption.[19] Prices, by contrast, provided the signal for individuals to make their own choices, and inequality of outcome rewarded people who made the right decisions (or incentivised improvement, if they made the wrong ones).[20] In this sense, the role of the state was to establish the infrastructure for economic competition between private agents, and to provide limited, non-redistributive, social welfare (i.e. that which did not interfere with the rewards and pricing central to market competition).[21] As Foucault suggests, for early neoliberal theorists the market and its governance requirements thus constituted *the raison d'être* and limit of the state, but markets were not to be laissez-faire.[22] Unlike proponents of classical liberalism, neoliberal thinkers did not see the market as a natural phenomenon. From their perspective, states would be required to establish frameworks for economic activity, and to constantly monitor and intervene to guarantee competition (for instance, to prevent unfair practices) and manage the environment required for enterprise (e.g. by supporting education). This work would be ongoing as capital consistently produced newer and newer circumstances and arrangements.[23]

Over the post-war decades, neoliberal critiques of state and economy were promoted by international networks of economists, political scientists and philosophers through think-tanks, business organisations, journalism, and academia.[24] Core ideas and languages changed over this period. At the height of the Cold War, figureheads like the American economist Milton Friedman amplified a rhetoric of laissez-faire and economic primacy, even if this looked very different from eighteenth- and nineteenth-century variants.[25] Likewise, post-war neoliberal thinkers moved economic analyses into new realms.[26] Paramount in the British case were critiques of areas previously seen as distinct from private enterprise: state bureaucracy and professionally delivered welfare. According to such analyses, state employees and welfare professionals were not altruistic or service-oriented so much as self-interested and unaccountable.[27] Slowly, neoliberal critique concerning the efficiency of markets, the moral and political importance of competition, and the regulative role and limits of the state seeped into British political discourse, and Conservative politicians in particular engaged earnestly with these ideas from the 1970s onwards.[28] Arguments about the degenerative effects of the state on British life were central to crisis narratives around supposed political consensus, providing the platform for the 1979 Conservative election victory.[29]

Into the 1980s and 1990s, neoliberalism was but one ideological framework within which the Conservative Party developed its thinking.[30] All government policy was subject to the dynamics of British politics, from the electorate's attachment to redistributive welfare (embodied in the NHS) to ministerial individuality and constraints imposed by previous policy decisions.[31] Indeed, a leaked government think-tank paper in 1982 proposed remaking health services on an insurance basis. It provoked such political backlash that future policy groups consistently dismissed the idea, and the Prime Minister felt it necessary to insist that the NHS was 'safe in our hands'.[32] Nonetheless, over the 1980s and 1990s, neoliberalism as a rationality for organising the state slowly gained influence, even if providing only a set of analytical principles rather than a dominant grand plan.[33] Thus the Conservative governments of 1979–97 reformed union rights and social security, arguing that such changes would enhance labour market functionality and restore the political bulwark of market choice and democratic decision-making.[34] They denationalised firms and industries to reduce public ownership and promote market competition, establishing the state in a monitoring and regulatory role.[35] Such ideas even entered into the provision of welfare services. In housing, alongside the 'right to buy' council house scheme, the Thatcher administrations repositioned the central state as a distributor of public funds and local councils as 'strategic enablers' for alternative providers. Compulsory competitive tendering was introduced for delivering new projects, and even non-profit housing associations had to compete for fixed grants on new builds and raise private finance for social housing projects.[36]

In healthcare, neoliberal reforms built upon earlier impulses and tools that had been introduced to control costs and assist planning. Furthering practices of oversight and priority-setting developed under Labour governments, between 1982 and 1983 Conservative administrations instituted a review of financial auditing of NHS bodies, created a host of performance indicators (to enable cross-authority comparisons on resource use), and introduced annual performance reviews of health authorities.[37] As noted, parliamentary scrutiny committees provided a cross-party prompt in this direction.[38]

The first major change in policy, though one intended to support reviews and efficiency measures, was the introduction of general management into the NHS. Consensus management teams were replaced by individual managers at each level of the health service, ensuring 'responsibility drawn together in one person, at different levels of the organisation, for planning, implementation and control of performance'.[39] The reforms followed a six-month review of the NHS conducted by a small team of senior civil servants and business leaders, led by Roy (later Sir Roy) Griffiths, then managing director of Sainsbury's supermarkets.[40] The resulting report, whilst very respectful of clinicians and the NHS, echoed public choice theorists by suggesting that it 'cannot be said too often that the National Health Service is about delivering services to people. It is not about organising systems for their own sake.' The solution to inwardly focused professionals and bureaucrats emerged from the argument that there were 'clear similarities between NHS management and business management'. Thus the NHS could be subject to the same sorts of management roles and strategies as certain forms of profit-oriented organisation: managers would be concerned with 'levels of service, quality of product, meeting budgets, cost improvement, productivity, motivating and rewarding staff, research and development, and the long-term viability of the undertaking', all of which, 'in the private sector … would normally be carefully monitored against pre-determined standards and objectives'.[41] As well as undertaking 'real output measurement, against clearly stated management objectives and budgets', managers were charged with enrolling clinicians more effectively into management (and doctors were invited to become managers themselves).[42] Doctors – whose decisions allegedly 'dictate[d] the use of all resources' – would help to set priorities, establish measurements of output in terms of patient care, and 'accept the management responsibility that comes with clinical freedom.'[43] Expressing ideas of what scholars would call 'new public management', Griffiths thus suggested that incorporating accounting and managerial techniques from 'private'-sector bodies would help reorient the NHS to efficient 'public' service.[44]

Following Griffiths, the government embarked on a broader remaking of the health service in line with neoliberal and new public management analyses.[45] The Conservatives laid out the initial direction of travel in 1986 and 1987, with consultative and programme papers for reforms to primary healthcare.[46] Here the government discussed target-based, pay-for-performance elements of GP work, as well as strategies to reduce resource-wasting variations in care.[47] Under the new plans, Family Practitioner Committees, previously administrative agencies, would be reconstituted as managerial bodies. Through specified performance indicators and annual reports from GPs, the committees (later renamed Family Health Services Authorities, FHSAs) could assess the quality and level of primary care provision. Furthermore, the committees would monitor variations in practice standards and care (e.g. differences in referrals) and be empowered to obtain independent professional advice to improve activity.[48]

These reforms were enforced, despite considerable resistance, in the 1990 GP contract.[49] Complementary changes to the dynamics of the NHS were introduced by the 1989 White Paper *Working for Patients* and the resultant 1990 NHS and Community Care Act.[50] Through these documents, the third Thatcher administration (1987–90) made alterations to the roles and funding of health authorities, hospitals, GPs, and the Department of Health, all structured by the belief that 'the Government's main task must be to set a national framework of objectives and priorities'. In turn, authorities and managers – although 'remaining accountable to the centre' – 'must then be allowed to get on with the task of managing'.[51] Under the new reforms, RHAs survived, but were expected to concentrate on the core managerial tasks of 'setting performance criteria', 'monitoring' and 'evaluating' performance in line with government objectives.[52] They retained responsibility for numerous operational roles (such as blood transfusion services), but were expected to delegate as much responsibility to districts as possible. In turn, District Health Authorities were to delegate as many operational functions to units (hospitals) as was feasible, whilst 'ensuring that the health needs of the[ir] populations ... are met'.[53]

Crucially, under the new arrangements District Health Authorities became purchasers of services as well as management bodies. RHAs received central funds, transferring money to districts according to assessed needs.[54] District authorities subsequently 'purchased' care for their patients from hospital 'providers', which might either be directly managed (through devolved management budgets) or exist as independent trusts (initially restricted to hospitals of over 250 beds), or might operate in another district (where superior services or rates might be offered) or work in the 'private sector'.[55] Management of activity came either through a mixture of standard-setting and performance review (in directly provided hospitals) or from contracting (in the case of trusts or private providers). Finally, GPs were also offered the opportunities to become 'fundholders'. If large enough (initially having at least 11,000 registered patients), a practice could apply to receive money for a defined range of non-acute services, and then 'purchase' care directly for patients from hospitals within or without its district.[56] As well as being a provider with a contract and payment for performance, it would also become a purchaser of services from secondary care institutions.

These reforms had a range of aims, not least to enable finance to flow with patients through the service and to depute operational – and thus political – accountability to non-governmental parts of the state.[57] Moreover, whilst undoubtedly challenging pre-existing relationships and laying foundations for expanded private involvement in service delivery, the government's rejection of charges and insurance options meant that the reforms respected two significant principles of the NHS: central funding by taxation and universal access – a core of the supposed 'post-war consensus' – remained intact.[58]

Underpinning these changes, however, was an analysis consonant with contemporary neoliberal values. The introduction of stricter monitoring and accountability practices would prevent state-employed professionals from empire-building and direct their energies to meeting 'legitimate' objectives, namely providing service within available budgets. Some of this surveillance was to be undertaken at the institutional level, through reviews of practices and health authorities. However, self-review would also be performed by doctors through mandated clinical audit, with the aim of 'learning lessons', and potentially identifying and correcting costly variations in care.[59] Regulated competition, now incorporated into state services, was also intended to ensure the most efficient use of state resources and maximise quality within a given capacity. The 'best' hospitals would supposedly attract funding from GPs and District Health Authorities, whilst contracting and fixed budgeting for institutions would encourage innovation and clinical efficiency.[60] Finally, the intended efficiency savings would facilitate reduced taxation and lower 'inflationary spending', freeing capital for politically and economically desirable entrepreneurial activity. Notably, the state in this vision was not 'rolled back'. Instead, through the use of contracting, targets, review, and financial deputation, the central state had the potential to extend government influence further into individual units, and from here to third-sector and private providers.[61] Such trends were also manifest in areas like education, with the 1988 Education Reform Act enabling individual schools to opt out of local authority management and funding, but only at the cost of a national curriculum, results tables, competition for places, target-setting, and external audit.[62]

The reforms of the 1980s and early 1990s supported the management of medical labour in numerous ways, with legislative documents referring to clinical protocol, guidelines, and audit. Conceptually, professional management fitted neatly with the managerialism of neoliberal analyses. As with performance management and dispersed statecraft, guidelines disaggregated and codified the tasks of clinical workers, and audits subjected work and outcomes to supposedly objective measurement against pre-stated, quantified performance indicators.[63] Of course, although clear conceptual cross-overs exist, there is nothing inherently neoliberal about establishing guidelines or setting and auditing targets. Socialist regimes and social democratic planning operate through similar practices.[64] Nonetheless, within the neoliberal-inspired reforms of the early 1990s, the management of professional labour became tied to projects to introduce accountability practices for bureaucracies and to foster competition and market activity in public life. In terms of medicine, guidelines and auditing not only provided potential tools for judging professional work and reducing costly variations in care. They also provided mechanisms through which contracting could take place, and new providers be brought into contact with state finance. For the Department of Health, then, promoting managerial technologies in medicine could serve multiple purposes and smooth the implementation of broader projects to remake the state and its major services.

The effective implementation of government reforms relied upon co-operation from medical professionals. Politically, the response from the major professional bodies, individual doctors, and their allies within Parliament and the media was overwhelmingly critical. Many critics argued that the government sought to 'destabilise the NHS and replace it with a commercial' alternative.[65] Yet opposition on structural elements of reform masked support for elements of professional management. For instance, one contributor to the *BMJ* suggested that 'the notion of health care being bought and sold as a market commodity' raised 'fundamental questions about the possible lack of safety nets within a restructured health service'. Nonetheless, the author continued by declaring that 'the need for greater accountability is incontestable'.[66] Likewise, the well-known socialist GP Julian Tudor Hart strongly criticised the government's proposals for potentially distorting good medical practice, but his critiques of 'paying for means rather than ends' in the GP contract did not condemn targets or incentivised work per se.[67]

For all the rancour, the third Thatcher administration and first Major administration (1990–92) passed legislation and imposed contracts, and thought turned to how to make the best of the new dynamics. More importantly, a cross-over of interest in the management of professional labour enabled elite professional bodies, specialist practitioners and researchers, the Department of Health, and the NHS to construct a consensus around managerial policy. Neoliberal critique may have brought government to the table, but pre-existing professional interests in management were essential to making managerial policy.

Managing diabetes and its professionals under British neoliberalism

Diabetes management was heavily influenced by the NHS reforms. Before the internal market, financial stringency was a challenge and potential opportunity for innovators. We noted in Chapter 4 how neoliberal politics interacted with the management of retinopathy. Policy support for statistical indication linked to cost reduction, moreover, provided opportunities for reformers and planners in other areas. In Manchester, for instance, pioneers of new diabetes centres – institutions dedicated to more patient-centred, multi-disciplinary care than outpatient clinics – used political drives for audit and reduced inpatient costs to their advantage. Through statistical analyses and the promise of savings, innovators garnered political support for organisational change.[68] Likewise, physicians in the South-East Thames Region formed a diabetes group to facilitate the construction of a strategic plan. The group used Hospital Activity Analysis data and questionnaires to calculate the costs and activities associated with diabetes care, making the case for better forward projections and expanded staffing. Once again, they justified such activity on the grounds of reduced costs.[69]

Diabetes management, however, was also tied into neoliberal reforms and concerns evoked in government discussion of 'quality'.[70] As noted in the Introduction, diabetes care formed a central plank in the 1990 GP contract, which had been designed to improve the management of chronic disease. The contract built on pre-existing models of GP mini-clinics in diabetes and other conditions (see Chapter 2) and reinforced professional interest in systematic, managed care (Chapter 3). Moreover, the contract was predicated on the rationale that improved clinical practice could achieve public health aims of secondary prevention of

Making managerial policy 225

long-term sequelae (Chapter 1). Unlike professionally designed schemes, however, the government contract attached financial incentives to practice-based disease management. In exchange for payment, GPs engaged in performance management relationships with FHSAs. Practitioners would develop protocols with fellow professionals, and the relevant FHSA would assess care against agreed criteria to determine financial recompense. The new arrangements, therefore, reflected the mix of projects supporting managed medicine. One the one hand, cognisant of the conflict over contemporaneous organisational change, the government left protocol and audit as the responsibility of local professionals. Doctors assumed control of developing and managing new tools, which the state encouraged through funding and providing platforms for exchange.[71] On the other hand, the government tried to connect management of clinical labour with performance management structures designed to promote public health and efficiency savings. Despite potential conflict, and practitioners' anxieties that incentives might produce adverse effects, these interests formed the basis of managerial policies, and diabetes provided a key area of intervention.[72]

Government interest in diabetes thus partially derived from the condition's financial and humanitarian costs and its place within a broader landscape of worrisome chronic diseases. However, political focus on diabetes (and other chronic conditions) also underlined how government support for professional management gravitated towards conditions in which the infrastructure and momentum for managed practice had previously been established. As noted in earlier chapters, practitioners had experimented with local protocol for systematic care since the 1970s, whilst elite specialists and professional bodies had been producing national guidelines and undertaking audit of diabetes management for over a decade. The BDA and Royal Colleges had thus repositioned themselves as guarantors of quality structured care, and sought to produce guidance to inform local practice. Moreover, the infrastructure for professional co-operation was also already in place. The RCP and BDA, for instance, had developed close connections, auditing national provision of staffing and facilities of diabetes during the mid-1980s.[73] With both agencies interested in clinical audit, the Department of Health was able to facilitate ongoing developments, for instance funding a joint BDA–Royal College working group exploring routine audit of process and outcome in the early 1990s.[74] Similarly, the Department could also use funding to local centres of innovation – such as Manchester – as a means to further develop managerial tools.[75]

Indeed, the link between protocol and payment in the 1990 contract undoubtedly reflected the pre-existing 'good sense' surrounding diabetes treatment and built such developments into the performance-related system.

International trends also accelerated the creation of managerial structures, and opportunities for professional–state co-operation, in British diabetes care. As noted in Chapter 5, the St Vincent Declaration of 1989 was integral here. The Declaration set out basic quantified targets for the care and prevention of diabetes to be applied across national contexts, and resulted from a conference of leading specialists, researchers, and civil servants held under the aegis of the European regions of the International Diabetes Federation and the WHO.[76] The British government signed the Declaration, which generated new national infrastructure. For instance, in 1992, the BDA and the health departments of England, Wales, Scotland, and Northern Ireland formed a joint St Vincent Taskforce to develop the auditing and care arrangements necessary to meet the proposed targets. The group comprised medical and nursing professionals, as well as healthcare purchasers, providers, and patient representatives. Some leading professionals even hoped that the Taskforce would be able to assist health authorities in their contracting duties, as purchasing bodies lacked relevant expertise. Once again, funding such work in diabetes was simpler than in other areas of care because of the infrastructure for co-operation already in place.

The management of diabetes care, however, could also provide something of a model for the management of other conditions and areas of healthcare. Such a sentiment was expressed in the second report of the Clinical Standards Advisory Group (CSAG), published in 1994.[77] CSAG was a multi-disciplinary, statutory body with a rotating membership composed of nominees from the Royal Colleges and other leading professional bodies.[78] It was charged with making investigations into, and providing recommendations to government on, standards of care within given subjects. Created during intense conflict over NHS reforms, it was declared by politicians, members of the profession, and policy analysts to be an attempt to broker peace between professional bodies and the government.[79] Although potentially indicating the government's acceptance that the profession should set, monitor, and control its own standards, the Group's name and purpose also indicated a broad consensus over the need for more active surveillance and management of professional labour.

The Group's second report was on diabetes care, and was researched and written by a specially chosen Diabetes Committee whose broad membership included both medical and nursing specialists as well as generalists, such as administrative officers, a nationally prominent GP, directors of public health, and leading figures within the RCP.[80] The Committee followed the remit laid out in Parliament: to 'advise on standards of clinical care for people with diabetes', work which would entail 'reviews of existing statements of clinical standards, of the standards specified in NHS contracts, and of arrangements for auditing the delivery of services to contracted standards, in a representative sample of NHS districts and boards'.[81] Thus, upon creation, the Committee formed a sub-group (complete with co-opted members) to review nineteen existing international, American, and British standards, and to construct its own standards document.[82] This document served as a benchmark for multi-disciplinary groups which then visited providers, purchasers, clinical teams, GPs, and 'consumer representatives' to assess provision in eleven health districts of different sizes, locations, and reputations. From these visits, the Committee produced site reports, and the parent body published the Committee's own standards document and anonymised findings, along with its recommendations and the government's response, in a final report.

The relationship between diabetes and neoliberal healthcare reforms was visible, firstly, in the very terms of reference for the Committee. The Secretary of State for Health requested analysis of standards within contracts, as well of the infrastructure in place for auditing contracts against those standards. Such demands were perhaps a reaction to broader concerns that integrated chronic disease care might have been disrupted by the 1990s reforms, and to the impenetrable 'wall' erected 'between the purchasing and provider role of the District Health Authority'.[83] In fact, worries about lost contracting expertise were so great that the NHS Executive in England commissioned guidance on needs assessment by one of the CSAG authors, and endorsed 'a small number of existing clinical guidelines' on diabetes in order to help purchasers draw up contracts.[84] (And such decisions, once again, marked points of convergence between professional visions of self-management and performance management of the health service.)

Secondly, connections between NHS reforms, diabetes, and professional management can be seen in how the exercise itself acted as a local and national review of care. The Committee produced its own standards document, and the Group's findings influenced care in at least some of the locales visited (see below). Finally, the report itself articulated the possible attraction of diabetes as a conduit for further managerial developments. 'This study has shown', the authors noted, 'that standards of care can be assessed against a consensus document.' 'Our approach', they went on, 'would appear to be a useful model for assessing provision of care for other diseases of public health importance.'[85] It was a sentiment whose importance was amplified by the mixture of specialists and generalists on the Diabetes Committee, confirming the novelty of such managerial approaches at a systemic level as well as their applicability elsewhere.

Enrolling the neoliberal state and creating managerial consensus in diabetes care

Although there were areas of cross-over between elite professional endeavours to construct non-punitive technologies of medical management and neoliberal state programmes for professional and health authority performance management, these projects were by no means in complete alignment. Moreover, despite diabetes care providing an attractive proposition for the state to pursue its managerial interests, professionals themselves were central in promoting and co-constructing managerial instruments and policy around the condition. This is notable in the histories of both the St Vincent Declaration and the CSAG report on diabetes, as well as the creation of a later NSF for diabetes in Britain.

The creation of the St Vincent Declaration was, for instance, pointedly political. The event owed much to the work of, amongst others (including British epidemiologist Hilary King), Professor Harry Keen, an internationally renowned British diabetologist. Keen felt that an international initiative to improve diabetes care – one backed by the WHO – would pressure national governments into more concertedly addressing the growing challenge of diabetes at a clinical and public health level.[86] Furthermore, this political orientation was embodied in the form of the Declaration. Although the contents of the Declaration had been left to experts, and despite precedent in the WHO 'Health for All' initiative in 1979, there had been debate during drafting as to whether target-setting was appropriate (especially in the absence of baseline data) and what particular targets should be chosen.[87] However, targets were adopted specifically because those involved feared the Declaration would be toothless without them. In the event, the conference adopted a mixture of quantified outcome targets (for instance, halving the rate of gangrene amputations in five years) and specific process and structure objectives, such as establishing 'monitoring and control systems using state of the art information technology for quality assurance'.[88] Those who worked on the Declaration and its subsequent projects felt that it probably did not affect practice at the point of individual exchanges between clinical teams and patients. Crucially, though, the Declaration did provide political tools and momentum with which bodies like the BDA could lobby government, and through which individual practitioners could encourage local doctors and NHS authorities to take up auditing and guideline practices.[89] Moreover, professional lobbying was central to convincing the government to support the Declaration and to create subsidiary working groups. Interviewees who worked in relation to St Vincent, for instance, recalled civil servants' hesitancy about signing the Declaration. They noted departmental concern about 'special pleading', the idea that if the Minister for Health agreed to specific programmes for diabetes then the government would be open to similar claims for a host of conditions. Eventually, after concerted pressure, the UK did sign, creating a path for the creation of various groups for guideline and audit development schemes.[90]

Post-war policy networks also secured political support for the CSAG review of diabetes standards. The review emerged, in part, from the fate of diabetes within the Major government's public health initiative, *The Health of the Nation*. This programme continued the work of *Working for Patients* in laying out a role for the state as provider of a 'strategic framework' for public health, based on managerial principles of calculated target-setting and continuous performance assessment.[91] The centre would develop objectives, and, freed from the burden of delivering services day-to-day, health authorities could use contracts to achieve them.[92] Initial consultation produced sixteen areas for possible intervention, including diabetes. Reflecting a growing faith in guidelines and auditing, the suggested diabetes targets included 'the proportion of GP practices within a FHSA area who follow protocols agreed locally between hospital clinicians and primary care staff'.[93]

Despite the BDA submitting persuasive arguments for diabetes, the subsequent White Paper adopted fourteen quantified targets for five key areas: coronary heart disease and stroke, cancer, mental illness, HIV/AIDS and sexual health, and accidents.[94] The Major government suggested that these five areas met three key criteria, being areas of considerable premature death and avoidable ill-health, in possession of known effective interventions, and amenable to target-setting and monitoring.[95] Critics of the programme have suggested, by contrast, that alongside being causes of considerable NHS expenditure, the subjects chosen also contained historic trends favourable to future improvement for which the government might take credit.[96] Regardless of the reasoning, diabetes was omitted from the programme. However, interviewees who had close connection with the BDA suggested that the CSAG review of diabetes services was something of a 'sop' for the omission of diabetes from *The Health of the Nation*. The government was aware of needing to offer a concession, and influential figures within the CSAG parent group had colleagues' interests in mind when pushing for diabetes as an area of standards investigation.[97] The Group agreed, and the Diabetes Committee then pulled together leading figures in the field of diabetes management to drive the work forward.[98]

In this sense, rather than professionals being enrolled into state projects, specialists and elite professional bodies used the state to engage in activities that fitted their own priorities, or at least to co-operate with the state in a way that would better manage British medicine and its populations.[99] As subsequent projects remained predicated upon professional expertise, participants believed that their work would improve care and empower professionals to manage their own practice, not only in ways that facilitated quality-assurance mechanisms, but also in ways with resource implications that conflicted with state concerns about costs. One site review from the CSAG report, for instance, provided the grounds for local institutions to hire a consultant diabetologist where previously one had not been in place.[100] Equally, as indicated above, one interviewee involved in policy work recalled how reports like the CSAG's provided a means for the BDA to make the case for further government or health authority activity, with changes probably increasing short-term financial costs.[101]

As well as on professional and state co-operation, managerial policy for diabetes care also depended on the ways in which specialists moved between different bodies to produce a broad consensus on the core elements of 'quality' care. The existence of such consensus in diabetes care could be seen within the CSAG report, which suggested that 'within [the standards documents reviewed] there is a large measure of agreement on what constitutes care of acceptable quality'.[102] This overlap made it easier for the Diabetes Committee's sub-group to compile its own standards document, one which was wide-ranging in its focus but contained common elements discussed in Chapter 5, including lists of tests to be performed at medical and annual review, reflections on possible audit measures, recommendations for quantified performance indicators for patients, and discussion of the need for guidelines, registers, and recall-mechanisms.[103] In part, the commonality between extant standards documents reflected the broader 'good sense' about quality diabetes care discussed in earlier chapters. Yet this good sense – and its embodiment in the documentation of various agencies – was the product of elite practitioners and academics moving between bodies that produced standards and guidelines. Members of the CSAG, for instance, were involved in shaping the St Vincent Declaration and pioneered its subsequent work on audit. They also helped produce Royal College and BDA guidelines on diabetes management, worked on NHS Executive projects, and operated on many of the guideline committees formed and funded by the Department of Health.[104] Influential figures were also connected through training and research with other major figures in the field, such as Harry Keen, John Nabbarro, or Robert Tattersall.[105] Specific proposals and documents, in other words, emerged out of both broader political contexts and well-defined intellectual and policy communities.

Moving between different levels of the health services, and different arenas of discussion and governance, helped these figures to align recommendations of local and regional NHS authorities, elite professional bodies, international organisations, and lay-professional and state-sponsored agencies. They thus provided sufficient agreement for managerial recommendations and infrastructures to emerge, and mediated potentially conflicting agendas.[106] Using government funding and activity, certain elite specialists and professional bodies helped set national standards and, through their production of tools for management, sat at the forefront of quality regulation and governance. At the same time, through its resources and support, the government sought to use this repositioning to its own advantage, encouraging professional management in ways that furthered neoliberal drives for accountability and financial control. Undoubtedly, there were tensions and conflicts. Governments did not always support the findings of committees. They could refuse proposals that had resource implications or required direct government intervention in service provision. Equally, different aims and political realities could undermine government efforts to impose forms of performance management or contain costs. Despite these conflicts, though, co-operation between state agencies and elite professionals laid the foundation for future political and structural transformations and the creation of more managed medical labour.

Conclusion: NSFs and the making of managerial policy

The structure of the NHS came under further scrutiny after the mid-1990s. The election of a Labour government in 1997 ended eighteen years of Conservative government and brought new analyses of the service to the fore. The Blair administrations ended fundholding and internal markets, but kept the division between purchasers and providers and enhanced primary-care influence over the service. New policy established the Primary Care Group – which brought together GPs and other primary healthcare providers in an area as budget managers – as the fulcrum of the service, and softened mechanisms of competition in favour of co-operation and long-term contracting. The new government also encouraged mixed-sector capital projects to increase hospital capacity.[107]

Despite such changes, both Conservative and Labour governments from the early 1990s onwards retained an emphasis on guideline, audit, and healthcare management. Structurally, the Royal Colleges, elite specialist bodies, and ad hoc statutory groups had to share their role in producing guidance and undertaking review with new state agencies that reflected the growing rhetoric around Evidence-Based Medicine. During the late 1990s, independent Evidence-Based Medicine organisations like the Cochrane Centre were joined by state-sponsored agencies such as the National Institute for Clinical Excellence (NICE), Commission for Health Improvement, and National Audit Office.[108] New agencies could disrupt existing expert networks. For instance, one interviewee disliked the pressure for targets emerging from these agencies. A disagreement over the standardising drives of NICE meant that the interviewee was not involved in NICE guideline production work, despite great experience in this area.[109] Nonetheless, the emphasis of these agencies remained on providing guidance and undertaking review to ensure that local systems were set up to inform 'best practice'.[110]

In terms of diabetes, the continuing political and professional support for managing medicine can be seen from the creation of an NSF for diabetes between 2001 and 2002. Once again, diabetes was at the forefront of managerial policy, with the diabetes NSF one of five initial frameworks designed to set national standards for care and provide strategic advice on achieving such standards.[111] The diabetes framework built on a belief in managerial technologies as central to 'driv[ing] up quality and tackl[ing] variations in care', although, marking a slight break with earlier standards, it was also oriented towards patient experience and empowerment.[112] The framework itself laid out twelve objectives for the NHS and discussed their implications for service providers and doctors, alongside providing a plan for how these objectives could be met.[113] It also found support in new contract arrangements for GPs established under the QOF in 2004, through which complex financial incentives were developed for diabetes management (and chronic disease management more broadly) and payment was closely related to process and outcome assessment.[114] As of 2018, both the QOF and the NSF are still in use, the QOF in formal contracting, the NSF indirectly, providing the basis for Diabetes UK's policy work.[115]

Although the NSF appeared a striking innovation, interviewees involved in its creation underlined the importance of previous political work on diabetes to its construction, praising the policy networks, conceptual frameworks, and techniques developed over preceding decades. They recalled, for instance, the work of leading figures like Harry Keen and George Alberti (then President of the RCP of London), and lobbying from agencies like Diabetes UK.[116] Through slow concerted pressure and more light-touch conversations with ministers, civil servants, and the Chief Medical Officer, these actors were able to gain political momentum that was maintained by consecutive Ministers for Health.[117] Figures at the heart of this work and close to the External Reference Group that compiled the standards and delivery documents recalled using the intelligence and documents accumulated through the political efforts of the previous decade.[118] Indeed, the NSF itself directly made reference to 'build[ing] upon the vision of the St Vincent Declaration.'[119]

The developments laid out in this chapter, and those proceeding it, provided the groundwork for approaches to diabetes – and British medicine more broadly – that have lasted through to the present day. Although, if focusing on contemporary infrastructure, we might suggest that the rise of managerial medicine was 'incomplete' by the mid-1990s, the principles, practices, and techniques of medicine that we have traced throughout the post-war period had nonetheless become the foundation for policy and professional practice. By the end of the 1990s, new actors were making managerial policy. None, however, questioned the idea that the structure and review of medical rhythms, decision-making, and outcomes were essential to guaranteeing quality care. By the start of the present century, the management of medical practice was an increasingly naturalised feature of the health services. Diabetes care, moreover, had been at the forefront of such developments.

Notes

1. N. Timmins, *The Five Giants: A Biography of the Welfare State* (London: Fontana Press, 1996), p. 465. Initially, becoming a self-governing trust was voluntary, but by 1997, only 5 per cent of services remained directly managed: C. Webster, *The National Health Service: A Political History* (Oxford: Oxford University Press, 1998), p. 198.
2. J. Lewis, 'The medical profession and the state: GPs and the GP contract in the 1960s and 1990s', *Social Policy and Administration*, 32:2 (1998), 132–50.
3. On the limits to innovation: R. Klein, *The New Politics of the NHS: From Creation to Reinvention*, 5th edition (Oxford: Radcliffe, 2006), pp. 140–86.
4. C. Webster, *The Health Services since the War*, vol. I: *Problems of Health Care: The National Health Service before 1957* (London: HMSO, 1988), pp. 133–96, 223; Timmins, *The Five Giants*, p. 381.
5. Klein, *The New Politics of the NHS*, pp. 35–8, 58–66.
6. T. Cutler, 'Managerialism *avant la lettre*? The debate on accounting in the NHS hospitals in the 1950s', in V. Berridge and K. Loughlin (eds.), *Medicine, the Market, and the Mass Media: Producing Health in the Twentieth Century* (London: Routledge, 2005), pp. 124–45.
7. G. Rivett, *From Cradle to Grave: Fifty Years of the NHS* (London: King's Fund, 1997), pp. 111–12.
8. C. Webster, *The Health Services since the War*, vol. 2: *Government and Health Care: The British National Health Service, 1958–1979* (London: HMSO, 1996), appendix 3.10, p. 809.
9. Klein, *The New Politics of the NHS*, pp. 54–8.
10. G. O'Hara, *From Dreams to Disillusionment: Economic and Social Planning in the 1960s* (Basingstoke: Palgrave Macmillan, 2007).
11. Rivett, *From Cradle to Grave*, p. 181.
12. See Chapter 2. On management: S. Snow, '"I've never found doctors to be a difficult bunch": doctors, managers and NHS reorganisations in Manchester and Salford, 1948–2007', *Medical History*, 57:1 (2013), 65–86.
13. Klein, *The New Politics of the NHS*, pp. 91–2.
14. R. Venugopal, 'Neoliberalism as concept', *Economy and Society*, 44:2 (2015), 165–87.

15 D. Stedman Jones, *Masters of the Universe: Hayek, Friedman, and the Birth of Neoliberal Politics* (Princeton: Princeton University Press, 2014), pp. 2–4.
16 M. Foucault, *The Birth of Biopolitics: Lectures at the Collège de France, 1978–79*, trans. G. Burchell, ed. M. Senellart (Basingstoke: Palgrave Macmillan, 2008), pp. 65–70; R. Pinker, 'New liberalism and the middle way', in R. Page and R. Silburn (eds.), *British Social Welfare in the Twentieth Century* (Basingstoke: Macmillan, 1999), pp. 80–104; E. P. Hennock, 'Poverty and social reforms', in P. Johnson (ed.), *Twentieth Century Britain: Economic, Social and Cultural Change* (London: Longman, 1994), pp. 79–93.
17 Stedman Jones, *Masters of the Universe*, pp. 2–4.
18 Ibid., pp. 37–72.
19 Ibid., pp. 47–66; J. Tomlinson, 'Planning: debate and policy in the 1940s', *Twentieth Century British History*, 3:2 (1992), pp. 156–8, 162–9.
20 Stedman Jones, *Masters of the Universe*, pp. 63–4; Foucault, *The Birth of Biopolitics*, p. 143.
21 Stedman Jones, *Masters of the Universe*, p. 76; Foucault, *The Birth of Biopolitics*, pp. 142–5.
22 Foucault, *The Birth of Biopolitics*, pp. 82–7, 117–20.
23 Ibid., pp. 133–4, 138–41, 161. Figures like Hayek also allocated states roles in maintaining stable currencies, whilst regulation also involved such things as health and safety: Stedman-Jones, *Masters of the Universe*, p. 67.
24 Stedman-Jones, *Masters of the Universe*, pp. 134–79; B. Jackson, 'The think-tank archipelago: Thatcherism and neoliberalism', in B. Jackson and R. Saunders (eds.), *Making Thatcher's Britain* (Cambridge: Cambridge University Press, 2012), pp. 43–61; N. Rollings, 'Cracks in the post-war Keynesian settlement? The role of organised business in Britain in the rise of neoliberalism before Margaret Thatcher', *Twentieth Century British History*, 24:4 (2013), 637–59.
25 Stedman-Jones, *Masters of the Universe*, pp. 100–3.
26 Foucault, *The Birth of Biopolitics*, pp. 239–316.
27 Stedman-Jones, *Masters of the Universe*, pp. 126–33.
28 For earlier Conservative interest: C. Muller, 'The Institute of Economic Affairs: undermining the post-war consensus', *Contemporary British History*, 10:1 (1996), 88–110.
29 See Chapter 4; C. Hay, 'Chronicles of a death foretold: the Winter of Discontent and the construction of the crisis of British Keynesianism', *Parliamentary Affairs*, 63:3 (2010), 446–70.
30 R. Lowe, *The Welfare State in Britain since 1945*, 3rd edition (Basingstoke: Palgrave Macmillan, 2005), pp. 29–32; A. Gamble, *The Free Economy and the Strong State: The Politics of Thatcherism*, 2nd edition (Basingstoke: Macmillan, 1994), pp. 34–68.

31 P. Pierson, *Dismantling the Welfare State? Thatcher, Reagan and the Politics of Retrenchment* (Cambridge: Cambridge University Press, 1994).
32 Webster, *The National Health Service*, pp. 154–5; M. Gorsky, '"Searching for the people in charge": appraising the 1983 Griffiths NHS Management Inquiry', *Medical History*, 57:1 (2013), 96.
33 Although it does not refer to 'neoliberalism', see discussion of principles, opportunism, and ministerial influence in Klein, *The New Politics of the NHS*, pp. 146–52.
34 J. Bradshaw, 'Social security', in D. Marsh and R. A. W. Rhodes (eds.), *Implementing Thatcherite Policies: Audit of an Era* (Buckingham: Open University Press, 1992), pp. 81–99; D. Marsh, 'Industrial relations', in Rhodes and Marsh (eds.), *Implementing Thatcherite Policies*, pp. 32–49; P. Addison, *No Turning Back: The Peacetime Revolutions of Post-War Britain* (Oxford: Oxford University Press, 2010), pp. 275–314.
35 M. Moran, 'The regulatory state', *Parliamentary Affairs*, 54 (2001), 19–34; D. Marsh, 'Privatization under Mrs Thatcher: a review of the literature'. *Public Administration*, 69 (1991), 459–80; A. Gamble, 'Privatization, Thatcherism, and the British state', *Journal of Law and Society*, 16:1 (1989), 1–20.
36 P. Kemp, 'Housing', in Rhodes and Marsh (eds.), *Implementing Thatcherite Policies*, pp. 65–80; I. Kirkpatrick, S. Ackroyd, and R. Walker, *The New Managerialism and Public Service Professions: Change in Health, Social Services and Housing* (Basingstoke: Palgrave Macmillan, 2005), pp. 135–7.
37 Klein, *The New Politics of the NHS*, pp. 115–16; Webster, *The National Health Service*, pp. 165–7. Scholars have criticised these attempts to establish performance indicators as adding little to efficiency management and excluding meaningful data relating to clinical performance: Rivett, *From Cradle to Grave*, p. 334.
38 S. Harrison, *National Health Service Management in the 1980s* (Aldershot: Avebury, 1994).
39 E. R. Griffiths to N. Fowler, 'NHS Management Inquiry', 23 October 1983, reproduced in ibid., pp. 158–77, quote at p. 166.
40 Gorsky, '"Searching for the people in charge"', pp. 87–107.
41 Griffiths, 'NHS Management Inquiry', p. 165.
42 Ibid., p. 167.
43 Ibid., p. 172.
44 Although 'private' and 'public' are colloquially used to designate profit-oriented business and tax-funded state agencies respectively, the terms have malleable histories. Most importantly, techniques such as budget and programme review were common in state agencies before the 1980s. Other practices, later imported from businesses, were not necessarily common, and the view of the 'private' sector from within government was highly specific: J. Clarke and J. Newman, *The Managerial State: Power,*

Making managerial policy 237

Politics and Ideology in the Remaking of Social Welfare (London: Sage, 1997), pp. 27–9, 56. On the internal consistency of new public management: Kirkpatrick et al., *The New Managerialism*, pp. 64–5.
45 For responses to Griffiths: Gorksy, '"Searching for the people in charge"', pp. 101–5.
46 Secretaries of State for Social Services, Wales, Northern Ireland, and Scotland, *Primary Health Care: An Agenda for Discussion*, Cmnd 9778 (London: HMSO, 1986); Secretaries of State for Social Services, Wales, Northern Ireland, and Scotland, *Promoting Better Health: The Government's Programme for Improving Primary Health Care*, Cm 249 (London: HMSO, 1987).
47 Secretaries of State for Social Services, *Promoting Better Health*, pp. 13–16, 23.
48 Ibid., pp. 23–4, 53–4.
49 Klein, *The New Politics of the NHS*, pp. 158–61; Lewis, 'The medical profession and the state', pp. 139–44.
50 Secretaries of State for Social Services, Wales, Northern Ireland, and Scotland, *Working for Patients*, Cm 555 (London: HMSO, 1989); National Health Service and Community Care Act 1990, c. 19.
51 Secretaries of State for Social Services, *Working for Patients*, p. 12.
52 Ibid., p. 13.
53 Ibid., p. 14.
54 Ibid., pp. 30–3.
55 Ibid., pp. 33–5; on the criteria and process of acquiring trust status: pp. 22–9.
56 Ibid., pp. 49–53.
57 Klein, *The New Politics of the NHS*, pp. 150–1. See also Clarke and Newman, *The Managerial State*, pp. 29–33.
58 Klein, *The New Politics of the NHS*, pp. 146–58.
59 Secretaries of State for Social Services, *Working for Patients*, pp. 39–42, 55–60.
60 Ibid., pp. 16, 20–4, 30–7.
61 Clarke and Newman, *The Managerial State*, pp. 29–33.
62 G. Whitty, 'The New Right and the national curriculum: state control or market forces', in M. Flude and M. Hammer (eds.), *The Education Reform Act, 1988: Its Origins and Implications* (London: Falmer Press, 1990), pp. 21–36.
63 Kirkpatrick et al., *The New Managerialism*, p. 59.
64 A. B. Kipnis, 'Audit cultures: neoliberal governmentality, socialist legacy, or technologies of governing?', *American Ethnologist*, 35:2 (2008), 275–89.
65 Hansard, HC, vol. 152, cols. 1027 and cols. 1037, 11 May 1989; Klein, *The New Politics of the NHS*, pp. 152–61; Timmins, *The Five Giants*, pp. 465–71

66 J. Bain, 'NHS review', *BMJ*, 298:6675 (1989), 746.
67 J. T. Hart, 'Coronary heart disease: preventable but not prevented?', *British Journal of General Practice*, 40:340 (1990), 441–2, esp. p. 441.
68 H. Valier and R. Bivins, 'Organization, ethnicity and the British National Health Service', in J. Stanton (ed.), *Innovations in Health and Medicine: Diffusion and Resistance in the Twentieth Century* (London: Routledge, 2002), pp. 46–7.
69 W. D. Alexander and South East Thames Diabetes Physicians Group, 'Diabetes care in a UK health region: activity, facilities, and costs', *Diabetic Medicine*, 5:6 (1988), 577–81.
70 On the politics of quality: I. Kirkpatrick and M. M. Lucio (eds.), *The Politics of Quality in the Public Sector: The Management of Change* (London: Routledge, 1995).
71 P. Day, R. Klein, and F. Miller, *A Comparative US–UK Study of Guidelines* (London: Nuffield Trust, 1998), pp. 22–7.
72 D. J. Paynton, 'The NHS bill, the GP contract, and diabetic care', *Diabetic Medicine*, 8:3 (1991), 286.
73 RCP of London and BDA, *The Provision of Medical Care for Adult Diabetic Patients in the United Kingdom* (London: BDA, 1984).
74 D. R. R. Williams, P. D. Home, and Members of a Working Group of the RCP and BDA, 'A proposal for continuing audit of diabetes services', *Diabetic Medicine*, 9:8 (1992), 759–64.
75 I. J. Bennett, C. Lambert, G. Hinds, and C. Kirton, 'Emerging standards for diabetes care from a city-wide primary care audit', *Diabetic Medicine*, 11:5 (1994), 489–92.
76 A-M. Felton and M. S. Hall, 'Diabetes – from St Vincent to Glasgow. Have we progressed in 20 years?', *British Journal of Diabetes and Vascular Disease*, 9:4 (2009), 142.
77 CSAG, *Standards of Clinical Care for People with Diabetes* (London: HMSO, 1994).
78 The parameters for the body – including composition – were laid out in a Statutory Instrument: The Clinical Standards Advisory Group Regulations 1991, No. 578, available at: https://www.legislation.gov.uk/uksi/1991/578/introduction/made (accessed April 2018).
79 J. Warden, 'Peace in our time', *BMJ*, 300:6736 (1990), 1359; Klein, *The New Politics of the NHS*, p. 161.
80 CSAG, *Standards of Clinical Care for People with Diabetes*, appendix 3, p. 34.
81 Ibid., p. 1.
82 Ibid., pp. 17–18, 34, appendix 1 and appendix 3.
83 Paynton, 'The NHS bill, the GP contract, and diabetic care'.
84 CSAG, *Standards of Clinical Care*, pp. 35–7, 36.
85 Ibid., p. 2.

86 Interview with Professor Whittaker conducted by the author; interview with Professor Davies conducted by the author. Professor Whittaker is a retired consultant diabetologist who worked within major centres of diabetes care and research between the 1970s and 2000s. Professor Davies is a retired epidemiologist and health authority member who worked within major centres of diabetes care and research between the 1970s and 2000s, as well as undertaking government advisory and university administration work.
87 Interview with Professor Davies.
88 Ibid. For the declaration: G. E. Reiber and H. King, *Guidelines for the Development of a National Programme for Diabetes Mellitus*' (Geneva: WHO, 1991), annex 5, p. 62.
89 Interview with Professor Davies; interview with Professor Whittaker; interview with B. Potts conducted by the author. Potts presently works in Diabetes UK, and previously worked within an audit advisory group during the 1990s. K. Piwernetz, P. D. Home, O. Snorgaard, M. Antsiferov, K. Staehr-Johansen, and M. Krans for the DiabCare Monitoring Group of the St Vincent's Declaration Steering Committee, 'Monitoring the targets of the St Vincent Declaration and the implementation of the quality management in diabetes care: the DiabCare initiative', *Diabetic Medicine*, 10:4 (1993), 371–7.
90 Interview with Professor Davies.
91 Department of Health, *The Health of the Nation: A Consultative Document for Health in England*, Cm 1523 (London: HMSO, 1991), p. iv.
92 Ibid., pp. iii–iv.
93 Ibid., pp. 84–5.
94 Department of Health, *The Health of the Nation: A Strategy for Health in England*, Cm 1986 (London: HMSO, 1992); WLA, MSS (10522), BDA, 'The Health of the Nation: response from the British Diabetic Association', October 1991.
95 Department of Health, *The Health of the Nation: A Strategy for Health in England*, pp. 15–20.
96 Klein, *The New Politics of the NHS*, p. 169; interview with Professor Whittaker.
97 Interview with Professor Davies.
98 Ibid.; interview with Professor Whittaker.
99 S. Pickard, 'The role of governmentality in the establishment, maintenance, and demise of professional jurisdictions: the case of geriatric medicine', *Sociology of Health and Illness*, 32:7 (2010), 1072–86. But interaction was a two-way street, and subject to government interests: S. Sheard, 'Quacks and clerks: historical and contemporary perspectives on the structure and function of the British medical civil service', *Social Policy & Administration*, 44:2 (2010), 193–207.

100 Interview with Professor Davies.
101 Interview with B. Potts.
102 CSAG, *Standards of Clinical Care*, p. 17.
103 Ibid., pp. 18–29.
104 Ibid., p. 35. Philip Home, Rhys Williams, and Colin Waine, for instance, had all worked either on St Vincent's projects, on Royal College guideline production, or in other departmental capacities, as well as on the CSAG: cf. ibid., p. 34: ibid., pp. 36–7; Piwernetz et al., 'Monitoring the targets of the St Vincent Declaration'; C. Waine, *Why Not Care for your Diabetic Patients?*, 2nd edition (London: RCGP, 1988).
105 Interview with Professor Davies; interview with Professor Whittaker.
106 On the importance of individuals moving across arenas of discussion and action to stabilise projects: B. Latour, *The Pasteurization of France*, trans. A. Sheridan and J. Law (Cambridge, MA: Harvard University Press, 1993).
107 Klein, *The New Politics of the NHS*, pp. 192–8.
108 S. Harrison and B. Wood, 'Scientific-bureaucratic medicine and UK health policy', *Policy Studies Review*, 17:4 (2000), 25–42.
109 Interview with Professor Whittaker.
110 Klein, *The New Politics of the NHS*, pp. 197–9.
111 G. Chapman, S. Adam, and D. Stockford, 'National Service Frameworks: promoting the public health', *Journal of Epidemiology and Community Health*, 55:6 (2001), 373–4.
112 Department of Health, *National Service Framework for Diabetes: Standards* (London: Department of Health, 2001), p. 11.
113 Ibid.; Department of Health, *National Service Framework for Diabetes: Delivery Strategy* (London: Department of Health, 2002).
114 A. Dixon, A. Khachatryan, A. Wallace, S. Peckham, T. Boyce, and S. Gillam, *Impact of Quality and Outcomes Framework on Health Inequalities* (London: King's Fund, 2011).
115 Interview with B. Potts.
116 Interview with Professor Davies; interview with B. Potts.
117 Interview with B. Potts.
118 Ibid.; interview with Professor Davies.
119 Department of Health, *National Service Framework for Diabetes: Standards*, p. 11.

Epilogue

The creation of the NSF for diabetes in the early 2000s marked the consolidation of managerial approaches to the disease and its professionals at a national level. The framework laid out clear standards for high-quality care and strategies for achieving them. The latter built upon the registers, recall systems, care protocols, guidelines, and practices of target-setting and audit – the technology of quality – through which professional bodies had sought to subject diabetes care to structure and review over the post-war period.[1] Although it introduced subtle changes to the prevailing consensus on diabetes management – for instance, developing primary preventive strategies and bringing professional management closer to performance management – even these innovations were closely tied to developments discussed in the preceding pages.

In concluding a book of 'contemporary history', it is tempting to bring the narrative up to date. In an earlier draft, this Epilogue surveyed the changes in diabetes care since the early 2000s, tracing the evolution of the QOF since 2004 and the growth of the National Diabetes Audit after 2005. However, in the following pages I want to set the developments in diabetes management explored over the preceding six chapters against changes in chronic disease care more generally, and to consider the story of British professional management in relation to international and present-day comparators. In so doing, this Epilogue returns to themes and questions laid out in the Introduction, reflecting on diabetes' historic position as a model chronic condition and drawing out the relationship between chronic disease and professional management in modern medicine.

Diabetes and chronic disease in the twentieth century

In the five decades after the Second World War, health systems in Europe and North America gradually adjusted their approaches to the challenges of long-term disease.[2] Through its focus on diabetes, this work has traced the actors, politics, and technologies central to such adjustments in a leading chronic condition. Two questions remain, however: to what extent did the developments in diabetes draw from, and feed into, broader changes in relation to chronic disease? And how far can diabetes stand analytically as a model chronic condition for historians?

In Britain, the innovations in chronic disease care discussed in the present work initially cut across decades of national and local policy, with institutions at every level of the health services having sought to marginalise patients with long-term complaints since at least the late nineteenth century.[3] Hospitals adopted exclusionary approaches despite chronic conditions having been widely diagnosed, discussed, and treated in earlier centuries.[4] Certain lifelong complaints, such as consumption and gout, had even attained cultural and literary importance, and chronic illness formed the subject for innumerable medical handbooks and textbooks.[5] As noted in Chapter 1, however, hospitals in the nineteenth and early twentieth centuries regularly sought to exclude chronic and incurable cases in order to stem the potential demand for care.[6] At this time, emerging health systems were increasingly shaped by the demands of scientific medicine and institutional efficiency; after community-based consultation, only the most acute and medically challenging cases were supposed to be referred to the hospital. Once there, patients were to provide cases for clinical and scientific research, and to receive technologically oriented diagnostic and therapeutic interventions until either cured, stabilised, or dead.[7] Within this framework, chronic patients were grouped with elderly and infirm persons, positioned as the responsibility of families, and considered drains on limited institutional resources.[8] Nonetheless, whilst such policies were effective enough to influence the life course and experiences of ill persons, by the turn of the twentieth century chronic patients were accumulating within (often stigmatised) institutions. Different countries developed different approaches to the care of such individuals. However, in the absence of efficacious or active treatment, institutionalisation was a common fate of long-term patients, who might spend days, months, or even years between institutional walls.[9]

As argued in the first three chapters, it was in relation to the quotidian management of individual conditions that local systems made their first adjustments to previous policies. Certainly, some early care structures for longer-term problems fitted neatly within earlier organisational paradigms. For instance, treatments for cancer required specialist technologies and careful institutional management that were emerging from new relations between laboratories, hospitals, medical schools, universities, national funding councils, and industry.[10] Indeed, as noted in Chapter 1, the early management of diabetes through scientific diet and insulin developed within this framework.[11] Equally, across the post-war period, healthcare teams devised an array of practices to care for long-term diseases, often focusing heavily on acute and potentially terminal episodes.[12] Several disease- and population-specific programmes even drew attention away from broader policy notions of 'chronic disease', underlining its position as a medical and political construct rather than a neutral category.[13]

As outlined within Chapters 2 and 3, however, healthcare teams treating many long-term conditions also devised ways of working that differed from traditional, acute disease-oriented approaches. Building on a series of technical and pharmacological innovations, after the 1920s clinicians and researchers devised long-term management programmes for a host of incurable conditions, from diabetes and hypertension to asthma, anaemia, and rheumatoid arthritis.[14] Though many such conditions differed in course, symptomology, and the quotidian work required of patients, new systems of care were nonetheless based in similar practices of surveillance, education, long-term intervention, and, increasingly, proactive organisation.[15] Moreover, though specialist clinics initially provided a valued site of care for most of these conditions, from the 1960s onwards management slowly extended into the community.[16] Specialists and hospital clinics did not disappear, but multi-disciplinary teams increasingly operated across primary and secondary sites of care.[17]

Such migration was not solely dependent upon pharmaceutical innovation. Moves away from the hospital were also facilitated by experimentation with instruments of monitoring and with systems of organisation that integrated new spaces and combinations of labour.[18] Crucially, medical and nursing practitioners involved in such developments did not produce materials and ways of working *de novo*, but often adapted existing tools and methods over time. It was through designing such programmes that more cohesive concepts of chronic disease emerged, providing a useful foundation for organising medical practice. Early innovations did not distinguish between whether a condition was considered to be communicable or not, or to be even a pathology at all.[19] Hospital clinics for diabetes in Edinburgh, for instance, were initially based on those held for lupus; shared record cards in some sites were likewise adapted from those used in antenatal care.[20] Over time, however, systems of treatment for diabetes provided an example for other long-term conditions, and *vice versa*. Insulin, for instance, provided a model of research and treatment for the use of methonium compounds in hypertension, and recommendations for primary care asthma clinics used equivalents in diabetes and hypertension as comparators.[21] Similarly, appeals for GPs to become involved in chronic disease care more broadly were predicated on the potentially preventive powers of structured disease management, forms of which were widespread in hypertension and epilepsy, as well as diabetes.[22] Indeed, the tools mobilised to structure diabetes management were being applied across long-term conditions. As one letter to the *BMJ* pointed out, by the mid-1980s the RCGP had 'increasingly … defin[ed] protocols for the care of serious chronic disease', and 'clinics for the care of asthma, hypertension, chronic arthritic disease, diabetes, and other chronic disorders' were 'becoming widespread in general practice'.[23] Diabetes may have provided inspiration for some practitioners considering how to integrate specialist and GP in managing long-term illness, but this was a problem common to the care of other chronic conditions.[24] Tackling this issue provided a foundation for practical debates about chronic disease management in the last quarter of the twentieth century.

As George Weisz has made clear, the meta-concept of chronic disease had less centrality in Britain than elsewhere in terms of national policy.[25] The NHS's universal coverage, combined with its collectivisation of financial risk across a national population, certainly provided British clinicians with an effective foundation on which to innovate and share models of chronic disease care in practice.[26] However, these same features also undermined the political cache of 'chronic disease' until later in the century.[27] There were some movements in this direction before the 2000s, and diabetes once again provided an important component of such policy.[28] As noted in Chapters 4-6, whilst single diseases and their complications had previously attracted policy attention, both the 1990 GP contract and the related programme *The Health of the Nation* (1994) aimed to address rising rates of chronic disease (and associated acute outcomes), albeit in different ways. The GP contract sought to prevent and better manage chronic disease in the practice surgery, bringing together developments in the primary care management of diabetes and other conditions within a single measure.

Likewise, *The Health of the Nation* built upon decades of government-supported health education, emerging first in relation to smoking and lung cancer during the 1950s and 1960s and then spreading to other risk factors for multiple conditions, such as alcohol consumption and obesity.[29] Although diabetes was excluded from *The Health of the Nation*, the government had signed up to international targets of diabetes prevention and management, and the risk-based, target-oriented approach could be seen reflected in the final shape of the NSF a few years later.

Chronic disease and the management of medical professionals

Shifts in diabetes management, therefore, formed part of a broader change in approach to chronic diseases, and often served as an exemplar in some respects. Although its history cannot serve as the history of all conditions discussed under the banner of 'chronic disease', the dynamics involved in its management may well prove illuminating to future research.

With regard to professionals, one subject that a growing historical literature on chronic disease has not discussed is the relationship between long-term disease management and managerial approaches to medicine.[30] The contemporary connections between chronic disease management and professional management have occasionally been raised in sociological work. For instance, in a wide-ranging, though unfortunately brief, article published in 2005, the sociologist Carl May proposed that the NHS had experienced an 'explosion' of chronic illness since the 1960s. The growth of such conditions, May suggested, produced surveillance-oriented, routine, and 'highly determinative patterns of professional labour', 'forms of professional work that are amenable to external regulation and governance'.[31] In an even shorter response, David Armstrong questioned whether, rather than producing forms of regulatory work, chronic illness provided 'the ideal construct on which these forms of social management can be practised'.[32] Although this brief exchange was extremely productive, no more extensive investigation took place, and no historical work has assessed the potential relationships between chronic disease and managed medical labour to ask where and how possible connections were made.

The present work has taken up this challenge, tracing the emergence of new forms of managed care in relation to both disease profiles and broader patterns of political, professional, cultural, and technological change. In agreement with May, it has suggested that increasing consultations for chronic diseases were an important motivator for service innovation. However, it has also warned against explaining this increasing workload as the product of an 'epidemiological transition', the result of a process in which the epidemiological prominence of acute infectious disease gives way to an 'explosion' of chronic illness.[33] As indicated above, long-term illness has been a common feature of disease experience since at least the eighteenth century, and a post-war increase in consultations for chronic diseases therefore needs to be viewed in relation to the control of common infections (increasing the visibility of other problems) and contextualised in the development of new methods of diagnosis, novel modes of community research, mutating disease boundaries and definitions, and the creation of new categories of illness following pharmaceutical innovation.[34] Equally, it should be remembered that rising demand for treatment became problematic only within a system of limited means, characterised by ethical imperatives of life-extension and equitable treatment.

Even in such a situation, as Armstrong notes, the shape of disease management programmes was not inevitable. Rather than chronic illnesses generating new forms of working, that is, practitioners actively forged routines of disease management. They developed instruments that regulated, monitored, and integrated – in short, that managed – patient and practitioner from within a pre-existing culture of bureaucratised care, propelled by (and fostering) anxieties over clinical standards. In fact, it was by combining new therapeutics and ways of working that many conditions were made chronic, and similarities between diverse patterns of symptoms were constructed.[35] Finally, although this routinised disease management invited external regulation and provided an ideal vehicle for testing local and national systems of managed medicine, this work has demonstrated how a series of competing political projects, financial pressures, and cultural concerns about professional accountability underpinned such developments. The roots of these developments can be traced throughout (and in some cases, before) the post-war period. Nonetheless, they came to a head during the 1980s and early 1990s, with Conservative governments – guided by neoliberal principles of statecraft – supporting the development of national instruments and policies of professional management. As the chronic condition with perhaps the longest history of quantification and bureaucratisation, diabetes provided a perfect testing ground for new managerial solutions, and was incorporated into early efforts to introduce performance-related pay and establish national standards of care.

Yet, despite the importance of a motivated central government in establishing managerial structures for medicine, medical professionals themselves drove the creation of managed medicine, using chronic diseases like diabetes as vehicles for such work. They developed the first systems of structured local care, introducing mechanisms for regulating and reviewing the temporality and content of clinical activity in order to integrate dispersed labour. Amid professional and popular anxiety about the quality of British medical practice, elite specialists and GPs also developed the first national guideline and audit systems, designed to inform local care and structure national provision. In doing so, these practitioners incorporated previously academic tools for research and healthcare assessment into routine care. Moreover, acting through statutory bodies associated with the NHS and the standard-setting bodies of the Royal Colleges, leading professionals also worked in concert with government agencies to devise policies and populate committees refining managerial mechanisms. Indeed, through well-connected patient organisations like the BDA, these specialists lobbied for diabetes to be at the forefront of new developments, and enrolled international organisations to enhance the power and legitimacy of managerial programmes.

The importance of professional activity to the development and character of managed medical care in Britain can be seen in a short comparison with developments internationally. Drives for protocol production and audit of care have been characteristic of modern medicine at least since the last quarter of the twentieth century, though with precursors in the nineteenth and early twentieth centuries.[36] To some extent, that is, the move towards management emerged as a logical corollary of the rationality underpinning the scientific medicines of laboratory and clinic, a manifestation of standards and efficacy assessment writ large.[37] Furthermore, international connections forged through philanthropic organisations, global health agencies (such as the WHO), and growing policy communities also help to explain similarities.[38] Yet the character of management in different countries also reflects differences in the structures, politics, and cultures of medicine across nation-states.

In the USA, for instance, multiple groups contributed to concerns about costs of healthcare in general, and chronic disease in particular.

Hospitals, organised medicine, politicians, and federal and state government bodies were not the only actors in US health policy. Post-war policy debates received considerable interest from lawyers, academics, pharmaceutical companies, insurance agencies, philanthropic and non-profit organisations, and consumer representatives.[39] In response to concerns over costs and insurance coverage, these agents also drove the development of managerial technologies. Whereas US physicians had been able to shape medical institutions to their needs during the first half of the twentieth century, their influence soon became contested.[40] Into the 1960s and beyond, US medicine experienced a proliferation of state schemes and federal funding for services. However, whereas Britain nationalised hospitals and contracted GPs *en masse*, public financing of health services in the USA focused on reimbursement and subsidy and became filtered through intermediaries. The result was an intensification of market-based provision and new forms of regulation.[41] Notably, large-scale (multi-hospital and cross-sector) corporate suppliers of health services came to dominate. They offered increasingly bureaucratic employment for doctors, and placed greater emphasis on the standardisation of practice than in Britain, primarily to facilitate payment and enhance cost-control.[42] Similarly, in an insurance-based market system, economic analyses were applied much more readily to healthcare than in Britain, and assessment of quality and value for money (often invoked in the name of the consumer) emerged earlier in the USA.[43]

In the absence of Britain's comparatively centralised medical and political institutions, therefore, US doctors were less able to negotiate institutional and cultural pressures, and their activity became managed (by themselves and others) through new forms of payment, regulation, and review.[44] Although academic and administrative clinicians moved to control managerial structures, the greater array of interests converging on managed care in the USA meant that managerialism was much more readily aligned with external agencies and cost-control than in Britain.[45] Although the relationships between chronic disease and professional management in the USA are only beginning to be examined, close links between long-term sickness, service costs, and healthcare reform might suggest at least indirect connections, especially in light of the role that health management organisations play in the care of chronic disease and their emphasis on guidelines and audit.[46] As with managerial medicine more broadly, further comparative histories are needed to throw the relationships between chronic disease and professional management into greater relief.[47]

Professionals, professionalism, and the state

What, then, does the emergence of professional management in postwar Britain say about the changing nature of professionalism? And what do more recent developments indicate about the shifting relationship between professionals and the state?

As the foregoing history of diabetes management shows, medical professionals in Britain were rarely united in the post-war period, and new forms of activity embodied in chronic disease care and professional management were contested. Like those in the USA, British academic clinicians and health service researchers, although often involved with teaching hospitals, assumed new managerial roles over medical practice when creating guidelines and audit systems for local and national implementation. Service reviews noted the resentment felt by some rank-and-file doctors at such interference, and practitioners highlighted the problems of being 'flooded' with guidelines in the medical press.[48] Moreover, through letters, articles, and satirical cartoons, these professionals highlighted the often contradictory nature of existing guidelines. They queried the strength and validity of evidence on which many protocols were based, and wondered how abstracted knowledge could be applied to the individual patient.[49] Conflict could also be reproduced at the local level. Numerous practitioners avoided participating in shared diabetes care schemes, whilst others only half-heartedly engaged.

The professional division that could have posed the most serious problems for the emergence of new approaches was one that had been intimately linked to the development of medical hierarchies in the nineteenth and early twentieth centuries: that between GP and consultant. This divide had been historically fuzzy. However, it was hardening in major cities by the 1900s, and GPs had registered complaints about the role of outpatient clinics in undermining their patient base.[50] As discussed in Chapter 2, the NHS consolidated divisions between community-based GPs and hospital-based clinicians, and its affirmation of the referral mechanism served simultaneously as a rationing device and a support to a rationalising division of labour.[51] Institutional divisions were also repeated nationally in terms of material interests, with hospital clinicians being employed and reimbursed in different ways from GPs.[52] Although Britain's new arrangements provided clearer distinctions between (and greater financial security for) the two sets of practitioners, the division between general practice and the hospital continued to be a source of tension into the post-war period.[53] GPs during the 1950s and 1960s complained of the dull nature of much of their work, disappointed that the most interesting cases and technologies remained the purview of the hospital. For their part, specialists remained wary of GPs, and some complained about their lack of medical competence.[54] Mutual distrust even threatened to disintegrate some community-based diabetes care schemes.

Yet chronic disease care and related forms of professional management provided areas of shared concern for clinicians and GPs at multiple levels of the profession. As noted in Chapters 1 and 2, extending diabetes management into primary care interested both GPs and hospital clinicians but for different reasons: GPs sought to diversify their clinical practice and move into preventive work, whereas hospital clinicians saw an opportunity to ease their workload and refocus on the most complex cases. Nonetheless, novel schemes provoked concerns about standards of care. Both GPs and hospital consultants feared the dangers of poor co-ordination and GPs' unfamiliarity with disease management processes. New records, protocol, and audit measures were first introduced as means to facilitate care across sites and practitioners, as well as to ensure that key processes were not missed. New technologies thus facilitated new ways of working by smoothing mistrust and co-ordinating activity.[55] Undoubtedly, some hospital clinicians saw such systems as a means to discipline the care of GPs. Yet several prominent schemes were designed through GP–consultant co-operation, indicating a mutual interest from both sides of the professional divide. Likewise, at the collective level, GPs had formed the College of General Practitioners (later the RCGP) during the 1950s to provide a vehicle for raising standards through organising research and improving education.[56] Over the 1970s and 1980s, this body championed practice organisation and proactive care, with diabetes and chronic disease management as central elements of its professional project. The College and its leading figures were keen proponents of structured general practice and shared care schemes, and received support from significant specialists in the field. Moreover, they collaborated with the other Royal Colleges, and with specialists in the BDA, to create guidelines and conduct service reviews of new programmes, highlighting how shared interests could transcend professional boundaries.

The coalescing of these institutions around technologies of management suggests that this period saw the emergence of new visions of professionalism in medicine. During the early twentieth century, the freedom for individual practitioners to make decisions regardless of external lay or medical figures was something of a hallmark of being a professional. Collective regulation of standards for qualification and discipline may have been essential features of professional status, but, as one distinguished physician proudly declared in 1926:

> There is no voice to which you must ... give heed that can inscribe on tables of stone a series of medical commandments, or that can compel your subscription to thirty-nine or some other number of articles. Whether for good or for ill, the life offered by medicine is a life of intellectual liberty where every honest man may hold his own convictions, express his own judgements, and follow his own policy; and this without fear either of authoritative censure or official excommunication. However dignified and commanding certain professional organizations may be, none of them has the skill or competence to discharge thunderbolts against the practitioner who chooses to exercise his right of private judgement.[57]

By the late twentieth century, elite practitioners and institutions clearly felt that such freedom was for 'ill'. Instead, they suggested, being a good professional meant embracing external guidance and being open to self-review and peer review.[58] This reworking of professionalism has continued into the twenty-first century, and various agencies within and without medicine have sought to construct professionalism around discourses of evidence, accountability, and productivity.[59] Individual professional autonomy certainly remains important to practitioners, and a significant proportion of newly qualified doctors are choosing occupations according to their control over working hours and conditions.[60] However, unaided clinical autonomy is no longer prized as it once was, and engaging with external input and critique has become essential to good practice. Undoubtedly, therefore, being a professional means something different at the beginning of the twenty-first century to what it did at the beginning of the twentieth, and the transformations in medical management reviewed in this book would appear to provide part of the reason for such a change.

To what extent do shifts in the outlook and practice of medical professionals reflect a colonisation of medical professionalism by the state and its construct of managerialism?[61] The present work would suggest that a division between professionalism, managerialism, and the state rests on faulty assumptions. The regulation of medical practice (often connected with 'managerialism') was a professional project from the 1970s onwards, and in some form can be traced further back, to the emergence of laboratory practices and clinical research in the late nineteenth century.[62] Its origins, therefore, rests with neither the state nor the creation of more formal health service management in the 1980s. Furthermore, until the mid-1990s managerial reforms of medicine remained under the purview of medical professionals. The state promoted professional projects for its own ends. However, audit remained individualised, and guidelines were generally produced by Royal Colleges.[63]

In the twenty years following the mid-1990s managerial trends have intensified, and the regulation of medicine has become less individually focused. Elite professionals, patients' organisations, and state bodies have placed a tighter mesh of guidance and surveillance around the NHS and its medical practitioners, encouraging greater convergence between professional and performance management strategies. The rise of Evidence-Based Medicine and its hierarchy of evidence has, for instance, placed greater stress on codification of norms and standardisation of practice.[64] Furthermore, sociological work by Ruth McDonald, Stephen Harrison, and others has suggested that changes made to the structure and financial arrangements of the NHS since 1997 encouraged medical professionals to increase their own emphasis on performance standards.[65] This has particularly been the case for primary care, where between 2001 and 2013 emphases on target-oriented pay strengthened, the NHS moved to contracting organisations (rather than individual GPs), and indicative budgeting encouraged the creation of contracting consortia.[66] These shifts altered the dynamics of primary care, with GPs even in collegiate practices assuming monitoring roles, reviewing their own work and the work of fellow practitioners in order to ensure standards were met. Similarly, the deputation of responsibility for purchasing and budgeting decisions to consortia boards established new forms of oversight and administrative relationships between primary care staff. Performance data, practice norms, peer review, and delegate visits for practices were used to encourage adherence, supported by accountability agreements and practice reviews of referral and prescribing.[67] The effects of recent changes from Primary Care Trusts to Clinical Commissioning Groups are not entirely clear. However, the 'scaling up' that the new changes involve may see such pressures increase.

In traditional sociological terms, therefore, it might be said that the relative power of the state has increased at the expense of the profession over the past twenty years. Given present trends, such dynamics are unlikely to change in the near future. However, though insightful, such a framing perhaps underplays the continued role of medical professionals themselves in creating managerial structures. Whilst undoubtedly aligned with projects to reduce state expenditure and ensure resource efficiency, healthcare governance also continues to be the product of negotiation between visions of how to manage the medical profession.[68] It should be stressed, moreover, that scholars over the past two decades have highlighted a range of ways in which doctors could ameliorate pressures for conformity. Into the present century, doctors appealed to traditional forms of therapeutic individualism – the idea that familiarity with individual patients and drugs should inform prescribing – and integrated protocols with personal knowledge.[69] GPs thus incorporated such tools primarily when they supported experience and ongoing medical work, or simplified tasks and pre-existing practices.[70] Even with the added scrutiny that more recent NHS arrangements brought to care, discourses and perceptions of voluntarism have been central to making them work.[71] Setting norms and monitoring performance has undoubtedly become a central part of medicine, and certain discourses of professionalism have equated 'vocation' (doing what is best for clients) with adherence to guidelines and review practices.[72] However, such transformations have been consciously undertaken and multi-directional, and doctors have yet to be completely trapped within Weber's iron cage of modernity.[73]

The past, present, and future of diabetes care and professional management

Historical perspective may provide useful context and points of departure for prognostication, but drawing definitive conclusions from history is something of a fool's errand. Nonetheless, if asked what the future might hold for diabetes care – in the absence of radical breakthroughs to cure or prevent the condition – I would say it is likely that structures for professional management will be central to whatever innovations are to come. Many of the features that fostered structured care and professional oversight in the post-war period remain in the present. The NHS continues to be subject to financial constraints.

There are, moreover, considerable political pressures to reform the service's structures in pursuit of integrated and more efficient care.[74] Equally, in recent years commissioning and contracting practices have been extended across the health and social services, and auditing bodies have firmly established themselves as essential parts of clinical government.[75] Partly as a result of financial squeezes and extension of oversight machinery, we are still subject to regular medical and public health scandals, holding anxieties about professional performance and competence in place. Such concern has even found cultural outlets in popular prime-time television dramas, and is reinforced by those audits and reviews that highlight divergence from agreed standards of care.[76] In terms of diabetes, reviews of care by parliamentary bodies and patient organisations have encouraged the development of new frameworks and action plans.[77] As in the 1970s and 1980s, therefore, the potential 'failure' of existing governance frameworks has been productive of more intensified varieties of the same system.[78] Medical professionals and academics have also been central to this managerialisation, and a whole raft of institutions and career trajectories are invested in the pursuit of 'best practice'. In the absence of significant structural, political, or cultural change, it is safe to assume that managerial approaches to diabetes care (and British medicine more broadly) are here to stay for the foreseeable future.

Perhaps the big question overhanging any assessment of the future is 'are such systems beneficial?' Would the continued existence of managerial systems be a bad thing for patients and practitioners? Modern historians are not generally used to passing explicit moral comment on their subjects.[79] In the account preceding this Epilogue, for example, my interest has been to trace the changing contours of diabetes care in post-war Britain, and to consider the relationship between the management of chronic disease and emergence of systems for managing professional labour. I have legitimated such work in terms of historiographical benefit – opening vistas onto the dynamics of post-war British medicine and government, as well as providing useful insight into the histories and character of professionalism. Moreover, I have tried to explain the emergence and maintenance of such systems in relation to political, cultural, institutional, technological, and epistemological factors, and thus without recourse to appeals of their self-evident or universal benefit.[80] Indeed, I have suggested that what was beneficial for one set of professionals could have negative or unintended consequences for others, including patients.

However, historians are often closer to their work than they usually admit, and in producing this book I have found it difficult to completely disentangle myself from normative questions. The research for this work coincided with diagnoses of diabetes in my family, and as part of writing the manuscript I have been fortunate enough to interview actors involved with structures for managing the health service and its professionals. As a result of these experiences, I have come to appreciate the potential value of managerial technologies.[81] Practitioners themselves want reassurance that they are providing the most efficacious treatment for their patients, and – within the current capacities of therapeutics and the health services – it is certainly useful for patients, political bodies, and healthcare teams to know that specific tests or consultations are important, and whether crucial actions have been missed. Depending on one's political position, moreover, data on the performance of welfare services can help to improve policy and hold governments (as well as medical teams and institutions) to account.[82] On a personal level, the geographical inequalities in amputations for patients with diabetes in my home region of East Anglia have provided a stark warning that improvements need to be made in areas of deprivation or rural provision.[83]

Yet an overwhelming focus on management systems can also have negative consequences. On a macro-level, it can divert attention away from the factors underpinning inequalities. We may be aware of the connections between economic and social marginalisation on the one hand and higher rates of diabetes prevalence and morbidity on the other because of the surveillance and analytic systems at the heart of managerialism.[84] However, this inequality will not be properly addressed through technical solutions alone, by refining managerial frameworks to refocus professional attention on specified groups. If certain structures (of employment or discrimination) are simultaneously subjecting populations to increased risks and excluding them from mainstream institutions, then they will not come under the care of health services in the first place.[85] Undoubtedly the connections between marginality and morbidity are complex, but they will probably require fundamental changes in income distribution, social organisation, physical environments, and embedded cultural practices to produce more equitable outcomes. A political emphasis on management to the exclusion of broader thinking can, therefore, be dangerous in itself.

Furthermore, in the absence of significant institutional support and resourcing, an emphasis on new forms of working and auditable accountability at a micro-level can result in either a 'gaming' of the system, formalistic 'box-ticking', or an unhelpful skewing of priorities.[86] In such situations, all parties in medical encounters become unsatisfied and no-one receives the care they need. This is to say little about how intensive emphasis on performing routine tasks can result in simple bureaucratic fatigue (as discussed in Chapter 3), or how undue stress on targets and performance can result in serious problems of anxiety, depression, and physical ill-health in professionals.[87] To speak from experience with teaching staff in Britain's new academy system, the results can be personally devastating and professionally problematic: if work environments become so unwelcoming that we struggle to recruit professionals willing to work in them, everyone will lose out, and systems will become further impaired.

As this book has tried to highlight, those persons experimenting with, or promoting the use of, professional management tools have never intended these outcomes. In terms of diabetes care, prominent figures in policy creation see managerial systems as part of broader solutions, even if large-scale economic change remains outside the purview of acceptable policy, as during the post-war decades.[88] Nonetheless, in terms of the future, considerations like those above should allow us to pause and think about potential over-investment in systems of professional management as routes to quick technical fixes. Although by no means providing a guide to what we should do, this work and the historical and sociological materials on which it draws do suggest that emphasis on singular policy fixes is unlikely to be successful.[89]

In reflecting further on the past, or at least our framings of it in the form of history, this work has contributed to a growing body of literature on diabetes care, chronic disease management, and medical governance. It has suggested that historical perspectives can give new meaning to contemporary analysis, and proposed that histories of disease and technologies of management can provide new and important insight into twentieth-century Britain. Such work is by no means complete, and further research remains. Perhaps in years to come, broader comparative perspectives will reveal different avenues for investigation and interpretation. At the very least, however, it is hoped that this close analysis of managing diabetes has provided new light in which to view the history of managed medicine.

Notes

1. Department of Health, *National Service Framework for Diabetes: Delivery Strategy* (London: Department of Health, 2002), pp. 13–21. The NHS in Scotland had a similar 'Scottish Diabetes Framework', tailored to its unique institutional arrangements.
2. G. Weisz, *Chronic Disease in the Twentieth Century: A History* (Baltimore: Johns Hopkins University Press, 2014). Cf. D. Fox, *Power and Illness: The Failure of American Health Policy* (Berkeley: University of California Press, 1993).
3. As noted in Chapter 1, the NHS retained this exclusionary mentality so far as bed admission was concerned.
4. P. Jasen, 'Breast cancer and the language of risk, 1750–1950', *Social History of Medicine*, 15:1 (2002), 17–43, esp. pp. 21–35; A. Mackintosh, 'The patent medicines industry in late Georgian England: a respectable alternative to both regular medicine and irregular practice', *Social History of Medicine*, 30:1 (2017), 22–47, esp. 29–31. On the use and limitations of death certification for such assessments: A. Hardy, '"Death is the cure of all diseases": using the General Register Office cause of death statistics for 1837–1920', *Social History of Medicine*, 7:3 (1994), 472–92.
5. R. Porter and G. S. Rousseau, *Gout: The Patrician Malady* (New Haven: Yale University Press, 2000); C. Timmermann, 'Chronic illness and disease history', in M. Jackson (ed.), *The Oxford Handbook of the History of Medicine* (Oxford: Oxford University Press, 2011), pp. 395–401; Weisz, *Chronic Disease in the Twentieth Century*, pp. 2–7.
6. J. Szabo, *Incurable and Intolerable: Chronic Disease and Slow Death in Nineteenth-Century France* (New Brunswick: Rutgers University Press, 2009).
7. D. Fox, *Health Policies, Health Politics: The British and American Experience, 1911–1965* (Princeton: Princeton University Press, 1986); S. Sturdy and R. Cooter, 'Science, scientific management and the transformation of medicine in Britain, c.1870–1950', *History of Science*, 36:4 (1998), 421–66; C. Lawrence, *Rockefeller Money, The Laboratory and Medicine in Edinburgh, 1919–1930: New Science in an Old Country* (New York: University of Rochester Press, 2005).
8. Szabo, *Incurable and Intolerable*.
9. Ibid.; Weisz, *Chronic Disease in the Twentieth Century*; A. Levene, 'Between less eligibility and the NHS: the changing place of Poor Law hospitals in England and Wales, 1929–39', *Twentieth Century British History*, 20:3 (2009), 322–45.
10. R. M. M. Domenech and C. Casañeda, 'Redefining cancer during the interwar period: British Medical Officers of Health, state policy, managerialism and public health', *American Journal of Public Health*, 97:9 (2007),

1563–71; Fox, *Power and Illness*, pp. 52–5; M. Edwards, *Control and the Therapeutic Trial: Rhetoric and Experimentation in Britain, 1918–48* (Amsterdam: Rodopi, 2007).
11 C. Sinding, 'Making the unit of insulin: standards, clinical work, and industry', *Bulletin of the History of Medicine*, 76:2 (2002), 231–70; Lawrence, *Rockefeller Money*.
12 J. Stanton, 'The cost of living: kidney dialysis, rationing and health economics in Britain, 1965–1996', *Social Science & Medicine*, 49:9 (1999), 1169–82; A. Nathoo, *Hearts Exposed: Transplants and the Media in 1960s Britain* (Basingstoke: Palgrave Macmillan, 2009); C. Timmermann and E. Toon (eds.), *Cancer Patients, Cancer Pathways: Historical and Sociological Perspectives* (Basingstoke: Palgrave Macmillan, 2012).
13 Timmermann and Toon (eds.), *Cancer Patients, Cancer Pathways*; P. Bridgen and J. Lewis, *Elderly People and the Boundary between Health and Social Care, 1946–91: Whose Responsibility?* (London: Nuffield Trust, 1999); Weisz, *Chronic Disease in the Twentieth Century*.
14 R. B. Tattersall, *Diabetes: The Biography* (Oxford: Oxford University Press, 2009); C. Feudtner, *Bittersweet: Diabetes, Insulin, and the Transformation of Illness* (Chapel Hill: University of North Carolina Press, 2003); J. A. Greene, *Prescribing by Numbers: Drugs and the Definition of Disease* (Baltimore: Johns Hopkins University Press, 2007); M. Jackson, *Asthma: The Biography* (Oxford: Oxford University Press, 2009), esp. pp. 183–8; H. K. Valier, 'The politics of scientific medicine in Manchester, c.1900–1960' (PhD dissertation, University of Manchester, 2002), pp. 169–74.
15 On the differing rhythms of long-term illness: K. Charmaz, *Good Days, Bad Days: The Self in Chronic Illness and Time* (New Brunswick: Rutgers University Press, 1991). Contemporary discussions explicitly noted the differences between specific conditions: C. E. Bucknall, C. Robertson, F. Moran, and R. D. Stevenson, 'Management of asthma in hospital: a prospective audit', *BMJ*, 296:6637 (1988), 1639. Nonetheless, for similarities in approach see chapters on diabetes, hypertension, anaemia, and asthma in J. Fry and G. Sandler, *Common Diseases: Their Nature, Presentation, and Care*, 5th edition (London: Kluwer Academic, 1993).
16 Fry and Sandler, *Common Diseases*, 5th edition; A. Foulkes, A.-L. Kinmouth, S. Frost, and D. Macdonald, 'Organised personal care – an effective choice for managing diabetes in general practice', *JRCGP*, 39:11 (1989), 444–7.
17 Bucknall et al., 'Management of asthma in hospital', 1637–9; K. Jones, 'Asthma – still a challenge for general practice', *JRCGP*, 39:6 (1989), 254–6.
18 V. L. Osbourne and D. G. Beevers, 'A comparison of hospital and general practice blood pressure readings using a shared-care record card', *JRCGP*, 31:6 (1981), 345–50; M. D. Moore, 'Reorganising chronic disease

management: diabetes and bureaucratic technologies in post-war British general practice', in M. Jackson (ed.), *The Routledge History of Disease* (London: Routledge, 2017), pp. 453–72.
19 P. Weindling, 'From infectious to chronic diseases: changing patterns of sickness in the nineteenth and twentieth centuries', in A. Wear (ed.), *Medicine in Society: Historical Essays* (Cambridge: Cambridge University Press, 1992), p. 315. For a history that draws comparative points across supposed aetiological lines: Timmermann, 'Chronic illness'.
20 'Scotland', *The Lancet*, 140:3599 (1924), 460–1; C. E. Upton, 'Diabetic community care', *The Practitioner*, 215:1284 (1975), 83.
21 C. Timmermann, 'Hexamethonium, hypertension and pharmaceutical innovation: the transformation of an experimental drug in post-war Britain', in C. Timmermann and J. Anderson (eds.), *Devices and Designs: Technology and Medicine in Historical Perspective* (Basingstoke: Palgrave Macmillan, 2006), pp. 166–7; Jones, 'Asthma', p. 256.
22 M. Lawrence, 'All together now', *JRCGP*, 38:7 (1988), 296–302, esp. p. 297; Foulkes et al., 'Organised personal care', p. 444.
23 E. Martin, 'What price academic general practice?', *BMJ*, 292:6537 (1986), 1736.
24 'Moving towards clinical integration', *BMJ*, 2 6402 (1976), 964; A. J. Snowden, T. A. Sheldon, and G. Alberti, 'Shared care in diabetes', *BMJ*, 310:6973 (1995), 142–3.
25 Weisz, *Chronic Disease in the Twentieth Century*.
26 Cf. the USA: Fox, *Power and Illness*.
27 Weisz, *Chronic Disease in the Twentieth Century*.
28 Moore, 'Reorganising chronic disease management'.
29 See Chapters 1 and 2.
30 Of course, it might be worth speaking of 'histories of chronic diseases', given that historians have tended to examine chronic illnesses through 'biographies' and single-disease studies (like the present work): Timmermann, 'Chronic illness', p. 393.
31 C. May, 'Chronic illness and intractability: professional–patient interactions in primary care', *Chronic Illness*, 1:1 (2005), 15–20, quotation at p. 17.
32 D. Armstrong, 'Chronic illness: epidemiological or social explosion', *Chronic Illness*, 1:1 (2005), 26–7, quotation at p. 27.
33 Though, *contra* Armstrong, and in line with the introduction, such change was probably part of the picture. 'Transition' theory emerged from global policy interest in fertility control: G. Weisz and J. Olsyznko-Gryn, 'The theory of epidemiologic transition: the origins of a citation classic', *Journal of the History of Medicine and the Allied Sciences*, 65:3 (2010), 287–326. In its most basic form, transition has been taken to refer to the shifting fertility and mortality profiles of given societies, in which (a) high birth rates

and high mortality rates give way to low birth rates and low mortality rates, and (b) acute infectious diseases of childhood give way to non-communicable, chronic, and degenerative diseases of middle and old age as predominant causes of death. On the utility and applicability of transition theory historically: Weindling, 'From infectious to chronic diseases', pp. 305–9; M. Worboys and F. Condrau, 'Epidemics and infections in nineteenth century Britain', *Social History of Medicine*, 20:1 (2007), 147–58; G. Mooney, 'Infectious diseases and epidemiologic transition in Victorian Britain? Definitely', *Social History of Medicine*, 20:3 (2007), 595–606; M. Worboys and F. Condrau, 'Final response: epidemics and infections in nineteenth-century Britain', *Social History of Medicine*, 22:1 (2009), 165–71; A. Mercer, *Infections, Chronic Disease, and the Epidemiological Transition: A New Perspective* (Rochester: University of Rochester Press, 2014).

34 Weisz, *Chronic Disease in the Twentieth Century*; D. Armstrong, 'Chronic illness: a revisionist account', *Sociology of Health and Illness*, 36:1 (2014), 15–27; C. Timmermann, 'A matter of degree: the normalization of hypertension, c.1940–2000', in W. Ernst (ed.), *Histories of the Normal and the Abnormal: Social and Cultural Histories of Norms and Normativity* (London: Routledge, 2006), pp. 245–61; Greene, *Prescribing by Numbers*; Feudtner, *Bittersweet*.

35 Feudtner, *Bittersweet*.

36 S. Timmermanns and M. Berg, *The Gold Standard: The Challenge of Evidence-Based Medicine and Standardization in Health Care* (Philadelphia: Temple University Press, 2003); G. Weisz, A. Cambrosio, P. Keating, L. Knaapen, T. Schlich, and V. J. Tournay, 'The emergence of clinical practice guidelines', *Milbank Quarterly*, 85:4 (2007), 691–727; S. Reverby, 'Stealing the golden eggs: Ernest Amory Codman and the science and management of medicine', *Bulletin of the History of Medicine*, 55:2 (1981), 156–71.

37 D. Armstrong, 'Clinical sense and clinical science', *Social Science and Medicine*, 11:11–13 (1977), 599–601.

38 Lawrence, *Rockefeller Money*; S. Sheard, *The Passionate Economist: How Brian Abel-Smith Shaped Global Health Policy and Social Welfare* (Bristol: Policy Press, 2013).

39 Fox, *Power and Illness*; Greene, *Prescribing by Numbers*.

40 P. Starr, *The Social Transformation of American Medicine* (New York: Basic Books, 1982).

41 R. Stevens, *In Sickness and in Wealth: American Hospitals in the Twentieth Century* (New York: Basic Books, 1989); Fox, *Power and Illness*.

42 Starr, *The Social Transformation of American Medicine*; D. Light and S. Levine, 'The changing character of the medical profession: a theoretical overview', *Milbank Quarterly*, 66:2 (1988), 10–32; Stevens, *In Sickness and in Wealth*.

43 D. Irvine, *A Doctor's Tale: Professionalism and Public Trust* (Abingdon: Radcliffe Medical Press, 2003). The classic in this regard is: A. Donabedian, 'Evaluating the quality of medical care', *Milbank Memorial Fund Quarterly*, 44:3, part 2 (1966), 166–203. Assessment of quality was also broader in the USA and, given its basis in social sciences, should be distinguished from health service assessment and audit of efficacy, which had a strong history in Britain.
44 Stevens, *In Sickness and in Wealth*; Light and Levine, 'The changing character of the medical profession', pp. 10–20. For instance, Starr discusses the fragmentation of the profession in relation to American Medical Association membership and corporations: Starr, *The Social Transformation of American Medicine*, pp. 398, 427.
45 E. Freidson, 'The changing nature of professional control', *Annual Review of Sociology*, 10 (1984), 1–20. Cf. P. Day, R. Klein and F. Miller, *A Comparative US–UK Study of Guidelines* (London: Nuffield Trust, 1998).
46 Weisz, *Chronic Disease in the Twentieth Century*, esp. pp. 234–8. For the entanglements of managed care and a specific long-term sickness: K. Wailoo, *Dying in the City of the Blues: Sickle Cell Anemia and the Politics of Race and Health* (Chapel Hill: University of North Carolina Press, 2001), pp. 219–24.
47 Day et al., *A Comparative US–UK Study of Guidelines*. This study suggested that in the mid- to late 1990s, the most consistently used guidelines by managed care organisations related to common chronic conditions: diabetes, asthma, hypertension, lower back pain, and chronic headaches: pp. 51, 57.
48 Interview with Professor Davies conducted by the author; A. Hibble, D. Kanka, D. Pencheon, and F. Pooles, 'Guidelines in general practice: the new Tower of Babel?', *BMJ*, 317:7162 (1998), 862–3, quotation at p. 862.
49 For instance, in one cartoon, a practitioner and patient are seen in the consulting room, with the doctor confronting a handful of guidelines. The caption reads: 'Let's see, how shall we monitor your blood pressure this time?': D. Evans and A. Haines (eds.), *Implementing Evidence-Based Changes in Healthcare* (Abingdon: Radcliffe Medical Press, 2000), p. 236. See also G. Feder, 'Clinical guidelines in 1994', *BMJ*, 309:6968 (1994), 1457–8; A. Saha, 'Clinical guidelines', *BMJ*, 310:6980 (1995), 670. Such complaints also came from within academic medicine itself: Snowden et al., 'Shared care in diabetes'.
50 A. Digby, *The Evolution of British General Practice, 1850–1948* (Oxford: Oxford University Press, 1999), pp. 287–305, esp. pp. 289–91; Sturdy and Cooter, 'Science, scientific management and the transformation of medicine in Britain', pp. 427–8, 432–6.
51 G. Rivett, *From Cradle to Grave: Fifty Years of the NHS* (London: King's Fund, 1998), p. 82.

52 Ibid., p. 35; for more detail on the early history of doctors' pay: pp. 80–2, 89–90, 99–102.
53 G. Weisz, *Divide and Conquer: A Comparative History of Medical Specialization* (Oxford: Oxford University Press, 2006), p. 181. But cf. G. Smith and M. Nicolson, 'Re-expressing the division in British medicine under the NHS: the importance of locality in general practitioners' oral histories', *Social Science and Medicine*, 64:4 (2007), 938–48.
54 See Chapter 2.
55 Timmermanns and Berg, *The Gold Standard*.
56 Rivett, *From Cradle to Grave*, pp. 90–1.
57 C. O. Hawthorne, 'The freedom of medicine', *BMJ*, 2:3432 (1926), 705–8, quotation at p. 706.
58 RCGP, *What Sort of Doctor? Assessing Quality of Care in General Practice* (London: RCGP, 1985).
59 L. Jones and J. Green, 'Shifting discourses of professionalism: a case study of general practitioners in the United Kingdom', *Sociology of Health and Illness*, 28:7 (2006), pp. 940–1; J. Evetts, 'A new professionalism? Challenges and opportunities', *Current Sociology*, 59:4 (2011), 406–22; F. Moffatt, P. Martin, and S. Timmons, 'Constructing notions of health care productivity: the call for a new professionalism?', *Sociology of Health and Illness*, 36:5 (2014), 686–702.
60 Jones and Green, 'Shifting discourses of professionalism'.
61 This has been something of a key question in sociology: D. Numerato, D. Salvatore, and G. Fattore, 'The impact of management on medical professionalism: a review', *Sociology of Health and Illness*, 34:4 (2012), 626–44.
62 Armstrong, 'Clinical sense and clinical science'; Edwards, *Control and the Therapeutic Trial*; H. Valier and C. Timmermann, 'Clinical trials and the reorganization of medical research in post-Second World War Britain', *Medical History*, 52:4 (2008), 493–510.
63 Day et al., *A Comparative US–UK Study of Guidelines*, pp. 11–46.
64 Timmermanns and Berg, *The Gold Standard*.
65 S. Harrison and G. Dowswell, 'Autonomy and bureaucratic accountability in primary care: what English general practitioners say', *Sociology of Health and Illness*, 24:2 (2002), 208–26.
66 R. McDonald, K. Checkland, S. Harrison, and A. Coleman, 'Rethinking collegiality: restratification in English general medical practice 2004–2008', *Social Science and Medicine*, 68:7 (2009), 1199–1200.
67 Ibid., pp. 1201–5.
68 R. Flynn, 'Clinical governance and governmentality', *Health, Risk and Society*, 4:2 (2002), 155–73. In this sense, the governmentality practices that govern rank-and-file practitioners enact reflect the aims of not just political actors, but medical professionals.

69 D. Armstrong, 'Clinical autonomy, individual and collective: the problem of changing doctors' behaviour', *Social Science and Medicine*, 55:10 (2002), 1771–7.
70 K. Checkland, 'National Service Frameworks and UK general practitioners: street level bureaucrats at work?', *Sociology of Health and Illness*, 26:7 (2004), 951–75.
71 McDonald et al., 'Rethinking collegiality'.
72 Cf. T. J. Johnson, *Professions and Power* (London: Macmillan, 1972).
73 M. Weber, *The Protestant Ethic and the Spirit of Capitalism*, trans. E. Parsons (London: Routledge: 2001).
74 D. Campbell, 'NHS cash squeeze forces hospitals to postpone non-urgent operations', *The Guardian*, 16 November 2017, available at: https://www.theguardian.com/society/2017/nov/16/lincolnshire-nhs-enforces-three-month-wait-for-surgery (accessed February 2018); A. Charles, 'Accountable care explained', *The King's Fund*, 18 January 2018, available at: https://www.kingsfund.org.uk/publications/accountable-care-explained (accessed February 2018).
75 H. Buckingham and J. Rees, 'The context for service delivery: third sector, state and market relationships 1997–2015', in J. Rees and D. Mullins (eds.), *The Third Sector Delivering Public Services: Developments, Innovations, and Challenges* (Bristol: Policy Press, 2016), pp. 41–62; House of Commons Committee of Public Accounts, *Department of Health: The Management of Adult Diabetes Services in the NHS*, HC 289 (London: HMSO, 2012).
76 D. Campbell, 'Mid Staffs hospital scandal: the essential guide', *The Guardian*, 6 February 2013, available at: https://www.theguardian.com/society/2013/feb/06/mid-staffs-hospital-scandal-guide (accessed February 2018); British Broadcasting Corporation, *Trust Me* (2017).
77 NHS England, *Action for Diabetes* (London: NHS, 2014), available at: https://www.england.nhs.uk/2014/01/tackling-diabetes-2014/ (accessed February 2018).
78 M. Power, *The Audit Society: Rituals of Verification* (Oxford: Oxford University Press, 1999).
79 There have, however, been notable exceptions, and an influential conduit for bringing history and policy together has been the History & Policy collaboration, founded in 2002: http://www.historyandpolicy.org (accessed April 2018).
80 In this sense, I have followed a model of practice developed within histories of science: S. Shapin and S. Schaffer, *Leviathan and the Air Pump: Hobbes, Boyle and the Experimental Life* (Princeton: Princeton University Press, 1985).
81 I am particularly grateful to my interviewees for insightful discussion as to the motivations for, and benefits of, managerial systems.

82 Once again, I am grateful to Dr Emily Andrews for her incisive comments on data collection and its use in tracking performance. For a non-party-political approach: Institute for Government, 'Performance Tracker', *Institute for Government*, 2018, available at: https://www.instituteforgovernment.org.uk/publications?field_themes_tid=374 (accessed February 2018).

83 'Did you know diabetes is leading cause of foot amputation? Healthwatch Suffolk calls for greater awareness', *East Anglian Daily Times*, 15 March 2017, available at: www.eadt.co.uk/news/did-you-know-diabetes-is-leading-cause-of-foot-amputation-healthwatch-suffolk-calls-for-greater-awareness-1-4933296 (accessed February 2018).

84 NICE, 'Type 2 diabetes prevention: population and community-level interventions', *NICE Guidance*, May 2011, available at: https://www.nice.org.uk/guidance/ph35/chapter/2-Public-health-need-and-practice (accessed February 2018).

85 Health outcomes and attendance at health services are often worse for minority ethnic and socio-economically deprived communities, as well for persons experiencing significant instability, such as homelessness: M. Evandrou, J. Falkingham, Z. Feng, and A. Vlachantoni, 'Ethnic inequalities in limiting health and self-reported health in later life', *Journal of Epidemiology and Community Health*, 70:7 (2016), 653–62; L. A. V. Marlow, J. Wardle, and J. Waller, 'Understanding cervical screening non-attendance among ethnic minority women in England', *British Journal of Cancer*, 113:5 (2015), 833–9; A. Gilani, 'The challenges of managing diabetes in hard-to-reach-groups', *Diabetes and Primary Care*, 16:4 (2014), 206–11; M. Marmot, J. Allen, P. Goldblatt, T. Boyce, D. McNeish, M. Grady, and I. Geddes, *Fair Society, Healthy Lives: The Marmot Review* (London: The Marmot Review, 2010). Though much can be done to improve the accessibility of services in different ways, particularly by listening to affected populations, focusing on services themselves will address only some of the complex factors underpinning these issues. For an overview of research in this area: W. Ahmad and H. Bradby (eds.), *Ethnicity, Health and Health Care: Understanding Diversity, Tackling Disadvantage* (Oxford: Blackwell, 2008).

86 The classic discussion about targets and activity in recent years has been in education, where an emphasis on examination results has resulted in 'teaching to test', rather than for knowledge and skills: K. Sellgren, 'Teaching to the test gives "hollow understanding"', *BBC News*, 11 October 2017, available at: www.bbc.co.uk/news/education-41580550 (accessed February 2018). For examples in health: G. Bevan and C. Hood, 'What's measured is what matters: targets and gaming in the English public health system', *Public Administration*, 84:3 (2006), 517–38.

87 L. D. Berg, E. H. Huijbens, and H. G. Larsen, 'Producing anxiety in the neoliberal university', *Canadian Geographer*, 60:2 (2016), 168–80. Of course, this can be extended to all workers and persons living under forms of audit-related precarity, such as those being constantly reassessed for disability benefit: T. Schrecker and C. Bambra, *How Politics Makes us Sick: Neoliberal Epidemics* (Basingstoke: Palgrave Macmillan, 2015).

88 See the mix of prevention and monitoring in the NSF. On the decline of structural solutions in post-war public health: D. Porter, *Health Citizenship: Essays in Social Medicine and Biomedical Politics* (Berkeley: University of California Press, 2011), pp. 154–81.

89 In many ways, this returns us to the classical debates about technical fixes and horizontal changes that have characterised many imperial, global, and national health challenges: M. Worboys, 'The discovery of colonial malnutrition between the wars', in D. Arnold (ed.), *Imperial Medicine and Indigenous Societies* (Manchester: Manchester University Press, 1988), pp. 208–25; A. Hardy, 'Beriberi, vitamin B1 and world food policy, 1925–1970', *Medical History*, 39:1 (1995), 61–77. For an interrogation of the idea of a technological fix: L. Rosner (ed.), *The Technological Fix: Visions, Trials, and Solutions* (London: Routledge, 2004).

Bibliography

Films
British Broadcasting Corporation, *Trust Me* (BBC, 2017).

Archival sources

The National Archives, London (TNA)
BD 18/793, Diabetic services: general correspondence.
FD 7/2606, Medical Research Council: Committees, Working Parties and Conferences, Registered Files (D Series), Royal College of Physicians Standing Committee on Endocrinology and Diabetes.
FD 23/1442, British Diabetic Association, University Group Diabetic Programme (UGDP): details of setting up the Working Party on Oral Hypoglycaemic Agents in the Treatment of Diabetes and membership list.
MH 55/422, Supply of insulin by local authorities, 1923–26.
MH 133/271, Birmingham diabetes survey.
MH 150/953, Hospital eye service: facilities for the detection and treatment of diabetic retinopathy; proposed pilot project.
MH 160/416, Consideration of records for diabetic clinics.

National Records of Scotland, Edinburgh (NRS)
HH48/112/5, 'National Health Service: Management Executive Letter', 1996.
HH98/242, National Medical Consultative Committee, 1985.
HH98/453, National Medical Consultative Committee, 1986–87.
HH98/454, National Medical Consultative Committee, 1986–87.
HH98/631, National Medical Consultative Committee, 1985–86.
HH98/632, National Medical Consultative Committee, 1986.

Royal College of General Practitioners Archives, London
MSS, B Fry C6-1.

Wellcome Library Archive, London (WLA)
EPH546, R. D. Lawrence, 'The Line-Ration Scheme', c.1951.
EPH546, British Diabetic Association, 'Basic exchange list for diabetics', c.1967.
MSS (10522), British Diabetic Association, 'The Health of the Nation: response from the British Diabetic Association', October 1991.
P9997, Nutritional Subcommittee of the British Diabetic Association, 'Dietary recommendations for the 1980s – a policy statement by the British Diabetic Association', 1982.
P10503, British Diabetic Association, Royal College of Physicians, and Royal College of General Practitioners, 'Guidelines: good practice in the diagnosis and treatment of non-insulin dependent diabetes mellitus' (London: Royal College of Physicians, 1993).
PP/ASH/A/3, British Diabetic Association Committee on Blindness, 1967–69.
SA/CMO/C/60 – Box 27, Royal College of Obstetricians and Gynaecologists, 'Recommendations on the principles and organisation of general practitioner maternity units and their relation to specialist maternity units', 1962.

Internet sources (live)

Barry, E., S. Roberts, S. Finer, S. Vijayaraghavan, and T. Greenhalgh, 'Time to question the NHS diabetes prevention programme', *BMJ*, 2015, available at: www.bmj.com/content/351/bmj.h4717 (accessed September 2017).
Campbell, D., 'Mid Staffs hospital scandal: the essential guide', *The Guardian*, 6 February 2013, available at: https://www.theguardian.com/society/2013/feb/06/mid-staffs-hospital-scandal-guide (accessed September 2017).
Campbell, D., 'NHS cash squeeze forces hospitals to postpone non-urgent operations', *The Guardian*, 16 November 2017, available at: https://www.theguardian.com/society/2017/nov/16/lincolnshire-nhs-enforces-three-month-wait-for-surgery (accessed February 2018).
Cao, B., F. Bray, H. Beltrán-Sánchez, O. Ginsburg, S. Soneji, and I. Soerjomataram, 'Benchmarking life expectancy and cancer mortality: global comparison with cardiovascular disease 1981–2010', *BMJ*, June 2017, available at: http://www.bmj.com/content/357/bmj.j2920 (accessed April 2018).
Charles, A., 'Do the public still trust doctors and nurses?', *The King's Fund*, 7 December 2015, available at: https://www.kingsfund.org.uk/blog/2015/12/public-trust-doctors-nurses (accessed January 2018).
Charles, A., 'Accountable care explained', *The King's Fund*, 18 January 2018, available at: https://www.kingsfund.org.uk/publications/accountable-care-explained (accessed February 2018).

Coman, J., 'Margaret Thatcher: 20 ways that she changed Britain', *The Guardian*, 14 April 2013, available at: https://www.theguardian.com/politics/2013/apr/14/margaret-thatcher-20-changes-britain (accessed May 2017).

Diabetes UK, *Diabetes: Facts and Figures*, version 4, Diabetes UK, May 2015, available at: https://www.diabetes.org.uk/Documents/Position%20statements/Facts%20and%20stats%20June%202015.pdf (accessed June 2015).

Diabetes UK, 'Risk Score', *Diabetes UK*, 2015, available at: https://riskscore.diabetes.org.uk/start (accessed September 2017).

Did you know diabetes is leading cause of foot amputation? Healthwatch Suffolk calls for greater awareness', *East Anglian Daily Times*, 15 March 2017, available at: www.eadt.co.uk/news/did-you-know-diabetes-is-leading-cause-of-foot-amputation-healthwatch-suffolk-calls-for-greater-awareness-1-4933296 (accessed February 2018).

Institute for Government, 'Performance Tracker', *Institute for Government*, 2018, available at: https://www.instituteforgovernment.org.uk/publications?field_themes_tid=374 (accessed February 2018).

Joseph, Sir K., Speech given at Edgbaston, 19 October 1974, *Margaret Thatcher Foundation*, available at: www.margaretthatcher.org/document/101830, (accessed April 2017).

NHS Health and Social Care Information Centre, *National Diabetes Audit: Report for the Audit Period, 2003/04*, 2005, available at: https://digital.nhs.uk/catalogue/PUB02598 (accessed September 2017).

National Institute for Health and Care Excellence, 'Type 2 diabetes prevention: population and community-level interventions', *NICE Guidance*, May 2011, available at: https://www.nice.org.uk/guidance/ph35/chapter/2–Public-health-need-and-practice (accessed February 2018).

Sellgren, K. '"Teaching to the test gives "hollow understanding"', *BBC News*, 11 October 2017, available at: www.bbc.co.uk/news/education-41580550 (accessed February 2018).

Thatcher, M., 'My kind of Tory Party?', *Daily Telegraph*, 30 January 1975, *Margaret Thatcher Foundation*, available at: www.margaretthatcher.org/document/102600, (accessed April 2017).

Thatcher, M., Speech given in Derby, 2 May 1975, *Margaret Thatcher Foundation*, available at: www.margaretthatcher.org/document/102458 (accessed April 2017).

Thatcher, M., 'It's your freedom they hate', *Sunday Express*, 23 November 1975, *Margaret Thatcher Foundation*, available at: www.margaretthatcher.org/document/102808 (accessed April 2017).

Thomas, J., '*Lives of the Fellows: David Aelwyn Williams*', Royal College of Physicians, 2009, available at: http://munksroll.rcplondon.ac.uk/Biography/Details/4780 (accessed March 2018).

Triggle, N., 'Diabetes care depressingly poor, says MPs', *BBC News*, 6 November 2012, available at: www.bbc.co.uk/news/health-20210823 (accessed May 2015).

Legislation

Chronically Sick and Disabled Persons Act 1970, c. 44.
The Clinical Standards Advisory Group Regulations 1991, No. 578, available at: https://www.legislation.gov.uk/uksi/1991/578/introduction/made (accessed April 2018).
National Health Service and Community Care Act 1990, c. 19.

Archived oral histories

Interview with J. Hill conducted by the University of Oxford, 1 October 2004, available at: www.diabetes-stories.com/transcript.asp?UID=19 (accessed April 2017).
Interview with H. Keen conducted by the University of Oxford, 21 November 2006, available at: www.diabetes-stories.com/interview.asp?UID=52 (accessed April 2014).
Interview with M. MacKinnon conducted by the University of Oxford, 23 April 2007, available at: www.diabetes-stories.com/interview.asp?UID=62 (accessed April 2017).
Interview with Shirley conducted by the University of Oxford, 23 March 2004, available at: www.diabetes-stories.com/interview.asp?UID=4 (accessed April 2017).
Interview with J. Wilson conducted by the University of Oxford, 11 December 2006, available at: www.diabetes-stories.com/interview.asp?UID=53 (accessed April 2017).

Published sources

'350,000 may have diabetes', *The Times*, 17 July 1962, p. 6.
Abel-Smith, B., *The Hospitals, 1800–1948: A Study in Social Administration in England and Wales* (Cambridge, MA: Harvard University Press, 1964).
Acheson, H. W. K., 'Medical audit and general practice', *The Lancet*, 305:7905 (1975), 511–13.
'Acute myocardial infarction and pre-existing diabetes', *The Lancet*, 322:8347 (1983), 451.
Addison, P., *The Road to 1945: British Politics and the Second World War* (London: Pimlico, 1994 [1975]).
Addison, P., *No Turning Back: The Peacetime Revolutions of Post-War Britain* (Oxford: Oxford University Press, 2010).

Ahmad, W., and H. Bradby (eds.), *Ethnicity, Health and Health Care: Understanding Diversity, Tackling Disadvantage* (Oxford: Blackwell, 2008).

Alberti, K. G. M. M., 'The role of diabetes', *BMJ*, 303:6805 (1991), 769.

Alexander, W. D., and South East Thames Diabetes Physicians Group, 'Diabetes care in a UK health region: activity, facilities, and costs', *Diabetic Medicine*, 5:6 (1988), 577–81.

Al Sayegh, H., and R. J. Jarrett, 'Oral glucose-tolerance tests and the diagnosis of diabetes: results of a prospective study based on the Whitehall survey', *The Lancet*, 314:8140 (1979), 431–3.

Andrews, C. T., 'A survey of diabetes in west Cornwall', *BMJ*, 1:5016 (1957), 427–33.

Annual Meeting, Oxford: Scientific Sections', *BMJ*, 2:5353 (1963), 371–6.

Armstrong, D., 'Clinical sense and clinical science', *Social Science and Medicine*, 11:11–13 (1977), 599–601.

Armstrong, D., *Political Anatomy of the Body: Medical Knowledge in Britain in the Twentieth Century* (Oxford: Oxford University Press, 1983).

Armstrong, D., 'Space and time in British general practice', *Social Science and Medicine*, 20:7 (1985), 659–66.

Armstrong, D., 'The rise of surveillance medicine', *Sociology of Health and Illness*, 17:3 (1995), 393–404.

Armstrong, D., 'Clinical autonomy, individual and collective: the problem of changing doctors' behaviour', *Social Science and Medicine*, 55:10 (2002), 1771–7.

Armstrong, D., 'Chronic illness: epidemiological or social explosion', *Chronic Illness*, 1:1 (2005), 26–7.

Armstrong, D., 'Chronic illness: a revisionist account', *Sociology of Health and Illness*, 36:1 (2014), 15–27.

Arney, W. R., and B. J. Bergen, *Medicine and the Management of Living: Taming the Last Great Beast* (Chicago: University of Chicago Press, 1985).

Arnold, D., 'Diabetes in the tropics: race, place, and class in India, 1880–1965', *Social History of Medicine*, 22:2 (2009), 245–61.

Arnold, D., 'British India and the "beri-beri problem", 1798–1942', *Medical History*, 54:3 (2010), 295–314.

Aronowitz, R. A., *Making Sense of Illness: Science, Society, and Disease* (Cambridge: Cambridge University Press, 1998).

Aveline, M. O., D. K. McCulloch, and R. B. Tattersall, 'The practice of group psychotherapy with adult insulin-dependent diabetics', *Diabetic Medicine*, 2:3 (1985), 275–82.

Bain, J., 'NHS review', *BMJ*, 298:6675 (1989), 746.

Ball, S., and A. Seldon (eds.), *The Heath Government, 1970–1974: A Reappraisal* (Longman: London, 1996).

Barry, N., 'Neoclassicism, the New Right and British social welfare', in R. M. Page and R. Silburn (eds.), *British Social Welfare in the Twentieth Century* (Macmillan: Basingstoke, 1999), pp. 55–80.

Becker, H. S., B. Geer, E. C. Hughes, and A. L. Strauss, *Boys in White: Student Culture and Medical School* (New Brunswick, NJ: Transaction Books, 1984 [1961]).
Begg, A. C., *Insulin in General Practice: A Concise Clinical Guide for Practitioners* (London: William Heinemann, 1924).
Benett, I., 'Diabetes mini-clinic', *JRCGP*, 37:307 (1988), 76–7.
Bennett, I. J., C. Lambert, G. Hinds, and C. Kirton, 'Emerging standards for diabetes care from a city-wide primary care audit', *Diabetic Medicine*, 11:5 (1994), 489–92.
Benson, T., 'Why general practitioners use computers and hospitals do not – part 1: incentives', *BMJ*, 325:7372 (2002), 1086–9.
Benson, T., 'Why general practitioners use computers and hospitals do not – part 2: scalability', *BMJ*, 325:7372 (2002), 1090–3.
Berg, L. D., E. H. Huijbens and H. G. Larsen, 'Producing anxiety in the neoliberal university', *Canadian Geographer*, 60:2 (2016), 168–80.
Berg, M., 'Practices of reading and writing: the constitutive role of the patient record in medical work', *Sociology of Health and Illness*, 18:4 (1996), 499–524.
Berg, M., 'Problems and promises of the protocol', *Social Science and Medicine*, 44:8 (1997), 1081–8.
Berlivet, L., '"Association or causation?" The debate on the scientific status of risk factor epidemiology, 1947–c.1965', in V. Berridge (ed.), *Making Health Policy: Networks in Research and Policy after 1945* (Amsterdam: Rodopi, 2005), pp. 39–74.
Berridge, V., *Marketing Health: Smoking and the Discourse of Public Health in Britain, 1945–2000* (Oxford: Oxford University Press, 2007).
Berridge, V., 'Medicine and the public: the 1962 report of the Royal College of Physicians and the new public health', *Bulletin of the History of Medicine*, 81:1 (2007), 286–311.
Berridge, V. (ed.), *Making Health Policy: Networks in Research and Policy after 1945* (Amsterdam: Rodopi, 2005).
Berridge, V., and K. Loughlin (eds.), *Medicine, the Market and the Mass Media: Producing Health in the Twentieth Century* (London: Routledge, 2005).
Better general practice', *The Lancet*, 263:6813 (1954), 659–60.
Bevan, G., and C. Hood, 'What's measured is what matters: targets and gaming in the English public health system', *Public Administration*, 84:3 (2006), 517–38.
Bijker, W. E., T. P. Hughes, and T. Pinch (eds.), *The Social Construction of Technological Systems: New Directions in the Sociology and History of Technology, Anniversary Edition* (Cambridge, MA: MIT Press, 2012 [1987]).
Bivins, R., 'Coming "home" to (post)colonial medicine: treating tropical bodies in post-war Britain', *Social History of Medicine*, 26:1 (2013), 1–20.
Black, N., and E. Thompson, 'Obstacles to medical audit: British doctors speak', *Social Science and Medicine*, 36:7 (1993), 849–56.

Bliss, M., *The Discovery of Insulin, 25th Anniversary Edition* (Chicago: University of Chicago Press, 2007).
Bloom, A., 'Photocoagulation for diabetic retinopathy', *The Lancet*, 308:7978 (1976), 206.
Bosanquet, N., and C. Salisbury, 'The practice', in I. Loudon, J. Horder, and C. Webster (eds.), *General Practice under the National Health Service, 1948–1997* (Oxford: Oxford University Press, 1998), pp. 45–64.
Bowker, G. C., and S. Star, *Sorting Things Out* (Cambridge, MA: MIT Press, 1999).
Bradshaw, C., and J. Spencer, 'Nurse-run diabetic clinics in general practice', *Diabetic Medicine*, 7:7 (1990), 572–3.
Bradshaw, J., 'Social security', in D. Marsh and R. A. W. Rhodes (eds.), *Implementing Thatcherite Policies: Audit of an Era* (Buckingham: Open University Press, 1992), pp. 81–99.
Brandt, A. M., and M. Gardner, 'The golden age of medicine?', in R. Cooter and J. Pickstone (eds.), *Companion to Medicine in the Twentieth Century* (Abingdon: Routledge, 2003), pp. 21–37.
Brick, D. L., J. Brick, and J. W. Richardson, 'Fining the doctor', *BMJ*, 2:4902, S.233 (1954), 241.
Bridgen, P., 'Hospitals, geriatric medicine, and the long-term care of elderly people, 1946–1976', *Social History of Medicine*, 14:3 (2001), 507–23.
Bridgen, P., and J. Lewis, *Elderly People and the Boundary between Health and Social Care, 1946–91: Whose Responsibility?* (London: Nuffield Trust, 1999).
British Diabetic Association, *Helping People Live with Diabetes* (London: British Diabetic Association, 1988).
British Diabetic Association', *BMJ*, 2:5315 (1962), 1251.
British Medical Association annual meeting, Cardiff, 1953: health visitor and the family doctor', *BMJ*, 2:4830 (1953), 276–84.
British Medical Association: scientific sections', *The Lancet*, 254:6567 (1949), 67–9.
Brown, H., 'Hand injuries', *BMJ*, 3:5927 (1974), 403–6.
Brownbridge, G., A. Evans, M. Fitter, and M. Platts, 'An interactive computerized protocol for the management of hypertension: effects on the general practitioner's clinical behaviour', *JRCGP*, 36:5 (1986), 198–202.
Buckingham, H., and J. Rees, 'The context for service delivery: third sector, state and market relationships 1997–2015', in J. Rees and D. Mullins (eds.), *The Third Sector Delivering Public Services: Developments, Innovations, and Challenges* (Bristol: Policy Press, 2016), pp. 41–62.
Bucknall, C. E., C. Robertson, F. Moran, and R. D. Stevenson, 'Management of asthma in hospital: a prospective audit', *BMJ*, 296:6637 (1988), 1637–9.
Bufton, M., and V. Berridge, 'Post-war nutrition science and policy making in Britain c.1945–1994: the case of diet and heart disease', in D. Smith and J. Phillips (eds.), *Food, Science, Policy and Regulation in the Twentieth Century:*

Bibliography

International and Comparative Perspectives (London: Routledge, 2000), pp. 207–22.

Burns-Cox, C. J., 'Early detection of diabetic retinopathy', *The Lancet*, 324:8404 (1984), 693–4.

Burrows, P. J., P. J. Gray, A.-L. Kinmonth, D. J. Payton, G. A. Walpole, R. J. Walton, D. Wilson, and G. Woodbine, 'Who cares for the patient with diabetes? Presentation and follow-up in seven Southampton practices', *JRCGP*, 37:295 (1987), 65–9.

Buxton, M. J., M. J. Sculpher, B. A. Ferguson, J. E. Humphreys, J. F. B. Altman, D. J. Spiegelhalter, A. J. Kirby, J. S. Jacob, H. Bacon, S. B. Dudbridge, J. W. Stead, T. G. Feest, H. Cheng, S. L. Franklin, P. Courtney, J. F. Talbot, R. Ahmed, and T. R. Dabbs, 'Screening for treatable diabetic retinopathy: a comparison of different methods', *Diabetic Medicine*, 8:4 (1991), 371–7.

Buxton, M. J., M. J. Sculpher, B. A. Ferguson, J. E. Humphreys, J. F. B. Altman, D. J. Spiegelhalter, A. J. Kirby, J. S. Jacob, H. Bacon, S. B. Dudbridge, J. W. Stead, T. G. Feest, H. Cheng, S. L. Franklin, P. Courtney, J. F. Talbot, R. Ahmed, and T. R. Dabbs, 'A relative cost-effectiveness analysis of different methods of screening for diabetic retinopathy', *Diabetic Medicine*, 8:7 (1991), 644–50.

Bynum, W. F., *Science and the Practice of Medicine in the Nineteenth Century* (Cambridge: Cambridge University Press, 1994).

Cairncross, A., *The British Economy since 1945: Economic Policy and Performance, 1945–1990* (Oxford: Blackwell, 1992).

Calnan, M., *Preventing Coronary Heart Disease: Prospects, Policies, and Politics* (London: Routledge, 2002 [1991]).

'"Calorie control" diabetic diet', *BMJ*, 1:4282 (1943), 143–4.

Cantor, D., 'The MRC's support for experimental radiology during the interwar years', in J. Austoker and L. Bryder (eds.), *Historical Perspectives on the Role of the MRC: Essays in the History of the Medical Research Council of the United Kingdom and its predecessor, the Medical Research Committee, 1913–1953* (Oxford: Oxford University Press, 1989), pp. 181–204.

Cantor, D., 'Introduction: cancer control and prevention in the twentieth century', *Bulletin of the History of Medicine*, 81:3 (2007), 1–38.

'Can we prevent it?', *The Lancet*, 288:7474 (1966), 1171–2.

Carter, O. C., 'The 100% issue', *BMJ*, 2:4354, S.103 (1944), 101–2.

Cartwright, A., *Patients and their Doctors: A Study of General Practice* (London: Routledge and Kegan Paul, 1967).

Central Health Services Council, *Report of the Central Health Services Council for the Year Ended December 31, 1952*, House of Commons Papers, 218 (London: HMSO, 1953).

Central Health Services Council, *Report of the Central Health Services Council for the Year Ended December 31, 1953*, House of Commons Papers, 190 (London: HMSO, 1954).

Central Health Services Council, *The Field Work of the Family Doctor: Report of the Sub-Committee* (London: HMSO, 1963).

Chapman, G., S. Adam, and D. Stockford, 'National Service Frameworks: promoting the public health', *Journal of Epidemiology and Community Health*, 55:6 (2001), 373–4.

Charmaz, K., *Good Days, Bad Days: The Self in Chronic Illness and Time* (New Brunswick: Rutgers University Press, 1991).

Checkland, K., 'National Service Frameworks and UK general practitioners: street level bureaucrats at work?', *Sociology of Health and Illness*, 26:7 (2004), 951–75.

Cherry, S., 'Regional comparators in the funding and oranisation of the voluntary hospital system, c.1860–1939', in M. Gorsky and S. Sheard (eds.), *Financing Medicine: The British Experience since 1750* (London: Routledge, 2006), pp. 59–76.

Chote, R., R. Crawford, C. Emmerson, and G. Tetlow, *IFS Briefing Note 5: Public Spending Under Labour* (London: Institute for Fiscal Studies: 2010), available at: https://www.ifs.org.uk/bns/bn92.pdf (accessed May 2017).

Clarke, G., 'History of the Royal College of Physicians of London', *BMJ*, 1:5427 (1965), 79–82.

Clarke, J., and J. Newman, *The Managerial State: Power, Politics and Ideology in the Remaking of Social Welfare* (London: Sage, 1997).

Cleave, T. L., G. D. Campbell, and N.S. Painter, *Diabetes, Coronary Thrombosis, and the Saccharine Disease*, 2nd edition (Bristol: John Wright & Sons, 1969).

Clift, B., and J. Tomlinson, 'Negotiating credibility: Britain and the International Monetary Fund, 1956–1976', *Contemporary European History*, 17:4 (2008), 545–66.

'Clinical diabetes mellitus', *JRCGP*, 15:4 (1968), 307–8.

Clinical Standards Advisory Group, *Standards of Clinical Care for People with Diabetes* (London: HMSO, 1994).

Clinicians must be involved in purchasing', *BMJ*, 306:6882 (1993), 935.

Clyne, M. B., J. Fry, E. J. Raffle, and W. Tait: 'Murder at the cross-roads', *The Lancet*, 273:7083 (1959), 1146–9.

Cochrane, A. L., 'A medical scientist's view of screening', *Public Health*, 81:5 (1967), 207–13.

Cochrane, A. L., *Effectiveness and Efficiency: Random Reflections on the Health Services* (London: Nuffield Provincial Hospitals Trust, 1972).

Cogwheel in Scotland', *BMJ*, 4:5841 (1972), 661–2.

Collings, J. S., 'General practice in England today: a reconnaissance', *The Lancet*, 255:6604 (1950), 555–79.

Collings, J. S., 'Group practice: existing patterns and future policies', *The Lancet*, 262:6775 (1953), 31–3.

'Continuing care in chronic disease', *BMJ*, 2:5404 (1964), 308.

Cook, C., 'Oral history – Walter Holland', *Journal of Public Health*, 26:2 (2004), 121–9.
Cooter, R., 'The politics of spatial innovation: fracture clinics in interwar Britain', in J. Pickstone (ed.), *Medical Innovations in Historical Perspective* (Basingstoke: Macmillan, 1992), pp. 146–64.
Corbett, J. T., 'Keeping records in general practice', *JRCGP*, 5:2 (1962), 270–4.
Corless, D., 'Diet in the elderly', *BMJ*, 4:5885 (1973), 158–60.
Craig, B. L., 'Hospital records and record-keeping c.1850–c.1950, part 1: The development of records in hospitals', *Archivaria*, 29:1 (1989), 57–87.
Craig, B. L., 'The role of records and of record-keeping in the development of the modern hospital in London, England and Ontario, Canada', *Bulletin of the History of Medicine*, 65:3 (1991), 376–97.
Crombie, D. L., 'Preventive medicine and presymptomatic diagnosis', *JRCGP*, 15:5 (1968), 344–51
Culley, A. R., 'The care of the aged and infirm and the chronic sick', *Public Health*, 60:5 (1947), 102–4.
Cutler, T., 'Dangerous yardstick? Early cost estimates and the politics of financial management in the first decade of the National Health Service', *Medical History*, 47:2 (2003), 217–38.
Cutler, T., 'Managerialism *avant la lettre*? The debate on accounting in the NHS hospitals in the 1950s', in V. Berridge and K. Loughlin (eds.), *Medicine, the Market, and the Mass Media: Producing Health in the Twentieth Century* (London: Routledge, 2005), pp. 124–45.
Daly, J., *Evidence-Based Medicine and the Search for a Science of Clinical Care* (Berkeley: University of California Press, 2005).
Davis, C., 'The health visitor as mother's friend: a woman's place in public health, 1900–14', *Social History of Medicine*, 1:1 (1988), 39–59.
Day, J., H. Humphries, and H. Alban-Davies, 'Problems of comprehensive shared diabetes care', *BMJ*, 240:6587 (1987), 1590–2.
Day, P., R. Klein, and F. Miller, *A Comparative US–UK Study of Guidelines* (London: Nuffield Trust, 1998).
Dean, M., *Governmentality: Power and Rule in Modern Society* (London: SAGE, 2010).
'Death of Proplist', *The Lancet*, 296:7679 (1970), 918.
Delamothe, T., 'Wanted: guidelines that doctors will follow', *BMJ*, 307:6898 (1993), 218.
Denham, M., 'The surveys of the Birmingham chronic sick hospitals, 1948–1960', *Social History of Medicine*, 19:2 (2006), 279–93.
Department of Health, *The Health of the Nation: A Consultative Document for Health in England*, Cm 1523 (London: HMSO, 1991).
Department of Health, *The Health of the Nation: A Strategy for Health in England*, Cm 1986 (London: HMSO, 1992).

Department of Health, *National Service Framework for Diabetes: Standards* (London: Department of Health, 2001).
Department of Health, *National Service Framework for Diabetes: Delivery Strategy* (London: Department of Health, 2002).
Department of Health and Social Security, Department of Education and Science, Scottish Office, and Welsh Office, *Prevention and Health,* Cmnd 7047 (London: HMSO, 1977).
Department of Health for Scotland, *Committee on Scottish Health Services,* Cmd 5204 (Edinburgh: HMSO, 1936).
Detection of diabetes', *BMJ,* 2:5151 (1959), 555–6.
'Detection of diabetes', *BMJ,* 1:5291 (1962), 1535–6.
Dewar, D., and W. Funnell, *A History of British National Audit: The Pursuit of Accountability* (Oxford: Oxford University Press, 2017).
'Diabetes and insulin', *BMJ,* 1:4662 (1950), 1122.
'Diabetes mellitus – incidence, causation, management', *Proceedings of the Royal Society of Medicine,* 55:3 (1962), 205–11.
'A diabetic clinic', *BMJ,* 1:3828 (1934), 906.
'Diabetic retinopathy', *The Lancet,* 296:7682 (1970), 1073–4.
Diack, L., and D. F. Smith, 'Professional strategies of Medical Officers of Health in the post-war period – 1: "innovative traditionalism": the case of Dr Ian MacQueen, MOH for Aberdeen, 1952–1974, a "bull-dog" with the "hide of a rhinoceros"', *Journal of Public Health Medicine,* 24:2 (2002), 123–9.
'Diagnosis of diabetes', *The Lancet,* 276:7153 (1960), 745–6.
Digby, A., *Making a Medical Living: Doctors and Patients in the English Market for Medicine, 1720–1911* (Cambridge: Cambridge University Press, 1994).
Digby, A., *The Evolution of British General Practice, 1850–1948* (Oxford: Oxford University Press, 1999).
Digby, A., and N. Bosanquet, 'Doctors and patients in an era of national health insurance and private practice', *Economic History Review,* 41:1 (1988), 74–94.
Dingwall, R. W. J., 'Collectivism, regionalism and feminism: health visiting and British social policy', *Journal of Social Policy,* 6:3 (1977), 291–315.
Dirks, N., *Castes of Mind: Colonialism and the Making of Modern India* (Princeton: Princeton University Press).
Dixon, A., A. Khachatryan, A. Wallace, S. Peckham, T. Boyce, and S. Gillam, *Impact of Quality and Outcomes Framework on Health Inequalities* (London: King's Fund, 2011).
Dixon, P. N., 'Work of a nurse in a health centre treatment room', *BMJ,* 4:5678 (1969), 292–4.
'Do anticoagulant drugs prevent complications?', *BMJ,* 4:5888 (1973), 352.
Doll, R., Monitoring the National Health Service', *Proceedings of the Royal Society of Medicine,* 66:8 (1973), 729–40.
Dollery, C. T., 'Constructive attack', *BMJ,* 2:5804 (1972), 56.

Domenech, R. M. M., and C. Casañeda, 'Redefining cancer during the interwar period: British Medical Officers of Health, state policy, managerialism and public health', *American Journal of Public Health*, 97:9 (2007), 1563–71.
Donabedian, A., 'Evaluating the quality of medical care', *Milbank Memorial Fund Quarterly*, 44:3, part 2 (1966), 166–203.
Donaldson, R. J., 'Multiple screening clinics', *Public Health*, 81:5 (1967), 218–21.
Doney, B. J., 'An audit of the care of diabetics in a group practice', *JRCGP*, 26:171 (1976), 734–42.
Dornan, T., and S. Vernon, 'Diabetes and the eye', in R. B. Tattersall and E. A. M. Gale (eds.), *Diabetes Clinical Management* (Edinburgh: Churchill Livingstone, 1990), pp. 263–79.
Doyle, B. M., *The Politics of Hospital Provision in Early Twentieth-Century Britain* (London: Pickering and Chatto, 2014).
Droller, H., 'An outbreak of hepatitis in a diabetic clinic', *BMJ*, 1:4400 (1945), 623–5.
Dudley, H., 'Necessity for surgical audit', *BMJ*, 1:5902 (1974), 275–7.
Dunleavy, P., and C. Hood, 'From old public administration to new public management', *Public Money and Management*, 14:3 (1994), 9–16.
Earl, C. J. C., 'Treatment of diabetics as hospital out-patients', *BMJ*, 1:3461 (1927), 831–3.
Eder, N. R., *National Health Insurance and the Medical Profession in Britain, 1913–39* (London: Garland, 1982).
Edwards, M., *Control and the Therapeutic Trial: Rhetoric and Experimentation in Britain, 1918–48* (Amsterdam: Rodopi, 2007).
'Effectiveness and Efficiency', *The Lancet*, 299:7752 (1972), 668–9.
Egan, D. F., 'Towards a new public health', *Public Health*, 79:4 (1965), 181–3.
Elliot, R. W., 'The prevention of illness in middle age', *Public Health*, 79:6 (1965), 317–25.
Evandrou, M., J. Falkingham, Z. Feng, and A. Vlachantoni, 'Ethnic inequalities in limiting health and self-reported health in later life', *Journal of Epidemiology and Community Health*, 70:7 (2016), 653–62.
Evans, D., and A. Haines (eds.), *Implementing Evidence-Based Changes in Healthcare* (Abingdon: Radcliffe Medical Press, 2000).
Evans, E. O., and I. McWhinney, 'General practitioner and the general hospital', *BMJ*, 1:5384 (1964), 688–90.
Eve, F. C., 'Diabetic treatment simplified', *BMJ*, 1:3362 (1925), 1033–5.
Evetts, J., 'New professionalism and new public management: changes, continuities, and consequences', *Comparative Sociology*, 8:2 (2009), 247–66.
Evetts, J., 'A new professionalism? Challenges and opportunities', *Current Sociology*, 59:4 (2011), 406–22.

Exton-Smith, A. N., and G. S. Crockett, 'The chronic sick under new management: experiences in starting a geriatric unit', *The Lancet*, 253:6563 (1949), 1016-18.
Ezedum, S., and D. Kerr, 'Collaborative care of hypertensives, using a shared record', *BMJ*, 2:6099 (1977), 1402-3.
Fairfield, L., 'Care of the chronic sick', *The Lancet*, 242:6267 (1943), 455-7.
Feder, G., 'Clinical guidelines in 1994', *BMJ*, 309:6968 (1994), 1457-8.
Felton, A.-M., M. S. Hall, 'Diabetes – from St Vincent to Glasgow. Have we progressed in 20 years?', *British Journal of Diabetes and Vascular Disease*, 9:4 (2009), 142-4.
Feudtner, C., 'The want of control: ideas, innovations, and ideals in the modern management of diabetes mellitus', *Bulletin of the History of Medicine*, 69:1 (1995), 66-90.
Feudtner, C., 'Pathway to health: juvenile diabetes and the origins of managerial medicine', in A. M. Stern and H. Markel (eds.), *Formative Years: Children's Health in the United States, 1880-2000* (Ann Arbor: University of Michigan Press, 2002), pp. 208-32.
Feudtner, C., *Bittersweet: Diabetes, Insulin, and the Transformation of Illness* (Chapel Hill: University of North Carolina Press, 2003).
Fissell, M. E., 'The disappearance of the patient's narrative and the invention of hospital medicine', in R. French and A. Wear (eds.), *British Medicine in an Age of Reform* (London: Routledge, 1991), pp. 91-109.
Fletcher, C. M., 'Inquiry into diabetic care', *BMJ*, 2:4357 (1944), 58.
Flynn, R., 'Clinical governance and governmentality', *Health, Risk and Society*, 4:2 (2002), 155-73.
Forsyth, G., and R. Logan, *Gateway or Dividing Line? A Study of Hospital Outpatients in the 1960s* (Oxford: Oxford University Press for the Nuffield Provincial Hospitals Trust, 1968).
Foucault, M., *Discipline and Punish: The Birth of the Prison*, trans. A. Sheridan (London: Penguin, 1991 [1975]).
Foucault, M., *The Birth of the Clinic: An Archaeology of Medical Perception*, trans. A. M. Sheridan-Smith (London: Routledge, 2010 [1973]).
Foucault, M., *The Birth of Biopolitics: Lectures at the Collège de France, 1978-79*, trans. G. Burchell, ed. M. Senellart (Basingstoke: Palgrave Macmillan, 2008).
Foulkes, A., A.-L. Kinmouth, S. Frost, and D. Macdonald, 'Organised personal care – an effective choice for managing diabetes in general practice', *JRCGP*, 39:11 (1989), 444-7.
Fox, D., *Health Policies, Health Politics: The British and American Experience, 1911-1965* (Princeton: Princeton University Press, 1986).
Fox, D., *Power and Illness: The Failure of American Health Policy* (Berkeley: University of California Press, 1993).

Francis, M., 'The Labour Party: modernisation and the politics of restraint', in B. Conekin, F. Mort, and C. Waters (eds.), *Moments of Modernity: Reconstructing Britain, 1945–1964* (London: Rivers Oram Press, 1999), pp. 152–70.
Freidson, E., 'The changing nature of professional control', *Annual Review of Sociology*, 10 (1984), 1–20.
Freidson, E., 'The reorganization of the medical profession', *Medical Care Research and Review*, 42:1 (1985), 11–35.
Freidson, E., *Profession of Medicine: A Study of the Sociology of Applied Knowledge* (Chicago: University of Chicago Press, 1988 [1970]).
French, D. G., 'Advances in general practice', *The Practitioner*, 183:1096 (1959), 513–18.
Friedman, E., E. Grable, and J. Fine, 'Central venous pressure and direct serial measurements as guides in blood volume replacement', *The Lancet*, 288:7464 (1966), 609–14.
Fry, J., 'Government and profession', *The Lancet*, 269:6970 (1957), 689–90.
Fry, J., 'General practice to-morrow', *BMJ*, 2:5416 (1964), 1064–7.
Fry, J., *Common Diseases: Their Nature, Incidence and Care*, 2nd edition (Lancaster: MTP Press Limited, 1979).
Fry, J., and G. Sandler, *Common Diseases: Their Nature, Presentation, and Care*, 5th edition (London: Kluwer Academic, 1993).
Fuller, J. H., M. J. Shipley, G. Rose, R. J. Jarrett, and H. Keen, 'Coronary-heart-disease risk and impaired glucose tolerance: the Whitehall study', *The Lancet*, 315:8183 (1980), 1373–6.
Functions review is vital', *BMJ*, 307:6895 (1993), 69.
Furdell, E. L., *Fatal Thirst: Diabetes in Britain until Insulin* (Leiden: Brill, 2009).
Gamble, A., *The Free Economy and the Strong State: The Politics of Thatcherism* (Durham, NC: Duke University Press, 1988).
Gamble, A., 'Privatization, Thatcherism, and the British state', *Journal of Law and Society*, 16:1 (1989), 1–20.
Gamble, A., *The Free Economy and the Strong State: The Politics of Thatcherism*, 2nd edition (Basingstoke: Macmillan, 1994).
Gedney, J., 'Reconstruction of general practice', *BMJ*, 290:6478 (1985), 1350.
Geiringer, E., 'Murder at the cross-roads or the decapitation of general practice', *The Lancet*, 273:7081 (1959), 1039–45.
Gibbins, R. L., and J. Saunders, 'Develop diabetic care in general practice', *BMJ*, 297:6642 (1988), 187–9.
Gilani, A., 'The challenges of managing diabetes in hard-to-reach-groups', *Diabetes and Primary Care*, 16:4 (2014), 206–11.
Gilliland, I. C., 'Registrars', *The Lancet*, 256:6640 (1950), 710–11.
Gorsky, M., '"Threshold of a new era": the development of an integrated hospital system in northeast Scotland, 1900–39', *Social History of Medicine*, 17:2 (2004), 247–67.

Gorsky, M., 'Local leadership in public health: the role of the Medical Officer of Health in Britain, 1872–1974', *Journal of Epidemiology and Community Health*, 61:6 (2007), 468–72.

Gorsky, M., 'Local government health services in interwar England: problems of quantification and interpretation', *Bulletin of the History of Medicine*, 85:3 (2011), 384–412.

Gorsky, M., '"To regulate and confirm inequality"? A regional history of geriatric hospitals under the English National Health Service, c.1948–1975', *Ageing & Society*, 33:4 (2013), 598–625.

Gorsky, M., '"Searching for the people in charge": appraising the 1983 Griffiths NHS Management Inquiry', *Medical History*, 57:1 (2013), 87–107.

Graham, G., 'The diet in diabetes', *BMJ*, 2:4307 (1943), 115–16.

Granshaw, L., '"Fame and fortune by means of bricks and mortar": the medical profession and specialist hospitals in Britain, 1800–1948', in L. Granshaw and R. Porter (eds.), *The Hospital in History* (London: Routledge, 1989), pp. 199–220.

Gray, A., and B. Jenkins, 'Policy analysis in British central government: the experience of PAR', *Public Administration*, 60:4 (1982), 429–50.

Gray, M., and G. Fowler (eds.), *Preventive Medicine in General Practice* (Oxford: Oxford University Press, 1983).

Greene, J. A., *Prescribing by Numbers: Drugs and the Definition of Disease* (Baltimore: Johns Hopkins University Press, 2007).

Grene, J. D., and J. M. Henderson, 'Automated recall in general practice', *JRCGP*, 21:107 (1971), 352–5.

Hall, S., 'The great moving right show', in S. Hall and M. Jacques (eds.), *The Politics of Thatcherism* (London: Lawrence and Wishart in Association with Marxism Today, 1983), pp. 19–39.

Hammersley, M., M. Holland, S. Walford, and P. Thorn, 'What happens to defaulters from a diabetic clinic?', *BMJ*, 291:6505 (1985), 1330–2.

Hampton, J., *Disability and the Welfare State in Britain: Changes in Perception and Policy, 1948–79* (Bristol: Policy Press, 2016).

Hampton, J. R., 'The end of clinical freedom', *BMJ*, 287:6401 (1983), 1237–8.

Hand, J., 'Marketing health education: advertising margarine and visualising health in Britain from 1964–c.2000', *Contemporary British History*, 31:4 (2017), 477–500.

Hand, J., '"Tucking your tummy in isn't the answer": visualising obesity as a public health concern in 1970s and 1980s Britain', in M. Jackson and M. D. Moore (eds.), *Balancing the Self: Medicine, Politics, and the Regulation of Health in the Twentieth Century* (forthcoming).

Hanlon, G., 'Professionalism as enterprise: service class politics and the redefinition of professionalism', *Sociology*, 32:1 (1998), 43–63.

Hanlon, G., 'Institutional forms and organizational structures: homology, trust and reputational capital in professional services firms', *Organization*, 11:2 (2004), 187–210.

Hardy, A., '"Death is the cure of all diseases": using the General Register Office cause of death statistics for 1837–1920', *Social History of Medicine*, 7:3 (1994), 472–92.

Hardy, A., 'Beriberi, vitamin B1 and world food policy, 1925–1970', *Medical History*, 39:1 (1995), 61–77.

Harrison, S., *National Health Service Management in the 1980s* (Aldershot: Avebury, 1994).

Harrison, S., and W. I. U. Ahmad, 'Medical autonomy and the UK state 1975 to 2025', *Sociology*, 34:1 (2000), 129–46.

Harrison, S., and G. Dowswell, 'Autonomy and bureaucratic accountability in primary care: what English general practitioners say', *Sociology of Health and Illness*, 24:2 (2002), 208–26.

Harrison, S., M. Moran, and B. Wood, 'Policy emergence and policy convergence: the case of 'Scientific-Bureaucratic Medicine' in the United States and United Kingdom', *British Journal of Politics and International Relations*, 4:1 (2002), 1–21.

Harrison, S., and C. Pollitt, *Controlling Health Professionals: The Future of Work and Organization in the NHS* (Buckingham: Open University Press, 1994).

Harrison, S., and B. Wood, 'Scientific-bureaucratic medicine and UK health policy', *Policy Studies Review*, 17:4 (2000), 25–42.

Hart, J. T., 'Specialization in general practice', *JRCGP*, 30:4 (1980), 216–19.

Hart, J. T., 'A new kind of doctor', *Journal of the Royal Society of Medicine*, 74:12 (1981), 871–83.

Hart, J. T., 'Coronary heart disease: preventable but not prevented?', *British Journal of General Practice*, 40:340 (1990), 441–2.

Hart, P. M., D. B. Archer, and A. B. Atkinson, 'Diabetic patients should continue to be assessed by direct ophthalmoscopy', *BMJ*, 312:7047 (1996), 1670.

Harvey, D., *A Brief History of Neoliberalism* (Oxford: Oxford University Press, 2005).

Hasler, J., 'The size and nature of the problem', in J. Hasler and T. Schofield (eds.), *Continuing Care: The Management of Chronic Disease*, 2nd edition (Oxford: Oxford University Press, 1984), pp. 1–13.

Hastings, S., 'Scientific freedom and social medicine', *BMJ*, 1:4290 (1943), 392–3.

Hatfield, F. S. E., 'Monitoring general practitioners', *JRCGP*, 26:171 (1976), 764.

Hawthorne, C. O., 'On peripheral neuritis and retinal changes in diabetes mellitus', *The Lancet*, 154:3970 (1899), 876–7.

Hawthorne, C. O., 'The freedom of medicine', *BMJ*, 2:3432 (1926), 705–8.
Hay, C., 'Whatever happened to Thatcherism?', *Political Studies Review*, 5:2 (2007), 183–201.
Hay, C., 'Chronicles of a death foretold: the Winter of Discontent and the construction of the crisis of British Keynesianism', *Parliamentary Affairs*, 63:3 (2010), 446–70.
Hayes, T. M., and J. Harries, 'Randomised controlled trial of routine hospital clinic care versus routine general practice care for type-II diabetics', *BMJ*, 289:6447 (1984), 728–30.
Hayward, R., *The Transformation of the Psyche in British Primary Care, 1870–1970* (London: Bloomsbury Academic, 2014).
Hedgecoe, A. M., 'Reinventing diabetes: classification, division, and geneticization of disease', *New Genetics and Society*, 21:2 (2002), 7–27.
Hennessey, P., *Whitehall* (London: Fontana Press, 1990).
Hennock, E. P., 'Poverty and social reforms', in P. Johnson (ed.), *Twentieth Century Britain: Economic, Social and Cultural Change* (London: Longman, 1994), pp. 79–93.
Hess, V., and J. A. Mendelsohn, 'Case and series: medical knowledge and paper technology, 1600–1900', *History of Science*, 48:3 (2010), 287–314.
Hibble, A., D. Kanka, D. Pencheon, and F. Pooles, 'Guidelines in general practice: the new Tower of Babel?', *BMJ*, 317:7162 (1998), 862–3.
'High carbohydrate diets in diabetes', *The Lancet*, 222:5740 (1933), 538.
Hill, R. D., 'Community care service for diabetics in the Poole area', *BMJ*, 1:6018 (1976), 1137–9.
Hill, R. D., *Diabetes Health Care: A Guide to the Provision of Health Care Services* (London: Chapman and Hall, 1987).
Hilton, M., *Consumerism in Twentieth-Century Britain* (Cambridge: Cambridge University Press, 2003).
Hilton, M., N. Crowson, J. McKay, and J.-F. Mouhot, *The Politics of Expertise: How NGOs Shaped Modern Britain* (Oxford: Oxford University Press, 2013).
Himsworth, H. P., 'Management of diabetes mellitus, part II', *BMJ*, 2:3942 (1936), 188–90.
Himsworth, H. P., 'Diet in the aetiology of human diabetes', *Proceedings of the Royal Society of Medicine*, 62 (1949), 323–6.
Himsworth, H. P., 'The syndrome of diabetes mellitus and its causes', *The Lancet*, 253:6551 (1949), 465–73.
Hodgkin, K., 'Good general practice without routine screening examinations', *JRCGP*, 11:S.1 (1966), 100–6.
Hoffenberg, R., *Clinical Freedom* (London: Nuffield Provincial Hospitals Trust, 1987).
Home, P., and S. Walford, 'Diabetes care: whose responsibility?', *BMJ*, 289:6447 (1984), 713–14.

Home, P. D., and W. M. G. Tunbridge, 'Appointments and turnover of consultants and senior registrars in diabetes and endocrinology in the UK, 1984 and 1985', *Diabetic Medicine*, 4:1 (1987), 79–82.
Honigsbaum, F., *The Division in British Medicine: A History of the Separation of General Practice from Hospital Care, 1911–1968* (London: Kogan and Page, 1979).
Horder, J., 'Alma Ata Declaration', *BMJ*, 286:6360 (1983), 191–4.
Horder, J., 'Conclusion', I. Loudon, J. Horder, and C. Webster (eds.), *General Practice under the National Health Service, 1948–1997* (Oxford: Oxford University Press, 1998), pp. 278–84.
Horobin, G., and J. McIntosh, 'Time, risk and routine in general practice', *Sociology of Health and Illness*, 5:3 (1983), 312–31.
House of Commons Committee of Public Accounts, *Department of Health: The Management of Adult Diabetes Services in the NHS*, HC 289 (London: HMSO, 2012).
Howell, J. D., *Technology in the Hospital: Transforming Patient Care in the Early Twentieth Century* (Baltimore: Johns Hopkins University Press, 1995).
Howlett, P., 'The "Golden Age", 1955–1973', in P. Johnson (ed.), *Twentieth Century Britain: Economic, Social and Cultural Change* (London: Longman, 1994), pp. 320–39.
Hull, A., 'Hector's house: Sir Hector Hetherington and the academization of Glasgow hospital medicine before the NHS', *Medical History*, 45:2 (2001), 207–42.
Hurwitz, B., C. Goodman, and J. Yudkin, 'Prompting the clinical care of non-insulin dependent (type-II) diabetic patients in an inner city area: one model of community care', *BMJ*, 306:6878 (1993), 624–5.
Hurwitz, B., and J. Yudkin, 'Diabetes care: whose responsibility?', *BMJ*, 289:6450 (1984), 1000–1.
Illich, I., *Limits to Medicine: Medical Nemesis – the Expropriation of Health* (Harmondsworth: Penguin, 1977).
'Impaired glucose tolerance and diabetes – WHO criteria', *BMJ*, 281:6254 (1980), 1512–13.
'Improvement of the N.H.S.', *The Lancet*, 269:6958 (1957), 41–2.
'Inquiry is urged into hospital queues', *The Times*, 13 August 1968, p. 2.
Ireland, J. T., W. S. T. Thomson, and J. Williamson, *Diabetes Today: A Handbook for the Clinical Team* (Aylesbury: HM+M, 1980).
Irvine, D., *A Doctor's Tale: Professionalism and Public Trust* (Abingdon: Radcliffe Medical Press, 2003).
Jackson, B., 'The think-tank archipelago: Thatcherism and neoliberalism', in B. Jackson and R. Saunders (eds.), *Making Thatcher's Britain* (Cambridge: Cambridge University Press, 2012), pp. 43–61.
Jackson, B, and R. Saunders (eds.), *Making Thatcher's Britain* (Cambridge: Cambridge University Press, 2012).

Jackson, J. G. L., *Employment Survey* (London: British Diabetic Association, 1961).
Jackson, J. G. L., 'R. D. Lawrence and the formation of the Diabetic Association', *Diabetic Medicine*, 13:1 (1996), 9–22.
Jackson, J. G. L., 'The formation of the Medical and Scientific Section of the British Diabetic Association', *Diabetic Medicine*, 14:10 (1997), 886–91.
Jackson, M., *Asthma: The Biography* (Oxford: Oxford University Press, 2009).
Jackson, M. '"Life begins at 40": self-help, marriage guidance, and the making of the midlife crisis in Britain and America', in M. Jackson and M. D. Moore (eds.), *Balancing the Self: Medicine, Politics, and the Regulation of Health in the Twentieth Century* (forthcoming).
Jackson, W. J., A. S. Paterson, C. K. M. Pong, and S. Scarparo, 'Doctors under the microscope: the birth of medical audit', *Accounting History Review*, 23:1 (2013), 23–47.
Jarrett, R. J., *Diabetes Mellitus* (London: Croom Helm, 1987).
Jarrett, R. J., H. Keen, J. H. Fuller, and M. McCartney, 'Treatment of borderline diabetes: controlled trial using carbohydrate restriction and phenformin', *BMJ*, 2:6091 (1977), 861–5.
Jarrett, R. J., H. Keen, J. H. Fuller, and M. McCartney, 'Worsening to diabetes in men with impaired glucose tolerance ("borderline diabetes")', *Diabetologia*, 16:1 (1979), 25–30.
Jasen, P., 'Breast cancer and the language of risk, 1750–1950', *Social History of Medicine*, 15:1 (2002), 17–43.
Jewson, N., 'Disappearance of the sick man from medical cosmology, 1770–1870', *Sociology*, 10:2 (1976), 225–44.
Johnson, R., 'Medical audit', *The Lancet*, 305:7908 (1975), 679.
Johnson, T. J., *Professions and Power* (London: Macmillan, 1972).
Jones, K., 'Asthma – still a challenge for general practice', *JRCGP*, 39:6 (1989), 254–6.
Jones, L., and J. Green, 'Shifting discourses of professionalism: a case study of general practitioners in the United Kingdom', *Sociology of Health and Illness*, 28:7 (2006), 927–50.
Jones, M., *Science Fiction Cinema and 1950s Britain: Recontextualizing Cultural Anxiety* (London: Bloomsbury, 2018).
Karnauchow, P. N., 'Medical audit', *The Lancet*, 305:7914 (1975), 1029–30.
Kassell, L., 'Casebooks in early modern England: medicine, astrology and written records', *Bulletin of the History of Medicine*, 88:4 (2014), 595–625.
Kavanagh, D., 'The postwar consensus', *Twentieth Century British History*, 3:2 (1992), 175–90.
Kavanagh, D., and P. Morris, *Consensus Politics from Attlee to Major*, 2nd edition (Oxford: Blackwell, 1995).
Keating, P., and A. Cambrosio, 'Cancer clinical trials: the emergence and development of a new style of practice', *Bulletin of the History of Medicine*, 81:1 (2007), 197–223.

Keen, H., 'The family doctor and the diabetic', *The Practitioner*, 194:1160 (1965), 244–9.
Keen, H., 'Diabetes detection', in G. Teeling-Smith (ed.), *Surveillance and Early Diagnosis in General Practice* (London: Office of Health Economics, 1966), pp. 19–24.
Keen, H., and S. Ng Tang Fui, 'The definition and classification of diabetes mellitus', *Clinics in Endocrinology and Metabolism*, 11 (1982), 283–7.
Keen, H., G. Rose, D. A. Pyke, D. Boyns, C. Chlouverakis, and S. Mistry, 'Blood sugar and arterial disease', *The Lancet*, 286:7411 (1965), 505–8.
Kemp, P., 'Housing', in D. Marsh and R. A. W. Rhodes (eds.), *Implementing Thatcherite Policies: Audit of an Era* (Buckingham: Open University Press, 1992), pp. 65–80.
Kemper, T. J., and S. R. Hayter, 'Audit of diabetes in general practice', *BMJ*, 302:6774 (1991), 451–3.
Kempi, V., W. Van der Linden, and C. Von Schéele, 'Diagnosis of deep vein thrombosis with ^{99m}Tc-streptokinase: a clinical comparison with phlebography', *BMJ*, 4:5947 (1974), 748–9.
Kerr, P., *Post-War British Politics: From Conflict to Consensus* (London: Routledge, 2001).
Kinnersley, P., P. Owen, C. Wilkinson, and J. Richards, 'Set menus and clinical freedom', *BMJ*, 303:6806 (1991), 857–8.
Kipnis, A. B., 'Audit cultures: neoliberal governmentality, socialist legacy, or technologies of governing?', *American Ethnologist*, 35:2 (2008), 275–89.
Kirkpatrick, I., S. Ackroyd, and R. Walker, *The New Managerialism and Public Service Professions: Change in Health, Social Services and Housing* (Basingstoke: Palgrave Macmillan, 2005).
Kirkpatrick, I., and M. M. Lucio (eds.), *The Politics of Quality in the Public Sector: The Management of Change* (London: Routledge, 1995).
Klein, R., 'Auditing the NHS', *BMJ*, 285:6343 (1982), 672–3.
Klein, R., 'The crises of the welfare states', in R. Cooter and J. Pickstone (eds.), *Medicine in the Twentieth Century* (Amsterdam: Rodopi, 2000), pp. 155–70.
Klein, R., *The New Politics of the NHS: From Creation to Reinvention*, 5th edition (Oxford: Radcliffe, 2006).
Kohner, E. M., and P. J. Barry, 'Prevention of blindness in diabetic retinopathy', *Diabetologia*, 26:3 (1984), 173–9.
Kratky, A. P., 'An audit of the care of diabetics in one general practice', *JRCGP*, 27:182 (1977), 536–43.
Laing, W., and Williams, R., *Diabetes: A Model for Health Care Management* (London: Office of Health Economics, 1989).
Larson, M. S., *The Rise of Professionalism: A Sociological Analysis* (Berkeley: University of California Press, 1977).
Latour, B., *The Pasteurization of France*, trans. Sheridan and J. Law (Cambridge, MA Harvard University Press, 1993).

Latour, B., *Reassembling the Social: An Introduction to Actor-Network-Theory* (Oxford: Oxford University Press, 2005).
Lawrence, C., 'Incommunicable knowledge: science, technology and the clinical art in Britain, 1850–1914', *Journal of Contemporary History*, 20:4 (1985), 503–20.
Lawrence, C., *Rockefeller Money, The Laboratory and Medicine in Edinburgh, 1919–1930: New Science in an Old Country* (New York: University of Rochester Press, 2005).
Lawrence, M., 'All together now', *JRCGP*, 38:7 (1988), 296–302.
Lawrence, R. D., *The Diabetic Life: Its Control by Diet and Insulin. A Concise Practical Manual for Practitioners and Patients*, 1st edition (London: J. & A. Churchill, 1925).
Lawrence, R. D., *The Diabetic Life: Its Control by Diet and Insulin. A Concise Practical Manual for Practitioners and Patients*, 6th edition (London: J. & A. Churchill, 1931).
Lawrence, R. D., 'Special clinics for diabetics', *BMJ*, 2:4262 (1942), 322.
Lawrence, R. D., 'Regional centres for the treatment of diabetes', *The Lancet*, 257:6668 (1951), 1318–19.
Lawrence, R. D., 'Regional diabetic services', *BMJ*, 2:4828 (1953), 160.
Lawrence, R. D., *The Diabetic Life: Its Control by Diet and Insulin and Oral Treatment by Sulphonyl-Ureas. A Concise Practical Manual*, 16th edition (London: J. & A. Churchill, 1960).
Lawrence, R. D., 'The beginning of the Diabetic Association in England', in D von Engelhardt (ed.), *Diabetes: Its Medical and Cultural History. Outlines, Texts, Bibliography* (New York: Springer-Verlag, c.1989 [1951], pp. 451–3.
Lean, M. E. J., and W. P. T. James, 'Prescription of diabetic diets in the 1980s', *BMJ*, 292:6524 (1986), 723–5.
Lescher, F. G., 'The modern treatment of diabetes mellitus and the use of zinc protamine insulin', *BMJ*, 1:4017 (1938), 13–14.
Levene, A., 'Between less eligibility and the NHS: the changing place of Poor Law hospitals in England and Wales, 1929–39', *Twentieth Century British History*, 20:3 (2009), 322–45.
Lewis, J., *What Price Community Medicine? The Philosophy, Practice and Politics of Public Health since 1919* (Brighton: Wheatsheaf, 1986).
Lewis, J., 'The medical profession and the state: GPs and the GP contract in the 1960s and 1990s', *Social Policy and Administration*, 32:2 (1998), 132–50.
Liebenau, J., 'The MRC and the pharmaceutical industry: the model of insulin', in J Austoker and L Bryder (eds.), *Historical Perspectives on the Role of the MRC: Essays in the History of the Medical Research Council of the United Kingdom and its Predecessor, the Medical Research Committee, 1913–1953* (Oxford: Oxford University Press, 1989), pp. 163–80.
Light, D., and S. Levine, 'The changing character of the medical profession: a theoretical overview', *Milbank Quarterly*, 66:2 (1988), 10–32.

Lister, J., *The Clinical Syndrome of Diabetes Mellitus* (London: H. K. Lewis, 1959).
Local Government Operational Research Unit, *Manchester's Old People: A Study for the Social Services Department*, 2nd edition (London: Royal Institute of Public Administration, 1972).
Local Government Operational Research Unit, *Identifying the Chronically Sick and Disabled in Reading* (London: Royal Institute of Public Administration, 1973).
Logan, R. F. L., *General Register Office Studies on Medical and Population Subjects*, 7 (London: HMSO, 1953).
Logan, R. F. L., 'Control of chronic disease in general practice and industry', *JCGP*, 11:S.1 (1966), 94–100.
'London diabetic clinics, provincial diabetic clinics', *Diabetic Journal*, 3:3 (1940), 32–4.
Loudon, I., and M. Drury, 'Some aspects of clinical care in general practice', in I. Loudon, J. Horder, and C. Webster (eds.), *General Practice under the National Health Service, 1948–1997* (Oxford: Oxford University Press, 1998), pp. 92–127.
Lowe, R., 'The Second World War, consensus and the foundation of the welfare state', *Twentieth Century British History*, 1:2 (1990), 152–82.
Lowe, R., *The Welfare State in Britain since 1945*, 3rd edition (Basingstoke: Palgrave Macmillan, 2005).
Löwy, I., 'The experimental body', in R. Cooter and J. Pickstone (eds.), *Companion to Medicine in the Twentieth Century* (Abingdon: Routledge, 2003), pp. 435–49.
Mackintosh, A., 'The patent medicines industry in late Georgian England: a respectable alternative to both regular medicine and irregular practice', *Social History of Medicine*, 30:1 (2017), 22–47.
MacLean, H., *Modern Methods in the Diagnosis and Treatment of Glycosuria and Diabetes* (London: Constable Co., 1922).
MacLean, H., *Modern Methods in the Diagnosis and Treatment of Glycosuria and Diabetes*, 5th edition (London: Constable Co., 1932).
MacKinnon, M., R. M. Wilson, C. A. Hardisty, and J. D. Ward, 'Novel role for specialist nurses in managing diabetes in the community', *BMJ*, 299:6698 (1989), 552–4.
Maksimov-Cox, D., 'The making of the clinical trial in Britain, 1910–1945: expertise, the state and the public' (PhD dissertation, University of Cambridge, 1997).
Malins, J., *Clinical Diabetes Mellitus* (London: Eyre & Spottiswoode, 1968).
Malins, J. M., 'Food and death rates from diabetes', *The Lancet*, 304:7890 (1974), 1201.
Malins, J. M., and J. M. Stuart, 'Diabetic clinic in a general practice', *BMJ*, 4:5780 (1971), 161.

'The management of diabetic out-patients', *The Lancet*, 231:5974 (1938), 509.

Marks, H., *The Progress of the Experiment: Science and Therapeutic Reform in the United States, 1900–1990* (Cambridge: Cambridge University Press, 1997).

Marland, H., 'A pioneer in infant welfare: the Huddersfield scheme, 1903–1920', *Social History of Medicine*, 6:1 (1993), 25–50.

Marlow, L. A. V., J. Wardle, and J. Waller, 'Understanding cervical screening non-attendance among ethnic minority women in England', *British Journal of Cancer*, 113:5 (2015), 833–9.

Marmot, M., J. Allen, P. Goldblatt, T. Boyce, D. McNeish, M. Grady, and I. Geddes, *Fair Society, Healthy Lives: The Marmot Review* (London: The Marmot Review, 2010).

Mars, S., 'Peer pressure and imposed consensus: the making of the 1984 *Guidelines of Good Clinical Practice in the Treatment of Drug Misuse*', in V. Berridge (ed.), *Making Health Policy: Networks in Research and Policy after 1945* (Amsterdam: Rodopi, 2005), pp. 149–84.

Marsh, D., 'Privatization under Mrs Thatcher: a review of the literature'. *Public Administration*, 69 (1991), 459–80.

Marsh, D., 'Industrial relations', in D. Marsh and R.A.W. Rhodes (eds.), *Implementing Thatcherite Policies: Audit of an Era* (Buckingham: Open University Press, 1992), pp. 32–49.

Marsh, D., and R. A. W. Rhodes (eds.), *Implementing Thatcherite Policies: Audit of an Era* (Buckingham: Open University Press, 1992).

Marshall, T. H., *Citizenship and Social Class and Other Essays* (Cambridge: Cambridge University Press, 1950).

Martin, E., 'What price academic general practice?', *BMJ*, 292:6537 (1986), 1736.

Martin, E., and S. Goodwin, 'Audit of diabetic care', *JRCGP*, 38:308 (1988), 123–4.

Martin, M., 'Medical knowledge and medical practice: geriatric medicine in the 1950s', *Social History of Medicine*, 8:3 (1995), 443–61.

May, C., 'Chronic illness and intractability: professional-patient interactions in primary care', *Chronic Illness*, 1:1 (2005), 15–20.

McDonald, R., K. Checkland, S. Harrison, and A. Coleman, 'Rethinking collegiality: restratification in English general medical practice 2004–2008', *Social Science and Medicine*, 68:7 (2009), 1199–1205.

McLaurin, S., and D. F. Smith, 'Professional strategies of Medical Officers of Health in the post-war period – 2: "progressive realism": the case of R. J. Donaldson, MOH for Teeside, 1968–1974', *Journal of Public Health Medicine*, 24:2 (2002), 130–5.

McWhinney, I., 'Medical audit in North America', *BMJ*, 2:5808 (1972), 277–9.

'A medical audit', *The Lancet*, 280:7251 (1962), 339–40.

Medical Research Council Working Party, 'MRC trial of treatment of mild hypertension: principal results', *BMJ*, 291: 6488(1985), 97–104.

Mercer, A., *Infections, Chronic Disease, and the Epidemiological Transition: A New Perspective* (Rochester: University of Rochester Press, 2014).
Michael, P., and C. Webster (eds.), *Health and Society in Twentieth-Century Wales* (Cardiff: University of Wales Press, 2006).
Micks, R. H., 'The diet in diabetes', *BMJ*, 1:4297 (1943), 598–600.
Millward, G., 'Social security policy and the early disability movement – expertise, disability and the government, 1965–77', *Twentieth Century British History*, 26:2 (2015), 274–97.
Millward, G., *Vaccinating Britain: Mass Vaccination and the Public since the Second World War* (Manchester: Manchester University Press, 2019).
Ministry of Health, *First Report of the Joint Working Party on the Organisation of Medical Work in Hospitals* (London: HMSO, 1967).
'Modern views on diabetes', *BMJ*, 2:4568 (1948), 209–10.
Moffatt, F., P. Martin, and S. Timmons, 'Constructing notions of health care productivity: the call for a new professionalism?', *Sociology of Health and Illness*, 36:5 (2014), 686–702.
Mold, A., *Making the Patient-Consumer: Patient Organisations and Health Consumerism in Britain* (Manchester: Manchester University Press, 2015).
Mold, A., '"Everybody likes a drink. Nobody likes a drunk: alcohol, health education, and the public in 1970s Britain', *Social History of Medicine*, 30:3 (2017), 612–36.
Mooney, G., 'Infectious diseases and epidemiologic transition in Victorian Britain? Definitely', *Social History of Medicine*, 20:3 (2007), 595–606.
Mooney, G., 'Diagnostic spaces: workhouse, hospital, and home in mid-Victorian London', *Social Science History*, 33:3 (2009), 357–90.
Moore, M. D., 'Harnessing the power of difference: colonialism and British chronic disease research, 1940–1975', *Social History of Medicine*, 29:2 (2016), 384–404.
Moore, M. D., 'Reorganising chronic disease management: diabetes and bureaucratic technologies in post-war British general practice', in M. Jackson (ed.), *The Routledge History of Disease* (London: Routledge, 2017), pp. 453–72.
Moore, M. D., 'Food as medicine: diet and diabetes management in twentieth-century Britain', *Journal of the History of Medicine and Allied Sciences*, 73:2 (2018), 150–67.
Moore, M. D., 'Balance and the "good diabetic" in Britain, c.1900–60', in M. Jackson and M. D. Moore (eds.), *Balancing the Self: Medicine, Politics, and the Regulation of Health in the Twentieth Century* (forthcoming).
Moran, M., 'The regulatory state', *Parliamentary Affairs*, 54 (2001), 19–34.
Morell, D., 'Introduction and overview', I. Loudon, J. Horder, and C. Webster (eds.), *General Practice under the National Health Service, 1948–1997* (Oxford: Oxford University Press, 1998), pp. 1–19.

Morgan, G. F., D. A. Cadman, P. H. Edwards, T. C. O'Dowd, and R. H. Davis, 'Diabetes care: whose responsibility?', *BMJ*, 289:6454 (1984), 1309–10.
Morris, J. N., 'Uses of epidemiology', *BMJ*, 2:4936 (1955), 395–401.
Morris, J. N., 'The prevention of disease in middle age', *Public Health*, 77:4 (1963), 237–40.
Morris, J. N., *Uses of Epidemiology*, 2nd edition (London: E. & S. Livingstone, 1964).
Morris, J. N., *Uses of Epidemiology*, 3rd edition (Edinburgh: Churchill Livingstone, 1975).
Morris, J. N., J. A. Heady, P. A. B. Raffle, G. C. Roberts, and J. W. Parks, 'Coronary heart disease and physical activity of work', *The Lancet*, 262:6795 (1953), 1053–7.
'Moving towards clinical integration', *BMJ*, 2:6402 (1976), 964.
Muller, C., 'The Institute of Economic Affairs: undermining the post-war consensus', *Contemporary British History*, 10:1 (1996), 88–110.
Murcott, A., 'Food and nutrition in post-war Britain', in J. Obelkevich and P. Catterall (eds.), *Understanding Post-War British Society* (London: Routledge, 1994), pp. 155–64.
Murphy, S., 'The early days of the MRC Social Medicine Research Unit', *Social History of Medicine*, 12:3 (1999), 389–406.
Nabarro, J., 'BDA present and future', *Diabetic Medicine*, 7:6 (1990), 476.
Nathoo, A., *Hearts Exposed: Transplants and the Media in 1960s Britain* (Basingstoke: Palgrave Macmillan, 2009).
National Audit Office, *The Management of Adult Diabetes Services in the NHS* (London: The Stationery Office, 2012).
'Neglect of the chronic sick', *The Lancet*, 248:6416 (1946), 240–1.
Newburgh, L. H., and J. W. Conn, 'A new interpretation of hyperglycaemia in obese middle-aged persons', *Journal of the American Medical Association*, 112:1 (1939), 7–11.
NHS England, *Action for Diabetes* (London: NHS, 2014), available at: https://www.england.nhs.uk/2014/01/tackling-diabetes-2014/ (accessed February 2018).
'NHS reorganisation, planning, and priorities', *BMJ*, 281:6250 (1980), 1300.
Numerato, D., D. Salvatore, and G. Fattore, 'The impact of management on medical professionalism: a review', *Sociology of Health and Illness*, 34:4 (2012), 626–44.
Oakley, A., 'Appreciation: Jerry [Jeremiah Noah] Morris, 1910–2009', *International Journal of Epidemiology*, 39:1 (2010), 274–6.
Oakley, W., 'The treatment of diabetes mellitus', *The Practitioner*, 157:942 (1946), 420–5.
Oakley, W. G., D. A. Pyke, and K. W. Taylor, *Diabetes and its Management*, 2nd edition (Oxford: Blackwell Scientific Publications, 1975).

Oakley, W. G., D. A. Pyke, and K. W. Taylor, *Diabetes and its Management*, 3rd edition (Oxford: Blackwell Scientific Publications, 1978).
Obelkevich, J., 'Consumption', in J. Obelkevich and P. Catterall (eds.), *Understanding Post-War British Society* (London: Routledge, 1994), pp. 141–54.
O'Donnell, S., 'Changing social and scientific discourses on type 2 diabetes between 1800 and 1950: a socio-historical analysis', *Sociology of Health and Illness*, 37:7 (2015), 1102–21.
Office of Health Economics, *The Common Illness of Our Time: A Study of the Problem of Ischaemic Heart Disease* (London: Office of Health Economics, 1966).
O'Hara, G., *From Dreams to Disillusionment: Economic and Social Planning in the 1960s* (Basingstoke: Palgrave Macmillan, 2007).
O'Hara, G., 'The complexities of "consumerism": choice, collectivism and participation within Britain's National Health Service, c.1961–1979', *Social History of Medicine*, 26:2 (2013), 288–304.
'One hundred and eighteenth annual meeting of the British Medical Association: aftercare by health visitors', *BMJ*, 2:4673 (1950), 268–94.
Oppenheimer, G. M., 'Profiling risk: the emergence of coronary heart disease epidemiology in the United States (1947–70)', *International Journal of Epidemiology*, 35:3 (2006), 720–30.
'Organization of out-patient departments', *BMJ*, S.1:2665 (1956), 55.
Osborne, T., 'Epidemiology as an investigative paradigm: the College of General Practitioners in the 1950s', *Social Science and Medicine*, 38:2 (1994), 317–26.
Osborne, T., 'Power and persons: on ethical stylisation and person-centred medicine', *Sociology of Health and Illness*, 16:4 (1994), 515–35.
Osbourne, V. L., and D. G. Beevers, 'A comparison of hospital and general practice blood pressure readings using a shared-care record card', *JRCGP*, 31:6 (1981), 345–50.
Oswald, N. T. A., 'A social health service without social doctors', *Social History of Medicine*, 4:2 (1991), 295–315.
'Panel conference: motions', *BMJ*, 2:4372, S.85 (1944), 91.
Pavy, F. W., *Researches on the Nature and Treatment of Diabetes* (London: John Churchill & Sons, 1869).
Paynton, D. J., 'The NHS bill, the GP contract, and diabetic care', *Diabetic Medicine*, 8:3 (1991), 286.
Pereira Gray, D., 'Postgraduate training and continuing education', in I. Loudon, J. Horder, and C. Webster (eds.), *General Practice under the National Health Service, 1948–1997* (Oxford: Oxford University Press, 1998), pp. 182–204.
Perkins, H., *The Rise of Professional Society: England since 1880* (London: Routledge, 1990).

Perry, M., 'Academic general practice in Manchester under the early National Health Service: a failed social experiment', *Social History of Medicine*, 13:1 (2000), 111–29.

'Photocoagulation for diabetic retinopathy', *The Lancet*, 308:7976 (1976), 77–8.

Pickard, S., 'The role of governmentality in the establishment, maintenance, and demise of professional jurisdictions: the case of geriatric medicine', *Sociology of Health and Illness*, 32:7 (2010), 1072–86.

Pickstone, J. V., *Medicine and Industrial Society: A History of Hospital Development in Manchester and its Region, 1752–1946* (Manchester: Manchester University Press, 1985).

Pierson, P., *Dismantling the Welfare State? Thatcher, Reagan and the Politics of Retrenchment* (Cambridge: Cambridge University Press, 1994).

Pietroni, R., 'Diabetes care: whose responsibility?', *BMJ*, 289:6450 (1984), 1001.

Pike, L. A., 'A general practitioner looks at diabetes', *Public Health*, 77:3 (1963), 165–9.

Pimlott, B., 'The myth of consensus', in L. M. Smith (ed.), *The Making of Britain: Echoes of Greatness* (Basingstoke: Macmillan, 1988), pp. 129–42.

Pinch, T., and W. E. Bijker, 'The social construction of facts and artifacts: or how the sociology of science and sociology of technology might benefit each other', in W. E. Bijker, T. P. Hughes, and T. Pinch (eds.), *The Social Construction of Technological Systems: New Directions in the Sociology and History of Technology*, Anniversary Edition (Cambridge, MA: MIT Press, 2012 [1987]), pp. 11–44.

Pinder, R., R. Petchey, S. Shaw, and Y. Carter, 'What's in a care pathway? Towards a cultural cartography of the new NHS', *Sociology of Health and Illness*, 27:6 (2005), 759–79.

Pinker, R., 'New liberalism and the middle way', in R. Page and R. Silburn (eds.), *British Social Welfare in the Twentieth Century* (Basingstoke: Macmillan, 1999), pp. 80–104.

Piwernetz, K., P. D. Home, O. Snorgaard, M. Antsiferov, K. Staehr-Johansen, and M. Krans for the DiabCare Monitoring Group of the St Vincent's Declaration Steering Committee, 'Monitoring the targets of the St Vincent Declaration and the implementation of the quality management in diabetes care: the DiabCare initiative', *Diabetic Medicine*, 10:4 (1993), 371–7.

Pope, C., 'Trouble in store: some thoughts on the management of waiting lists', *Sociology of Health and Illness*, 13:2 (1991), 193–212.

Pridham, J. A., 'Future trends in general practice', *JCGP*, 5:4 (1962), 537.

Porter, D., 'From social structure to social behaviour in Britain after the Second World War', *Contemporary British History*, 16:3 (2002), 58–80.

Porter, D., *Health Citizenship: Essays in Social Medicine and Biomedical Politics* (Berkeley: University of California Press, 2011).
Porter, R., and G. S. Rousseau, *Gout: The Patrician Malady* (New Haven: Yale University Press, 2000).
Porter, T. P., *Trust in Numbers: The Pursuit of Objectivity in Science and Public Life* (Princeton: Princeton University Press, 1995).
Power, M., *The Audit Society: Rituals of Verification* (Oxford: Oxford University Press, 1999).
Redhead, I. H., and J. J. A. Reid, 'Diabetic clinics and the general practitioner', *The Lancet*, 281:7273 (1963), 159–60.
Redmond, S., 'What diabetic care to expect', *Diabetic Medicine*, 7:6 (1990), 554.
Reedy, B. L. E., 'Morale and management in general practice', *JRCGP*, 16:1 (1968), 3–11.
Reiber, G. E., and H. King, *Guidelines for the Development of a National Programme for Diabetes Mellitus* (Geneva: World Health Organization, 1991).
Reid, J. J. A., 'Some public health aspects of diabetes mellitus', *Public Health*, 77:3 (1963), 145–57.
Reid, J. J. A., 'A new public health – the problems and the challenge', *Public Health*, 79:4 (1965), 183–96.
Reiser, S. J., *Medicine and the Reign of Technology* (Cambridge: Cambridge University Press, 1978).
'Retinal changes in diabetes', *The Lancet*, 246:6361 (1945), 114.
'Retinopathy', *The Lancet*, 299:7758 (1972), 1004.
Reverby, S., 'Stealing the golden eggs: Ernest Amory Codman and the science and management of medicine', *Bulletin of the History of Medicine*, 55:2 (1981), 156–71.
Rivett, G., *From Cradle to Grave: Fifty Years of the NHS* (London: King's Fund, 1998).
Roberts, M. J. D., 'The politics of professionalization: MPs, medical men, and the 1858 Medical Act', *Medical History*, 53:1 (2009), 37–56.
Robinson, E., C. Schofield, F. Sutcliffe-Brown, and N. Thomlinson, 'Telling stories about post-war Britain: popular individualism and the "crisis" of the 1970s', *Twentieth Century British History*, 28:2 (2017), 286–304.
Robinson, P. L., and E. T. Baker-Bates, 'A new diabetic chart', *BMJ*, 2:4790 (1952), 919–21.
Rollings, N., 'Poor Mr Butskell: a short life, wrecked by schizophrenia?', *Twentieth Century British History*, 5:2 (1994), 183–205.
Rollings, N., 'Cracks in the post-war Keynesian settlement? The role of organised business in Britain in the rise of neoliberalism before Margaret Thatcher', *Twentieth Century British History*, 24:4 (2013), 637–59.
Rosa, E. A., O. Renn, and A. M. McCright, *The Risk Society Revisited: Social Theory and Governance* (Philadelphia: Temple University Press, 2013).

Rose, N. 'Government, authority and expertise in advanced liberalism', *Economy and Society*, 22:3 (1993), 283–99.
Rosenfeld, S., *Common Sense: A Political History* (Cambridge, MA: Harvard University Press, 2011).
Rosner, L. (ed.), *The Technological Fix: Visions, Trials, and Solutions* (London: Routledge, 2004).
Rothstein, W., *Public Health and the Risk Factor: A History of An Uneven Medical Revolution* (New York: University of Rochester Press, 2003).
Royal College of General Practitioners, *The Future General Practitioner* (London: Royal College of General Practitioners, 1972).
Royal College of General Practitioners, *Prevention of Arterial Disease in General Practice: A Report of a Sub-Committee of the Royal College of General Practitioners' Working Party on Prevention*, Report from General Practice, 19 (London: Royal College of General Practitioners, 1981).
Royal College of General Practitioners, *What Sort of Doctor? Assessing Quality of Care in General Practice* (London: Royal College of General Practitioners, 1985).
Royal College of General Practitioners, *Diabetes Clinical Information Folder* (London: Royal College of General Practitioners, 1988).
Royal College of Physicians of London and British Diabetic Association, *The Provision of Medical Care for Adult Diabetic Patients in the United Kingdom* (London: British Diabetic Association, 1984).
Saha, A., 'Clinical guidelines', *BMJ*, 310:6980 (1995), 670.
Saks, M., 'Medicine and the counter culture', in R. Cooter and J. Pickstone (eds.), *Companion to Medicine in the Twentieth Century* (Abingdon: Routledge, 2003), pp. 113–24.
Sanders, L. J., 'From Thebes to Toronto and the 21st century: an incredible journey', *Diabetes Spectrum*, 15:1 (2002), 56–60.
Saunders, R., '"Crisis? What crisis?" Thatcherism and the seventies', in B. Jackson and R. Saunders (eds.), *Making Thatcher's Britain* (Cambridge: Cambridge University Press, 2012), pp. 25–42.
Schrecker, T., and C. Bambra, *How Politics Makes us Sick: Neoliberal Epidemics* (Basingstoke: Palgrave Macmillan, 2015).
Scotland', *The Lancet*, 140:3599 (1924), 460–1.
Scott, J. C., *Seeing Like a State: How Certain Schemes to Improve the Human Condition Have Failed* (New Haven: Yale University Press, 1998).
Scott, T., and A. Maynard, 'Will the new GP contract lead to cost effective medical practice?', Discussion Paper 82 (University of York, 1991).
Scottish Home and Health Department, Scottish Health Service Planning Council, *Report of the Working Group on the Management of Diabetes* (Edinburgh: HMSO, 1987).
Seaton, A., 'Against the "sacred cow": NHS opposition and the Fellowship for Freedom in Medicine, 1948–72', *Twentieth Century British History*, 26:3 (2015), 424–49.

Secretaries of State for Social Services, Wales, Northern Ireland, and Scotland, *Primary Health Care: An Agenda for Discussion*, Cmnd 9778 (London: HMSO, 1986).

Secretaries of State for Social Services, Wales, Northern Ireland, and Scotland, *Promoting Better Health: The Government's Programme for Improving Primary Health Care*, Cm 249 (London: HMSO, 1987).

Secretaries of State for Social Services, Wales, Northern Ireland, and Scotland, *Working for Patients*, Cm 555 (London: HMSO, 1989).

Selby, P., 'W(h)ither diabetes care?', *Diabetic Medicine*, 10:9 (1993), 791–2.

Senior Registrar, 'Consultant and specialist', *The Lancet*, 270:6990 (1957), 338–40.

Seymour, J., 'Not rights but reciprocal responsibility: the rhetoric of state health provision in early-twentieth century Britain', in A. Mold and D. Reubi (eds.), *Assembling Health Rights in Global Context: Genealogies and Anthropologies* (Oxford: Routledge, 2013), pp. 23–41.

Shapin, S., and S. Schaffer, *Leviathan and the Air Pump: Hobbes, Boyle and the Experimental Life* (Princeton: Princeton University Press, 1985).

Sharma, A., and A. Gupta (eds.), *The Anthropology of the State: A Reader* (Oxford: Blackwell, 2006).

Sheard, S., 'Quacks and clerks: historical and contemporary perspectives on the structure and function of the British medical civil service', *Social Policy & Administration*, 44:2 (2010), 193–207.

Sheard, S., *The Passionate Economist: How Brian Abel-Smith Shaped Global Health Policy and Social Welfare* (Bristol: Policy Press, 2013).

Sheard, S., 'Space, place and (waiting) time: reflections on health policy and politics', *Health Economics, Policy, and Law*, 13:3–4 (2018), 226–50.

Sheard, S., and L. Donaldson, *The Nation's Doctor: The Role of the Chief Medical Officer 1855–1998* (Abingdon: Radcliffe, 2005).

Sinding, C., 'Making the unit of insulin: standards, clinical work, and industry', *Bulletin of the History of Medicine*, 76:2 (2002), 231–70.

Sinding, C., 'Flexible norms? From patients' values to physicians' standards', in W. Ernst (ed.), *Histories of the Normal and the Abnormal: Social and Cultural Histories of Norms and Normativity* (London: Routledge, 2006), pp. 225–44.

Singh, B., M. Holland, and P. Thorn, 'Metabolic control of diabetes in general practice clinics: comparison with a hospital clinic', *BMJ*, 289:6447 (1984), 726–8.

Sleight, P., J. A. Spencer, and E. W. Towler, 'Oxford and McKinsey: Cogwheel and beyond', *BMJ*, 1:5697 (1970), 682–4.

Smith, G., and M. Nicolson, 'Re-expressing the division in British medicine under the NHS: the importance of locality in general practitioners' oral histories', *Social Science and Medicine*, 64:4 (2007), 938–48.

Snow, S., '"I've never found doctors to be a difficult bunch": doctors, managers and NHS reorganisations in Manchester and Salford, 1948–2007', *Medical History*, 57:1 (2013), 65–86.

Snowden, A. J., T. A. Sheldon, and G. Alberti, 'Shared care in diabetes', *BMJ*, 310:6973 (1995), 142–3.

Stacey, M., *Regulating British Medicine: The General Medical Council* (Chichester: John Wiley & Sons, 1992).

Standing Medical Advisory Committee of the Central Health Services Council, *The Standardization of Hospital Medical Records: Report of the Sub-Committee* (London: HMSO, 1965).

Stanton, J., 'The cost of living: kidney dialysis, rationing and health economics in Britain, 1965–1996', *Social Science & Medicine*, 49:9 (1999), 1169–82.

Starr, P., *The Social Transformation of American Medicine* (New York: Basic Books, 1982).

Stedman Jones, D., *Masters of the Universe: Hayek, Friedman, and the Birth of Neoliberal Politics* (Princeton: Princeton University Press, 2014).

Stevens, R., *In Sickness and in Wealth: American Hospitals in the Twentieth Century* (New York: Basic Books, 1989).

Stewart, J., 'Ideology and process in the creation of the British National Health Service', *Journal of Policy History*, 14:2 (2002), 113–34.

Stewart, J., 'The National Health Service in Scotland, 1947–74: Scottish or British', *Historical Research*, 76:193 (2003), 389–410.

Stewart, J. S., 'Cogwheel: a physician's view of a local version', *BMJ*, 4:5680 (1969), 420–3.

Stewart-Hess, C. H., 'The management of maturity onset diabetes in general practice', *JRCGP*, 23:137 (1973), 841–60.

Sturdy, S., 'The political economy of scientific medicine: science, education and the transformation of medical practice in Sheffield, 1890–1922', *Medical History*, 36:2 (1992), 125–59.

Sturdy S., and R. Cooter, 'Science, scientific management and the transformation of medicine in Britain, c.1870–1950', *History of Science*, 36:4 (1998), 421–66.

'Symposium on glaucoma', *BMJ*, 2:5404 (1964), 303.

'Symposium on the practical applications in general practice, public health and industry', *BMJ*, 2:5404 (1964), 306.

Szabo, J., *Incurable and Intolerable: Chronic Disease and Slow Death in Nineteenth-Century France* (New Brunswick: Rutgers University Press, 2009).

Tattersall, R. B., *Diabetes: The Biography* (Oxford: Oxford University Press, 2009).

Taylor, S., *Good General Practice: A Report on a Survey* (London: Oxford University Press, 1954).

'The teaching hospitals', *The Lancet*, 270:6989 (1957), 277–8.

Thane, P., 'Old age', in R. Cooter and J. Pickstone (eds.), *Companion to Medicine in the Twentieth Century* (Abingdon: Routledge, 2003), pp. 617–32.
Theriot, N. M., 'Negotiating illness: doctors, patients and families in the nineteenth century', *Journal of the History of Behavioural Sciences*, 37:4 (2001), 349–68.
Thorn, P. A., and R. G. Russell, 'Diabetic clinics today and tomorrow: mini-clinics in general practice', *BMJ*, 2:5865 (1973), 534–6.
'Thursday morning: opening remarks', *Public Health*, 81:5 (1966), 207.
Timmermann, C., 'A matter of degree: the normalization of hypertension, c.1940–2000', in W. Ernst (ed.), *Histories of the Normal and the Abnormal: Social and Cultural Histories of Norms and Normativity* (London: Routledge, 2006), pp. 245–61.
Timmermann, C., 'Hexamethonium, hypertension and pharmaceutical innovation: the transformation of an experimental drug in post-war Britain', in C. Timmermann and J. Anderson (eds.), *Devices and Designs: Technology and Medicine in Historical Perspective* (Basingstoke: Palgrave Macmillan, 2006), pp. 156–74.
Timmermann, C., 'Chronic illness and disease history', in M. Jackson (ed.), *The Oxford Handbook of the History of Medicine* (Oxford: Oxford University Press, 2011), pp. 393–410.
Timmermann, C., 'Appropriating risk factors: the reception of an American approach to chronic disease in the two German states, c.1950–1990', *Social History of Medicine*, 25:1 (2012), 157–74.
Timmermann, C., and E. Toon (eds.), *Cancer Patients, Cancer Pathways: Historical and Sociological Perspectives* (Basingstoke: Palgrave Macmillan, 2012).
Timmermanns, S., and M. Berg, *The Gold Standard: The Challenge of Evidence-Based Medicine and Standardization in Health Care* (Philadelphia: Temple University Press, 2003).
Timmins, N., *The Five Giants: A Biography of the Welfare State* (London: Fontana Press, 1996).
Tinker, A., 'Old age and gerontology', in J. Obelkevich and P. Catterall (eds.), *Understanding Post-War British Society* (London: Routledge, 1994), pp. 73–84.
Tomlinson, J., 'Why was there never a "Keynesian revolution" in economic policy?', *Economy and Society*, 10:1 (1981), 72–87.
Tomlinson, J., 'Planning: debate and policy in the 1940s', *Twentieth Century British History*, 3:2 (1992), 154–74.
Tomlinson, J., '"Liberty with order": Conservative economic policy, 1951–1964', in M. Francis and I. Zweiniger-Bargielowska (eds.), *The Conservatives and British Society* (Cardiff: University of Wales Press, 1996), pp. 274–88.
Tomlinson, J., *The Politics of Decline: Understanding Post-War Britain* (Harlow: Pearson Education, 2001).
'Towards medical audit', *BMJ*, 1:5903 (1974), 255–7.

Toye, R., 'Gosplanners versus thermostatters: Whitehall planning debates and their political consequences, 1945–49', *Contemporary British History*, 14:4 (2000), 81–106.

Tunbridge, R. E., 'Sociomedical aspects of diabetes mellitus', *The Lancet*, 262:6792 (1953), 893–9.

UK Prospective Diabetes Study Group, 'Intensive blood glucose control with sulphonylureas or insulin compared with conventional treatment and risk of complications in patients with type 2 diabetes (UKPDS 33)', *The Lancet*, 352:9131 (1998), 837–53.

'Undergraduate education conference, 7th May, 1961', *JCGP*, 5:2 (1962), 290–5.

Upton, C. E., 'Diabetic community care', *The Practitioner*, 215:1284 (1975), 83–6.

Uusitupa, M., 'Remission of type 2 diabetes: mission not impossible', *The Lancet*, 391:10120 (2018), 515–16.

Valier, H. K., 'The politics of scientific medicine in Manchester, c.1900–1960' (PhD dissertation, University of Manchester, 2002).

Valier, H., and R. Bivins, 'Organization, ethnicity and the British National Health Service', in J. Stanton (ed.), *Innovations in Health and Medicine: Diffusion and Resistance in the Twentieth Century* (London: Routledge, 2002), pp. 37–64.

Valier, H., and C. Timmermann, 'Clinical trials and the reorganization of medical research in post-Second World War Britain', *Medical History*, 52:4 (2008), 493–510.

Van Daelen, M., C. Van der Elst, and A. van de Ven, 'Risk management interconnections in law, accounting and tax', in M. van Daelen and C. Van der Elst (eds.), *Risk Management and Corporate Government: Interconnections in Law, Accounting and Tax* (Cheltenham: Edward Elgar, 2010), pp. 191–231.

Venugopal, R., 'Neoliberalism as concept', *Economy and Society*, 44:2 (2015), 165–87.

Waddington, I., *The Medical Profession in the Industrial Revolution* (Dublin: Gill and Macmillan, 1984).

Waddington, K., *Charity and the London Hospitals, 1850–1898* (Woodbridge: Boydell Press, 2000).

Waddington, K., *Medical Education at St Bartholomew's Hospital, 1123–1995* (Woodbridge: Boydell Press, 2003).

Wailoo, K., *Dying in the City of the Blues: Sickle Cell Anemia and the Politics of Race and Health* (Chapel Hill: University of North Carolina Press, 2001).

Waine, C., *Why Not Care for your Diabetic Patients?*, 2nd edition (London: Royal College of General Practitioners, 1988).

Waine, C., 'Diabetes and the NHS Bill', *Diabetic Medicine*, 8:3 (1991), 285.

Waine, C., *Diabetes in General Practice*, 3rd edition (London: Royal College of General Practitioners, 1992).

Walker, G. F., 'Reflections on diabetes mellitus: answers to a questionary', *The Lancet*, 262:6800 (1953), 1329–32.

Walker, J. B., 'Field work of a diabetic clinic', *The Lancet*, 262:6783 (1953), 445–7.

Walker, J. B., 'Diabetes in the community', *Public Health*, 77:3 (1963), 158–64.

Walker, J., 'Sociological implications of diabetes', *BMJ*, 2:4934 (1955), 317–19.

Walker, J., *Chronicle of a Diabetic Service* (London: British Diabetic Association, 1989).

Wall, R., 'Using bacteriology in elite hospital practice: London and Cambridge, 1880–1920', *Social History of Medicine*, 24:3 (2011), 776–95.

Wallace, S., and R. Gullan, 'Mild head injury: guidelines should be flexible', *BMJ*, 307:6901 (1993), 447–8.

Warden, J., 'Peace in our time', *BMJ*, 300:6736 (1990), 1359.

Warner, J. H., *The Therapeutic Perspective: Medical Practice, Knowledge and Identity in America, 1820–1885* (Cambridge, MA: Harvard University Press, 1986).

Warner, J. H., 'The history of science and the sciences of medicine', *Osiris*, 10 (1995), 164–93.

Warren, M. D., and A. Corfield, 'Mortality from diabetes', *The Lancet*, 301:7818 (1973), 1511–12.

Warren, M. W., 'Care of chronic sick: a case for treating chronic sick in blocks in a general hospital', *BMJ*, 2:4329 (1943), 822–3.

Weber, M., *The Theory of Social and Economic Organisation*, trans. A. M. Henderson and T. Parsons, ed. T. Parsons (New York: Free Press, 1966 [1947]).

Weber, M., *Economy and Society: An Outline of Interpretive Sociology*, vols. 1 and 2, ed. G. Roth and C. Wittich, trans. E. Fischoff et al. (Berkeley: California University Press, 1978).

Weber, M., *The Protestant Ethic and the Spirit of Capitalism*, trans. T. Parsons (London: Routledge: 2001).

Webster, C., *The Health Services Since the War, vol. 1: Problems of Health Care: The National Health Service before 1957* (London: HMSO, 1988).

Webster, C., 'Conflict and consensus: explaining the British health service', *Twentieth Century British History*, 1:2 (1990), 115–51.

Webster, C., *The Health Services Since the War, vol. 2: Government and Health Care: The British National Health Service, 1958–1979* (London: HMSO, 1996).

Webster, C., 'The politics of general practice', in I. Loudon, J. Horder, and C. Webster (eds.), *General Practice under the National Health Service, 1948–1997* (Oxford: Oxford University Press, 1998), pp. 20–44.

Webster, C., *The National Health Service: A Political History* (Oxford: Oxford University Press, 1998).

Weindling, P., 'From infectious to chronic diseases: changing patterns of sickness in the nineteenth and twentieth centuries', in A. Wear (ed.), *Medicine*

in *Society: Historical Essays* (Cambridge: Cambridge University Press, 1992), pp. 303–16.
Weisz, G., 'From clinical counting to Evidence-Based Medicine', in G. Forland, A. Opinel, and G. Weisz (eds.), *Body Counts: Medical Quantification in Historical and Sociological Perspectives* (Montreal: McGill University Press, 2005), pp. 377–93.
Weisz, G., *Divide and Conquer: A Comparative History of Medical Specialization* (Oxford: Oxford University Press, 2006).
Weisz, G., *Chronic Disease in the Twentieth Century: A History* (Baltimore: Johns Hopkins University Press, 2014).
Weisz, G., A. Cambrosio, P. Keating, L. Knaapen, T. Schlich, and V. J. Tournay, 'The emergence of clinical practice guidelines', *Milbank Quarterly*, 85:4 (2007), 691–727.
Weisz, G., and J. Olsyznko-Gryn, 'The theory of epidemiologic transition: the origins of a citation classic', *Journal of the History of Medicine and the Allied Sciences*, 65:3 (2010), 287–326.
Wells, H. G., 'Diabetics in sympathy', *The Times*, 15 Februrary 1934, p. 10.
Welshman, J., 'Growing old in the city: public health and the elderly in Leicester, 1948–74', *Medical History*, 40:1 (1996), 74–89.
Welshman, J., 'The Medical Officer of Health in England and Wales, 1900–1974: watchdog or lapdog?', *Journal of Public Health Medicine*, 19:4 (1997), 443–50.
Welshman, J., 'Inequalities, regions and hospitals: the Resource Allocation Working Party', in M. Gorsky and S. Sheard (eds.), *Financing Medicine: The British Experience since 1750* (Oxford: Routledge, 2006), pp. 221–41.
Welshman, J., and J. Walmers (eds.), *Community Care in Perspective: Care, Control and Citizenship* (Basingstoke: Palgrave Macmillan, 2007).
West, K.M., 'Hyperglycaemia as a cause of long-term complications', in H. Keen and J. Jarrett (eds.), *Diabetic Complications*, 2nd edition (London: Edward Arnold, 1982), pp. 13–18.
West, S., 'Notes on diabetic retinits', *The Lancet*, 183:4728 (1914), 1034–5.
'When wild ideas make sense', *BMJ*, 2:6204 (1979), 1532.
Whitty, G., 'The New Right and the national curriculum: state control or market forces', in M. Flude and M. Hammer (eds.), *The Education Reform Act, 1988: Its Origins and Implications* (London: Falmer Press, 1990), pp. 21–36.
Wilkes, E., and E. E. Lawton, 'The diabetic, the hospital and primary care', *JRCGP*, 30:213 (1980), 199–206.
Wilks, J. M., 'Diabetes – a disease for general practice', *JRCGP*, 23:126 (1973), 46–54.
Willems, D., 'Managing one's body using self-management techniques: practicing autonomy', *Theoretical Medicine and Bioethics*, 21:1 (2000), 23–38.

Bibliography

Williams, C. J. H., and T. A. Rathwell, 'Could the consultative document have its priorities wrong?', *BMJ*, 2:6041 (1976), 956–7.
Williams, D. R. R., P. D. Home, and Members of a Working Group of the Research Unit of the Royal College of Physicians and British Diabetic Association, 'A proposal for continuing audit of diabetes services', *Diabetic Medicine*, 9:8 (1992), 759–64.
Williams, D. R. R., C. Munroe, C. J. Hospesdales, and R. H. Greenwood, 'A three-year evaluation of the quality of diabetes care in the Norwich community care scheme', *Diabetic Medicine*, 7:1 (1990), 74–9.
Williamson, C., 'The quiet time? Pay-beds and private practice in the National Health Service: 1948–1970', *Social History of Medicine*, 28:3 (2015), 576–95.
Winner, L., 'Do artifacts have politics?', *Daedalus*, 109:1 (1980), 121–36.
Witts, L. J., 'Special clinics and planning', *BMJ*, 2:4259 (1942), 226.
Wojciechowski, M. T., 'Systematic care of diabetic patients in a general practice', *JRCGP*, 32:242 (1982), 531–3.
Worboys, M., 'The discovery of colonial malnutrition between the wars', in D. Arnold (ed.), *Imperial Medicine and Indigenous Societies* (Manchester: Manchester University Press, 1988), pp. 208–25.
Worboys, M., and F. Condrau, 'Epidemics and infections in nineteenth century Britain', *Social History of Medicine*, 20:1 (2007), 147–58.
Worboys, M., and F. Condrau, 'Final response: epidemics and infections in nineteenth-century Britain', *Social History of Medicine*, 22:1 (2009), 165–71.
Working Party of the College of General Practitioners, 'Diabetes survey', *BMJ*, 1:5291 (1962), 1497–503.
World Health Organization, *Diabetes Mellitus: Report of a WHO Expert Committee*, Technical Report Series, 310 (Geneva: World Health Organization, 1965).
World Health Organization, *WHO Expert Committee on Diabetes Mellitus: Second Report*, Technical Report Series, 646 (Geneva: World Health Organization, 1980).
World Health Organization, *Diabetes Mellitus: Report of a WHO Study Group*, Technical Report Series, 727 (Geneva: World Health Organization, 1985).
Wright, D., S. Mullally, and M. C. Cordukes, '"Worse than being married": the exodus of British doctors from the National Health Service to Canada, c.1955–75', *Journal of the History of Medicine and Allied Sciences*, 65:4 (2010), 546–75.
'The young chronic sick', *BMJ*, 1:5637 (1969), 134–5.
Yudkin, J. S., B. J. Boucher, K. E. Schopflin, B. T. Harris, H. R. Claff, N. J. D. Whyte, B. Taylor, D. H. Mellins, A. B. Wootliff, J. G. Safir, and E. J. Jones, 'The quality of diabetic care in a London health district', *Journal of Epidemiology and Community Health*, 34:4 (1980), 277–80.
Yudkin, J. S., B. Richter, and E. A. M. Gale, 'Intensified glucose lowering in type 2 diabetes: time for a reappraisal', *Diabetologia*, 53:10 (2010), 2079–85.

Index

accountability 5, 9, 54, 181–3, 184–7, 201–3, 218–19, 220–4, 231–2, 246–7, 251–3, 255–6
Alberti, George, Professor of Medicine, former President of the Royal College of Physicians 209 n.61, 233
antenatal care 129, 244
appointment systems 10, 117–18
  see also recall systems
asthma 22, 77 n.139, 99, 243–4
audit 2, 4, 5, 6, 7, 11, 18, 22, 24, 133–6, 137, 138–9, 182, 187, 192–3, 198–200, 201, 202–3, 207 n.39, 212 n.122, 219, 222–3, 224, 225–6, 227, 229, 231, 232, 247, 248–9, 250, 252, 254, 255–6, 261 n.43, 265 n. 87
autonomy
  clinical 5, 54, 186–8, 193–4, 195, 203, 207 n.43
  personal 182
  professional 5, 11–13, 54, 217, 251
  see also freedom

balance
  economic 8
  lifestyle 46
  physiological 19, 49, 63
  therapeutic 16–17, 48
borderline diabetes 61, 88, 95–6

British Diabetic Association (BDA) 10, 11, 15, 21–2, 24, 27, 50, 53–5, 60, 64, 91, 124–5, 133, 154, 155–7, 158, 159, 161, 167, 169, 176 n.97, 193, 196–8, 203, 211 n.96, 225–6, 229–30, 231, 247, 250

care team 3, 10, 22, 63–7, 91–2, 116–17, 121–2, 128, 131, 135–6, 188, 190–2
  see also dietician; district nurse; general practitioners; health visitors; nurses
Chief Medical Officer 107–8 n.59, 201, 216, 233
chronic disease management 98–9, 224–6, 232–3, 241–7, 247–8, 250
chronic sick 55–8
civil service 3, 7–8, 9, 11, 52, 54, 56, 58, 88, 156–9, 161, 162–3, 164–7, 168, 186, 215–16, 220, 226, 229, 233
clinical governance 151, 181, 203
clinical skill 3, 4, 7, 16, 83
Clinical Standards Advisory Group 226–8, 229–31
clinical trials 14, 51, 122, 134, 137, 153, 183, 187
classification of disease and 95, 96, 97–8

Index

treatment of diabetes and 17, 41 n.115, 59, 61, 95, 153–4, 156, 172 n.45
Cochrane, Archie, doctor and epidemiologist 183–4, 207 n.39
Cogwheel 89, 107–8 n.59, 184, 216
Cold War 59–60, 218
College of General Practitioners 74 n.91, 93, 250
  see also Royal College of General Practitioners
community diabetes care 65–7, 243, 250
  see also hospitals; shared care
community surveys 51, 58–9, 61, 73 n.82, 74 n.91, 88, 95–6, 246
complaints 182–3
computers 103–4, 119–20, 129, 131, 143 n.39
Conservative Party 7–8, 89, 160–1, 162, 164, 166, 217, 219, 232, 246
  the NHS and 1, 9, 185, 215, 217, 219–23
consultants 52, 56, 89, 119, 123, 138, 139, 158, 183, 186, 201, 216, 230
  relationships with GPs 12–13, 80, 82–3, 91–2, 103, 115, 129, 139, 249–50
continuity of care 66, 92, 94, 128

data
  diabetes management and 10, 64, 96, 125, 129, 133, 189, 198, 199–200, 224, 228–9
  health service management and 8–9, 89, 123, 133, 184, 215–17, 236 n.37, 252, 255
Department of Health 1–2, 199, 215–16, 221, 223, 224, 225, 226, 229, 231

Department of Health and Social Security 124, 150, 155–6, 156–9, 161, 162, 163, 164–7, 168, 182, 191–2
diabetes
  complications 2, 17, 18, 39 n.95, 80, 90–1, 98, 244–5
  costs of 11, 150, 163–4, 165–6
  relationship with control of blood glucose and metabolism 18, 49, 61, 63, 86, 88, 95–6, 97, 151
  retinopathy 95–6, 96–7, 151–6, 157–9, 162–7, 191, 198
  definition 15–17, 19
  diagnostic criteria 15–17, 60–1, 88, 95–6, 97, 189–90, 194
  patient self-care 2–3, 17, 21–2, 49, 53, 65–6, 116–17, 129, 197, 211 n.96
  prevalence 1, 10, 28 n.4, 59–61, 255
  treatment see balance; diet; insulin; oral hypoglycaemic agents
  types 14–15, 18–19, 39 n.95
diabetic outpatient clinics 3, 13–14, 21–2, 49, 50–1, 53–4, 65, 67–8, 79, 82, 83, 84–5, 90, 91, 92, 94, 97, 99, 102–3, 117–18, 119, 121, 124–5, 151, 155, 188, 190–1, 224, 243–4
  referral 50, 82, 83–4, 91, 92, 104, 131–2, 138, 191, 194
diet
  cause of diabetes and 1, 28–9 n.4
  challenges of 60, 64–5
  classification of patients and 18, 90, 92
  treatment programmes 16–17, 20, 39 n.95, 48–9, 152, 193
dietician 21, 63, 64, 65, 121, 128, 138, 190, 203
district nurse 47, 66, 92, 121, 190

economy 5, 8, 46, 57, 59, 88, 89, 99, 166, 167
elderly patients 55, 57, 64, 66, 67, 159, 173 n.58, 242
empire 51, 59
  medical knowledge and 17, 58, 189
  research networks and 44 n.157, 59, 208 n.55, 209 n.61
  techniques of government and 13, 265 n. 89
epidemiological research *see* epidemiology
epidemiologists 14, 15, 19, 55, 57, 58, 60, 61–2, 140, 155, 183, 207 n.39
epidemiology 19, 51, 58, 60–1, 95–7, 122–3, 165, 184
  see also community surveys
Evidence-Based Medicine 201–2, 232, 252

freedom
  clinical 184, 220
  economic 160, 217–18
  personal 211 n.96, 217–18
  professional 115, 132, 185, 201
Fry, John, general practitioner 185, 207 n.39

General Medical Council 11–12, 182, 205 n.10
general practice
  financing 82, 112 n.139, 185, 220–2
  ideologies of 93–4, 97–100, 128, 250
  professional esteem 82–3, 109 n.86
  research and 58, 74 n.91
general practitioners
  construction of managed medicine 2, 6, 118–19, 120, 123, 125–8, 129–31, 132–3, 135, 137–40, 185, 187, 194–6, 202, 227, 244, 247, 249–50
  diabetes care and 50, 82, 83–4, 85–8, 91–4, 97–9, 102–3, 106 n.34
  see also care team; diabetic outpatient clinics; shared care
  National Health Service and 1–2, 52–3, 81–2, 87, 128, 185, 186–7, 215–16, 220–1, 221–2, 224–5, 229, 232–3, 252
  relationship to hospital 12, 81–2, 93–4, 100, 105 n.12, 186, 222, 249
Griffiths management review 220
guidelines 204 n.1, 208 n.53
  criticisms of 7, 201–2, 207 n.39, 249
  emergence of 5, 7, 11, 22, 23–4, 89, 187, 188–93, 208 n.50, 225–6, 229, 232, 247, 248, 252
  health service reforms and 2, 223, 227, 229
  managing care and 4, 5, 184, 193–8, 227, 230–1, 232–3, 249
  see also protocols

Hart, Julian Tudor, general practitioner 98, 223–4
health economics 8, 11, 59–60, 90, 108 n.69, 164–6, 167, 183–5, 192, 201, 248
health economists *see* health economics
health service research 54, 135, 136, 163–4, 183, 249
health visitors 47, 65–6, 77 n.139, 92, 118, 121, 128, 190

Hospital Activity Analysis 184, 216, 224
hospitals
   clinical management in 3, 13–14, 133–4, 185, 186
   see also Cogwheel; Hospital Activity Analysis
   integrated diabetes care and 22, 65–6, 85–6, 91–3, 94, 97–8, 102, 121, 128–33, 139–40, 169, 192, 247
   National Health Service and 52, 53–4, 70 n.35, 87, 100–1, 207 n.46, 221–2
   service integration and 6, 12, 15, 18, 23, 51, 52–3, 65, 66, 100–1, 102, 123, 200, 243, 244, 254
hyperglycaemia *see* diabetes
hypertension 15, 20, 58–9, 61, 87, 98, 99, 111 n.122, 123, 131, 243, 244
   diabetes management and 95, 97, 98, 132
hypoglycaemia 17, 49, 66, 80, 88, 153, 195

impaired glucose tolerance 95
insulin 17, 22, 41 n.115, 48, 49, 50, 84, 116, 151, 243, 244
International Diabetes Federation 155, 200, 226

Joint Working Party on the Organisation of Medical Work *see* Cogwheel

Keen, Harry, diabetes specialist and epidemiologist 84, 85, 209 n.61, 228, 231, 233
ketonuria 16, 17, 18, 22, 48, 49, 125, 191, 197
Keynesianism 7, 160
King's Fund 90, 216

laboratories 3
   GP access 92, 106 n.34
   patient surveillance and 17, 18, 48, 50, 84, 119, 195
Labour Party 8, 52, 62, 76 n.120, 89–90, 99, 159, 162, 166, 169, 215, 217, 219, 232
Lawrence, Robin, diabetes specialist 19, 21, 53–4, 77 n.139
Local government 161
   hospitals 13, 50, 55–6
   public health departments 47, 53, 63, 65
   social services 56
   see also Medical Officer of Heath

Major, John, Prime Minister
   governments of 215, 224, 229–30
Malins, John, diabetes specialist 91, 93, 94, 159, 190
media 134, 182, 223
medical individualism 3, 5, 7, 12–13, 14, 37 n.72, 93–4, 96, 122, 123, 133–4, 153, 183–4, 185, 186–7, 194, 195, 200–1, 202–3, 251–2, 253
Medical Officer of Health 46–7, 53, 58, 61, 62, 66–7, 85, 87, 100–2
   see also local government
medical records 66, 139
   emergence of 17–18, 121–3
   managing care 3, 10, 63–4, 104, 124–31, 133–4, 137, 139, 250
   shared care records 129–31, 244
Medical Research Council 41 n.115, 122, 150, 156, 190
middle age 55, 58
Ministry of Health 41 n.115, 52, 53–4, 57, 79, 88, 89, 122, 124, 186, 188–9, 192, 215–16
   see also Department of Health; Department of Health and Social Security

Morris, Jerry, clinician and epidemiologist 60, 185, 206 n.32, 207 n.39

National Health Service
  costs 54, 88–90, 184–5, 215–17
  creation 50–3
  reforms 1–2, 24, 44 n.159, 99–102, 182–3, 219–24, 227
National Insurance 13, 50, 52, 122, 123
neoliberalism 2, 9, 29 n.6, 89, 160–1, 217–19
  health services and 6, 9, 169–70, 197, 211 n.96, 219–24, 224–5, 227–8, 231
New Right 5, 32 n.24, 169–70
Nuffield Provincial Hospitals Trust 90, 216
nurses 15, 18, 23, 64, 117
  care team and 50, 63, 65, 121, 128, 188, 190
  deputation 119, 126, 138, 191
  general practice and 87, 92
  specialists 103, 119, 138

ophthalmologists 121, 153, 155, 156–7, 158, 159, 165, 167, 191
Oral Hypoglycaemic Agent 92, 156, 172 n.45

Parliament 150, 156, 161, 169, 182, 184, 215, 223, 227
  legislation 6–7, 224
  select committees 162, 217, 219
patient consumerism 8, 90, 182–3, 197, 227, 248
Patients' Association 90, 108 n.69, 182

photocoagulation 97, 153–5, 156–7, 163
planning 9, 51, 88, 161, 223
  economic 8, 76 n.120, 160, 217–18
  health service 52, 53–4, 58, 88–9, 89–90, 100–1, 157, 159, 191–2, 216–17, 254
post-war consensus 7–8, 160–1, 219, 222
preventive healthcare 1, 19–20, 46–7, 53, 57, 62–3, 86–7, 98–9, 100–1, 244–5
  diabetes management and 1–2, 20–1, 27, 46, 60–1, 63, 86, 88, 94–8, 153–5, 158–9, 164, 165–6, 168–9, 224–5, 226, 241
  screening 47, 63, 86, 87–8, 97, 126, 154–5, 156–9, 161–2, 162–4, 165–6, 167, 189
  see also risk
productivity 59–60, 220, 251
professionalism 5, 13, 134, 193, 194, 200–3, 251–3
  identity 11, 12, 93, 201
  inter-professional conflict 12, 102–3, 183, 249–50
  professional regulation 4, 11–12, 14, 135, 183, 197, 198, 200–1, 202, 203, 217, 245–6, 248, 251
protocols 10, 136, 153, 198, 204 n.1
  emergence of 14, 91, 122–3, 131–2, 247, 250
  health service reforms and 2, 225–6
  managing care 104, 121, 132–3, 134, 138–9, 184, 187, 194, 195–6, 197, 199, 202–3, 244, 250, 253
  see also guidelines

Index

public health *see* chronic disease management; local government; Medical Officers of Health; preventive health care; risk

quality of care 2–4, 6, 115–16, 133–4, 186–7, 202–3, 220, 221–2, 224–5, 230–1, 261 n.43
  criticisms of 116, 134, 181–5, 187–8, 247
  quality assurance 137, 228–9, 230, 234, 241, 248
  see also standards of care

recall systems 3, 10, 104, 118–21, 125, 126, 134, 137, 231
Reid, J. R. R., Medical Officer of Health 46–7, 61, 63
risk 1, 4, 11, 97–9, 217, 244, 245, 255
  diabetes management and 20–1, 27, 61, 62–3, 85–6, 95–8, 132, 150, 154
  medical concepts of 19–20, 62, 86–8, 95
  routinisation 104, 138, 246
Royal Colleges 2, 6, 131, 133, 169, 192, 200, 201, 203, 225, 226, 232, 247, 250, 252
Royal College of General Practitioners 97–8, 99, 123, 128, 131, 132–3, 194–6, 202, 244, 250
Royal College of Physicians
  Edinburgh 43 n.145, 123
  London 22, 43 n.145, 83, 196, 199, 210 n.78, 225, 227
    Standing Committee on Endocrinology and Diabetes Mellitus 190–2, 198

scientific medicine 7, 13, 122, 242, 247
  laboratory practices 16–17, 252
  statistics 14, 96, 97, 153, 183, 189
Scotland
  British medicine and 23–4, 162–3, 168, 198–9, 226, 257
  health services in 52, 70 n.35, 72 n.67, 100–1, 198–9
  medical culture and politics of 23–4, 100–1, 192
Scottish Home and Health Department
  National Medical Consultative Committee 192–3, 198–9
social medicine 14–15, 35 n.56, 58, 60
social security 4, 8, 59–60, 160, 161, 162, 164, 165, 166, 218, 219
specialisation 12–13, 37 n.71, 56, 83–4, 122
  clinics *see* diabetic outpatient clinics
  diabetes specialists 11, 15, 21, 23–4, 51, 64, 90, 152, 157, 161, 168, 188, 190–1, 197, 209 n.61
  construction of professional management 2, 3, 6, 23–4, 139, 180–1, 192–3, 198–9, 200, 224, 225–8, 228–32, 247, 250
  relationships with GPs 17, 82, 85, 123, 139, 243, 244
standardisation 24, 38 n.87, 200
  care and 5, 18, 123, 125, 232, 248, 252
  categories and 154, 184, 189
  medical records and 122–3, 124–5
  units of medical work and 13, 14, 41 n.115, 184, 189

standards of care 1, 10, 13, 22, 50, 64, 68, 132, 135–6, 192, 196, 200–1, 202, 226
    concerns about 80, 93, 128–9, 246, 250
    published standards *see* guidelines; protocols
    see also quality of care
St Vincent Declaration 200, 226, 228–9, 231, 233
surveillance
    diabetes care and disease 3, 21, 22, 48–9, 58, 63, 97, 154, 169, 245
    patient 3, 22, 65–6, 85, 88, 91–2, 97, 117–21, 125–6, 128, 132–3, 191, 243
    health service and professionals and 128, 131, 197, 198–200, 207 n.39, 222, 226, 245–6, 252
shared care *see* community diabetes care; hospitals

Thatcher, Margaret, Prime Minister 160
    governments of 8, 9, 44 n.159, 103, 160, 162, 168, 215, 219, 221, 224

time
    economies of professional time 82, 87–8, 117
    management in medicine 10, 64, 92, 96, 117–19, 135
    waiting 80, 82, 90, 117, 119

United States of America 199
    health service reform 35 n.57, 60, 73 n.82
    management of medicine 5, 24, 36 n.65, 247–9

Wales
    British medicine and 23–4
    health services in 52, 70 n.35, 101
welfare state 4, 5, 7, 8, 55–6, 58, 59–60, 160–1
    expenditure 8, 58, 168, 203
    professionals 5, 13, 134, 217, 218
    services 57, 155, 161, 219, 255
    social security *see* social security
    see also post-war consensus
Whitehall 9, 216
    see also civil service; post-war consensus
World Health Organization 99, 189–90, 192, 226, 228, 247
    see also St Vincent Declaration

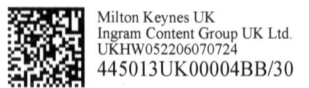

Milton Keynes UK
Ingram Content Group UK Ltd.
UKHW052206070724
445013UK00004BB/30

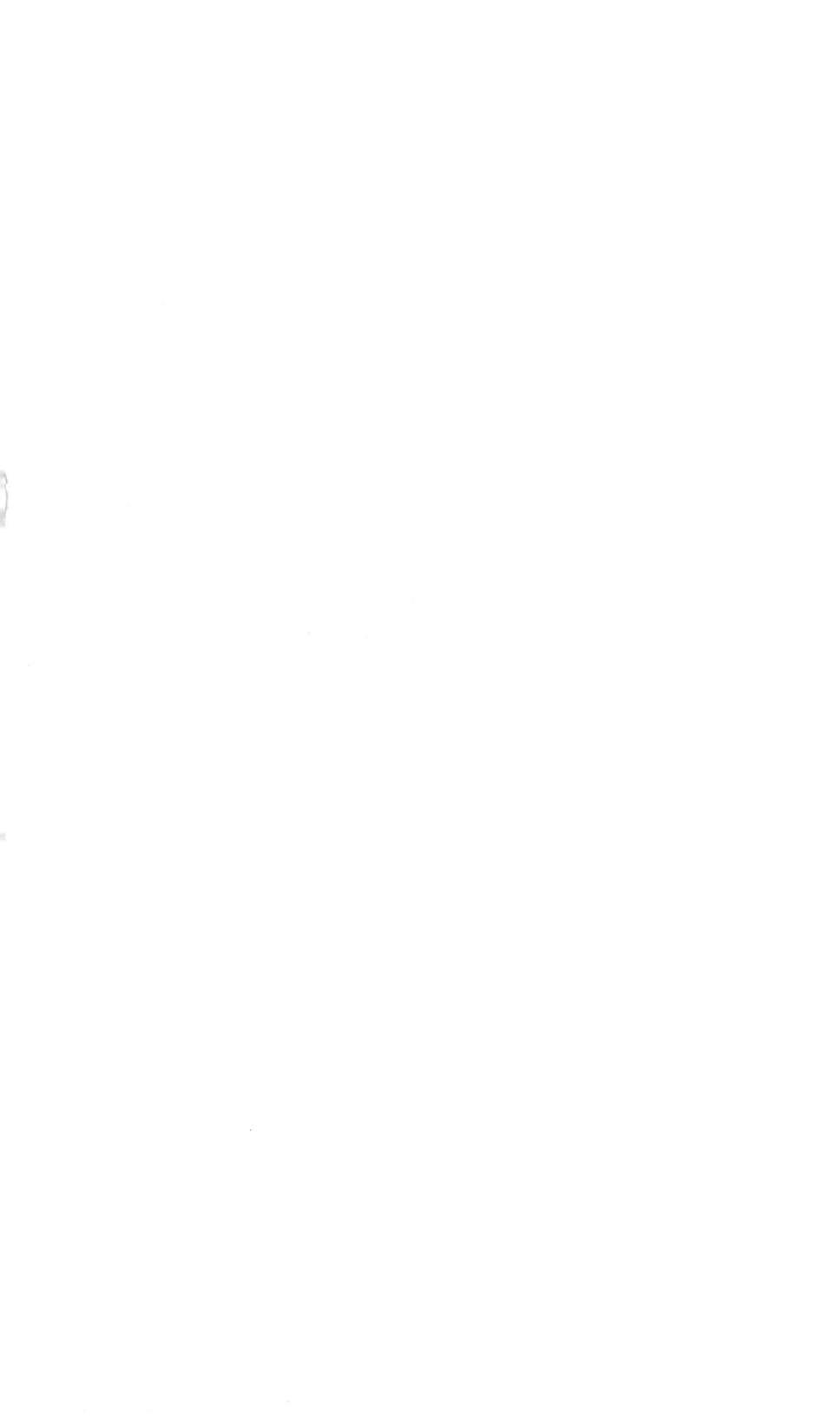